Preface

When I mentioned to my brother that I was about to finish this book, the first comment he made was something to the effect of, "What makes you an expert?!. You only have your own experiences to write about..." He was more or less right of course. However...

Which is why I went to the trouble in 2012 of compiling this reference guide for all fifty states, the District of Columbia, Puerto Rico, and more... The majority of it will be of no use to the reader, so I fervently recommend that you get the free edition from the Amazon Kindle lending library or pay the price of 99 cents for the Kindle edition. You will only need the information for the state or states pertinent to you, and I suspect this one is going to be a bit pricey in print.

I dedicate this book to both my wife for all her support

and to those unsung heroes out there who are currently

or have been family caregivers.

It is for you I wrote this one.

The

Caregiver's
Survival Guide
For Family Members
Reference Guide

Dave Coe, and others ©2012 on Amazon Kindle

Revised 2015

References Galore

-some actually useful...

In this section, you can find links to each state's programs for the care of your aging /and/or disabled adult family member. Depending upon the state and its programs, the two designations of senior, (aging, adult, etcetera), and disabled are sometimes more or less the same programs or not, with some programs over lapping, or not. If your loved one fits in both categories at least to some degree, then what may be available or dealt with under one (senior, disabled) might not be, or be a better way to go than the other category. As some of the state's websites are rather difficult to navigate, I have endeavored to do the best job possible to find the pertinent programs related to the in-home caregiving of a family member. The listings are alphabetically by state, and any actual program descriptions given are <u>directly copied,</u> and only slightly edited for relevance or form from the sites referenced. I make no promises about what you may or may not be able to achieve at these sites, but at least they are places to start.

It should also be noted that the number of states that actually provide direct support to family care givers is extremely limited (and severely limited as to your available assets in most cases), with the majority of states only offering assistance in restricted or transitional assistance categories such as situational in-home medical service or perhaps respite care for the caregiver. Caregiving services themselves are either community based or professional, and may or may not be covered by insurance or governmental (state or federal) full or partial payments. It is worth mentioning that there is a greater potential for assistance if your loved one is both disabled and elderly. The Americans With Disabilities Act seems to have helped there... You should also look for the sections on respite care. Respite care is most often provided by volunteers, and they usually come with verifiable references. Sometimes even a few hours off can be a godsend, and in many states, such as Kentucky, a caregiver is technically liable for any injury or death resulting from absence, such as that "quick trip to the store"...

Some state websites are relatively easy to navigate when looking for information relating to the caregiving of a loved one, such as California. Some however, such as New

Mexico, even confounded a pretty good web surfer like myself. The New Mexico official state web site suggests it has many services for both the senior and disabled populations, but I for one had very little success finding anything of real substance. This is why on some of the state pages compiled, you will see one web address followed by another and another and so on, without very little if anything specific being given in details. The follow-up pages just seemed to provide links to other pages. I did my best, folks. As to such categories as Native Americans, retired military, or others however, they may too be useful for your purposes. It is worth mentioning that sometimes you may find useful information for your particular caregiving situation on the sites of entirely different states. Skim through them, it might be worthwhile... Oh, and as I promised a section on Puerto Rico in this list: As nearly as I could find on four separate attempts, all medical activities in Puerto Rico involves Medicare and Medicaid. I have to suspect that I failed in this case, but I just couldn't find any other links. Sorry.

One note of caution, however, as to assistance of any kind: Very little happens with expediency! Excepting some services which are listed as say, emergency..., it can takes months to accomplish anything. Patience is usually needed in abundance, as is a good sense of humor, or at least the smarts to know that yelling at some poor clerk in the ... office is not going to get your case anywhere, and may put you and your loved one's needs at the bottom of the stack. So be cool, be tenacious, and remember if you are turned down for any given service, you can always apply again. As for the governmental options previously mentioned, Medicare I have been told, has over two hundred different programs for which you may apply. $3000.00 in liquid or available assets seems frequently to be the amount of demarcation, joint or legally shared monies trumps the single recipient (married persons cannot separate their assets), and set aside accounts for medical bills are considered in total (how much the current monthly balance is), not the amount devisable by twelve months. However, as I've heard from at least one worker (very unofficially), if the money is not in the bank...

In the end, your best help may come from the congregation of your church, mosque, or synagogue, perhaps a service organization (social or military,) or medical recovery group to which you or your loved one belongs. Resources are out there, folks; but you have to look.

Namaste, Aloha, Shalom, and good luck to you!

Alabama

Senior Citizen Resources: Alabama Department of Senior Citizens

Services	Support for Family Caregivers (CARES)

Services

- Caregiver Assistance
- Disaster Preparedness
- Elder Abuse
- Elder Law Helpline
- Insurance Counseling
- Legal Assistance
- Long Term Care Ombudsman
- Medicaid Waiver
- Medicare Fraud Prevention
- Nutrition & Wellness
- Personal Choices
- Senior Employment
- SenioRx /Wellness

Support for Family Caregivers (CARES)

Caregivers play a vital role in helping seniors maintain their health and independence. However, even though caregiving is rewarding, it can have a negative impact on the health and well-being of the caregiver. Caregiving has its greatest impact on the emotional health of caregivers. Caregivers of individuals with dementia and stroke survivors are at the highest risk for depression and anxiety disorders.

The National Family Caregiver Support Program (NFCSP) established in 2000, provides grants to States and territories, based on their share of senior citizens. This funding allows families to keep their loved ones at home for as long as possible thereby preventing premature nursing home placement. Alabama's allotment under the OAA amendment created the Alabama Cares Program. The Alabama Cares Program offers support for caregivers across the state by providing services through five basic areas:

(1) Information: provides public education, caregiver and provider training, health fairs, newsletters, brochures, and audio visual/written caregiver information.

(2) Assistance: provides outreach, case management, assessment, and information regarding resources and services.

(3) Counseling: provides support groups and trainings to assist and advise in areas of health, nutrition, financial literacy, and the role of care giving.

(4) Respite: provides temporary, substitute support of the care recipient to provide a brief period of relief/rest to the caregiver, help with personal care, homemaker services, adult day care, and skilled or unskilled services in the home.

(5) Supplemental Services: provides through a limited basis,

incontinence supplies, minor home modifications, assistive technology, home-delivered meals, emergency alarm response systems, nutritional supplements, chore services, and transportation.

Eligibility criteria for the Caregiver Program:

(1) A caregiver of any age, caring for an individual 60 years of age or older. The caregiver can also be caring for an individual who is under 60 years of age with Alzheimer's disease or a related dementia.

(2) A grandparent or relative caregiver, age 55 and older (not a parent) caring for a child 18 years of age or younger. Also, a grandparent age 55 or older providing care for a child with a severe disability of any age. Priority is given to those with the greatest social and economic need and family caregivers providing care and support to persons with Alzheimer's disease or other forms of dementia as well as related disorders.

To Contact Your Local Area Agency On Aging, Please Call:
1-800-AGELINE (1-800-243-5463)

Alaska

Commission on Aging http://www.alaskaaging.org/

http://www.alaskaaging.org/assets/youarenotalone.pdf

Alzheimer's Resource of Alaska (800) 478 1080 •

The Aging & Disability Resource Center (877) 625 2372

Kelda O. Barstad
Aging and Disability Resource Centers Program Manager
Division of Senior and Disabilities Services
550 W. Eighth Ave. Anchorage AK 99501
Direct: 907-269-4138 Fax: 907-269-8164
Front Desk: 907-269-3666

Kenai Peninsula IL Center
47255 Princeton Ave.
Soldotna, AK. 99669
Phone: 907-262-6333

Southeast AK IL Center
3225 Hospital Drive, Suite 300 Juneau, AK 99801
907-586-4920 1-800-478-7245

Municipality of Anchorage
825 L Street Anchorage, AK 99501
907-343-7770

Links: http://www.hss.state.ak.us/acoa/links.htm

Senior Benefits

Printable Senior Benefits Application (PDF)
Mail or fax your application to:
Senior Benefits Office
855 W. Commercial Drive,
Wasilla, AK 99654
Phone: 1-888-352-4150 or 352-4150;
Fax: 357-2561, toll-free 1-866-352-8539
Register to vote online! Or print out a registration form.
Consider Direct Deposit! Receive Public Assistance benefits easily and quickly through Direct Deposit.
Legislators keep, grow senior benefits:

Alaska lawmakers approved a new monthly cash benefit program for elders 65 and older on limited incomes in June 2007, and the new Senior Benefits Program started Aug. 1, 2007.
Three benefit amounts from $125 to $250 are offered, based on gross annual income (before any deductions are taken for taxes, Medicare premiums, etc.)
Assets, such as savings accounts, are not considered. Income limits are tied to the Federal Poverty guideline for Alaska and updated annually.
(Please see chart below.)

Senior Household Size	Senior Benefits Program Gross Annual Income Limit Effective 3/1/2011		
	$250 monthly payment	$175 monthly payment	$125 monthly payment
Individual	$10,200 ($850 per month)	$13,600 ($1,134 per month)	$23,800 ($1,984 per month)
Married Couple	$13,785 ($1,149 per month)	$18,380 ($1,532 per month)	$32,165 ($2,680 per month)

For more information or to apply, call the Senior Benefits Office toll-free at 1-888-352-4150, or 352-4150 in Mat-Su.

The program's new name clarifies that the private business Senior Care of Alaska, Inc. does not have any connection with senior benefits offered by the state. Seniors who want to apply for the Senior Benefits Program should **not** be referred to this business. If seniors have questions about the new program, they can contact the Senior Benefits Office at 1-888-352-4150 (statewide) or 352-4150 (in Wasilla).
Other senior resources that might be helpful:
Medicare Information Office, 1-800-478-6065, or 269-3680 in Anchorage.
Aging & Disability Resource Centers, 1-877-6AK-ADRC **(1-877-625-2372)**
The Division of Senior & Disabilities can also give you more information on state programs for seniors: 1-800-478-9996, or 269-3666 in Anchorage.

Chronic & Acute Medical Assistance (CAMA)

The Chronic & Acute Medical Assistance (CAMA) program is a state funded program designed to help needy Alaskans who have specific illnesses get the medical care they need to manage those illnesses. It is a program primarily for people age 21 through 64 who do not qualify for Medicaid benefits, have very little income, and have inadequate or no health insurance.

Frequently Asked Questions
How to Apply
Contact Us

Frequently Asked Questions

Who is Eligible?
To be eligible for CAMA, you must:

1. have a covered medical condition,
2. have no third party resources to cover treatment of that medical condition;
3. have very limited financial resources; and
4. be a U.S. Citizen or legal alien.

top of page ▲

What are the Covered Medical Conditions?

CAMA is available only if you have one of the following medical conditions:

- a terminal illness;
- cancer requiring chemotherapy;
- chronic diabetes or diabetes insipidus
- chronic seizure disorders;
- chronic mental illness;
- chronic hypertension.

top of page ▲

Verification of a Covered Medical Condition?

A physician or advanced nurse practitioner must verify that you have one of the covered medical conditions. A Certification of Medical Status (MED 11) form is used for this purpose. When completed, your health care provider submits the form directly to your public assistance caseworker.

top of page ▲

What Do You Mean By "Third Party Resources"?

CAMA is considered a last resort, meaning that you will not qualify for CAMA if you have a resource that covers treatment of your medical condition. If you have assistance available from a third party, you must use that resource. Third party resources that may be available to meet an individual's medical need include the following:

a. Coverage by a private medical or hospital insurance policy that will pay 100 percent of the cost of medical care;

b. Veteran's Administration, TRICARE, Office of Vocational Rehabilitation, Division of Mental Health and Developmental Disabilities, Medicaid, and Medicare and others;

c. Salvation Army, Red Cross, Lion's International, and other charitable organizations that meet the individual's medical need;

    d.   Payment for medical bills or medical insurance coverage available from another person who is liable;

    e.   Cash contributions from friends or relative intended to defray medical costs.

Eligibility to receive assistance from the U.S. Public Health Service through the Indian Health Service (IHS) is not considered an available resource for the purposes of determining initial eligibility for CAMA.

top of page ▲

Who Is Financially Eligible?

In addition to having a covered medical condition and no other resources to meet that health care need, you must meet the following financial eligibility requirements.

Your household income must be:

- $300 a month or less for one person
- $400 a month or less for two people
- add $100 for each additional person

You must have less than $500 in countable resources that could be used to pay medical bills. Countable resources include cash, bank/credit union accounts, or personal property. CAMA does not count your home, one vehicle, income producing property, property that is used for your job (boat, fishing gear, etc.), or a fishing permit.

top of page ▲

What Coverage is Available with the CAMA program?

For those who are eligible, CAMA pays for the following services:

1. prescription drugs and medical supplies, limited to 3 prescriptions per month and no more than a 30-day supply of any drug;
2. physician services; which are directly related to the medical condition that qualifies you for CAMA;
3. chemotherapy and radiation services for a recipient with cancer requiring

4. chemotherapy, if provided in an outpatient setting; and
   outpatient laboratory and X-ray services

top of page ⌃

How does CAMA work?

If you qualify for CAMA, you will be given a Recipient Identification Card (commonly called a "coupon") to give to your health care provider. A general description of CAMA covered services is printed on the face of the coupon. If you receive medical care for something that is not listed on the coupon, you will have to pay for the service yourself. Before you receive medical treatment, you must give the coupon to your doctor, clinic, or pharmacist. Your health care provider must be enrolled with the Department of Health and Social Services, Division of Health Care Services. They will send the bill to the state's contractor for payment. Payments are made directly to your health care provider.

A CAMA recipient does have a responsibility to share in the cost of the services received. There is a $1 co-payment on each prescribed drug or medical supply. You pay these charges directly to your health care provider and they will bill the CAMA program for the rest. Your health care provider may not ask you to pay more.

top of page ⌃

How to Apply

How do I apply for CAMA?

You can submit an application for CAMA at the nearest Division of Public Assistance office or with a fee agent living in your community. A completed application form, supporting documents, and an interview with a caseworker or local fee agent are required. You will be asked to bring the following supporting documents with you to your interview:

- papers that show your income such as tax forms, pay stubs, fish tickets, or a letter from the Internal Revenue Service saying that you do not pay taxes; and
- papers that show any other assets or resources like bank accounts.

At the interview, you will be given a form to take to your health care provider that is used to document and verify that you have one of the covered medical conditions. Your provider will return that form to your DPA caseworker. Your application and interview are confidential. No one will give out information about your health or financial status without your permission.

Your application will be reviewed and a notice will be sent to you within 30 days. If your application is approved, your benefits will start the month after you submitted your application. If your application is denied, you may have a right to appeal that decision at a fair hearing.

top of page ⌃

Contact Us

If you have any questions regarding the CAMA program, please contact the Division of Public Assistance office nearest you or the fee agent in your community.

More Information
If you have questions about CAMA eligibility, please contact dpapolicy@alaska.gov.

If you have questions about CAMA coverage, please call the Health Care Services Recipient Information Line at 1-800-780-9972

Adult Public Assistance (APA)

Adult Public Assistance Program was established in 1992 with the mandate to furnish financial assistance to needy aged, blind, and disabled persons and to help them attain self-support or self-care. People who receive APA financial assistance are over 65 years old or have severe and long term disabilities that impose mental and physical limitations on their day-to-day functioning.

APA Caseload Projection

APA caseload has steadily increased, a trend that is expected to continue. The increase may be attributed to a combination of state population growth, earlier identification of disabilities, increased longevity due in part to advances in medical technology, and the general aging of the Alaska population. The chart below illustrates this growth. Since 1990, the disabled caseload monthly average, including both physical and mental disabilities, has grown an average of 10% per year. The aged caseload average has grown approximately 6% per year between 1990 and 1995. Since 1995, however, the aged growth rate has slowed to 2% per year. The percentage of growth in the overall caseload during this period has averaged 7.2%.

Adult Public Assistance Income and Eligibility standards (pdf)

Average Benefit

APA provides financial assistance as its primary mission. In FY 2009, 16,869 households received $55.7 million in benefits.

Policy changes and Issues

The APA population is expected to continue to grow. To qualify for APA disability benefits, an individual must have a long term disability, therefore this population tends to remain beneficiaries of the APA program for their entire adult lives. Continued APA funding provides critical financial assistance to enable program participants to live as independently as possible.

APA beneficiaries touch many other state and federal programs. DPA is trying to better understand all the services this beneficiary group requires, the role of APA financial assistance and the best way to promote self support and self care for this population. To further this work, we have begun to engage with other DHSS Divisions and Departments that provide assistance to this population. Currently, there are a number of initiatives directed toward the adult disabled population underway. The Governor's Council on Disabilities and Special Education recently received funds from the Alaska Mental Health Trust Authority for an Employment Initiative Project. Through the Division of Vocational

Rehabilitation, these funds will be used to work with disabled adults, identify and overcome employment barriers, and assist clients to find and keep work. A research element will explore the demographics of this population, review adult public assistance programs and employment efforts in other states and evaluate the pilot project implemented by DVR.

The Division of Public Assistance has an Adult Public Assistance Project Team composed of staff from Division of Vocational Rehabilitation, Social Security Administration, Division of Medical Assistance, Division of Public Assistance, Disability Law Center, and the Division of Mental Health and Developmental Disabilities. This group is steering committee charged with developing a plan for a review of the Adult Public Assistance Program to determine both how the program can better serve Alaskans and develop a method to project future program costs

Personal Care Assistance Program

Personal Care Assistance (PCA) provides support for about 4,000 Alaskan seniors and individuals with disabilities. PCA services provide support related to an individual's activities of daily living (i.e. bathing, dressing, eating) as well as instrumental activities of daily living (i.e. shopping, laundry, light housework). PCA is provided statewide in Alaska through private agencies. The administration of the PCA program is overseen by the PCA Unit of Senior and Disabilities Services, Department of Health and Social Services.

- **Agency-Based PCA Program (ABPCA)** - Consumers may receive services through an agency that oversees, manages and supervises their care. ABPCA has been operational for over 10 years.
- **Consumer-Directed PCA Program (CDPCA)** - Each consumer may manage his or her own care by selecting, hiring, firing and supervising their own personal care assistant. The agency provides administrative support to the consumer and the personal care assistant. CDPCA became operational October 1, 2001.
  Both Agency-Based PCA services and Consumer-Directed PCA services are available in most communities in Alaska.

To properly use the save enabled PDF's. Right click on the link and save target as,

open the pdf in adobe reader. Fill out the form, when finished filling out the form ,go to file and choose save as. Then you can e-mail the saved PDF form or print it out to sign.

If there is a problem with a save enabled PDF please <u>contact me</u>

- **Changes in the Approval of Instrumental Activities of Daily Living (IADL) Under 7 AAC 43.755(14)**
  - o **IADL Shared Living Explanation**
  - o **<u>IADL Request For Additional Hours Form</u>**
- **Clarification Regarding Reinstatement of PCA Hours**

For additional information about the Personal Care Assistance Program use one of the following links:

Provider Resources:

Assessment Forms

- <u>PCA Consumer Assessment Tool/Personal Care Assessment Tool (CAT/PCAT)</u>
- <u>CAT/PCAT Authorized Services Plan</u>
- <u>Consumer CAT/PCAT Signature Form</u>
- <u>Request for Expedite</u>
- <u>Service Plan Amendment</u>

Application Forms For PCA Services

- <u>Authorization For Release Of Information</u>
- <u>Program Recipients Rights</u>
- <u>Consumer/Legal Representative Agreement</u>
- <u>Demographic Form (Intake Screening)</u>
- <u>Limited Power of Attorney</u>
- <u>Verification of Diagnosis</u>

Misc. Provider Forms

- <u>Request for Waiver of CPR FA Training</u>
- <u>Courses Acceptable for PCA CPR & FA Training</u>
- <u>First Aid Training Verification – Suggested Format</u>

- Notice Of Use Of Private Health Care Information
- Travel Request Form
- Request for Waiver of FA & CPR for PCA staff (pdf 15 KB)

PCA Training Information

- State-approved PCA Training Provider List
- PCA Training Instructor Approval Request Form (pdf 77 KB)

PCA Policies

- PCA Service Plans Policy Statement
- **10-1** Approval of IADL and Chore Services Policy - NULLIFIED by 12/14/2007 PCA Regulations
- **10-2** Cognitive Capacity - Money Management and Choice or Physical Disability Policy
- **10-3** Verification of Medical Diagnosis for PCA Services Policy -NULLIFIED by 2/22, 2011 by Policy Update)
- **10-4** Fair Hearings and Prior Authorizations Policy
- **10-5** PCA Managed Care
- **10-6** IADL: Shopping and Escort allowed extra time calculation
- **10-7** Determination of capability providing Instrumental Activities of IADL and/or Chore Services
- **10-8** Application Documents for Personal Care Assistance Services
- **10-9** Obtaining Medical Certification Form for Authorization of PCA and Older Alaskans/Adults with Physical Disabilities Waiver Services
- **10-10** Transfer of Services for Personal Care Assistance (PCA)
- **10-11** Authorization Start & End Dates (Rescinded 5/2011)

Memos, Procedures & Regulations

- CPR-FA Memo 2010
- PCA Program Regulation Implementation Memo 7 AAC 43.752(i)
- **PCA Program Memo Clarifying 7 AAC 43.775**
- Program Update Notice 2
- **PCA Regulations; 7AAC 125.010-7AAC 125.199**

If you are interested in receiving personal care services or want more information about becoming a Medicaid provider for this innovative program, please contact:

<u>PCA Unit Staff Contacts</u>

550 W. 8th St., Anchorage, Alaska 99501
Phone: (907) 269-3666 or (800) 478-9996
Fax: (907) 269-8164

Adult Protective Services

We are here to help you. Our services are voluntary. We will not force you to move or do anything against your own will. We are here to help you live in a safe and healthy environment and receive the services you need. Please contact our office if you need help or have any questions.

☑ **Report Harm done to a Vulnerable Adult**

- **Report of Harm form**
- <u>Authorization for Release of Information (enrollment, eligibility)</u>

Adult Protective Services helps to prevent or stop harm from occurring to vulnerable adults. Alaska law requires that protective services not interfere with the elderly or disabled adults who are capable of caring for themselves.
Vulnerable adults have a physical or mental impairment or condition that prevents them from protecting themselves or from seeking help from someone else.

Alaska law defines vulnerable adults to include adults 18 years of age or older, not just the elderly.

The harm they suffer may result from abandonment, abuse, exploitation, neglect or self-neglect. The following are examples of things to report:

ABANDONMENT is the desertion of a vulnerable adult by a caregiver.

ABUSE is the intentional or reckless non-accidental, non-therapeutic infliction of pain, injury, mental distress, or sexual assault.

EXPLOITATION is the unjust or improper use of another person or their resources for one's own benefit.

NEGLECT is the intentional failure of a caregiver to provide essential services.

SELF-NEGLECT is the act or omission by a vulnerable adult that results, or could result, in the deprivation of essential services necessary to maintain minimal mental, emotional, or physical health and safety.

⊡ **See Alaska Statute 47.24.010-.900 (Amended 1994)**

Examples of Adult Protective Services:

- Information and Referral
- Investigation of Reports
- Protective Placement
- Guardianship or Conservatorship Counseling
- Linking Clients to Community Resources
- Training and designation of local community resources to provide services.

For information and an application form about financial assistance for assisted living for adult protective services clients Use this link **(General Relief Application)**

- Assisted Living/General Relief Provider Resources
- Assisted Living Home Regulations
- Provider Agreement for Protection of Vulnerable Adults

⊡ Press Release From the Attorney General's Office
FOR IMMEDIATE RELEASE
May 20, 2009

"Operation False Charity" Law Enforcement Sweep

(Anchorage, AK) - Acting Attorney General Richard Svobodny, along with the Federal Trade Commission (FTC) and other law enforcers in at least 46 states, today announced "Operation False Charity," a nationwide, federal-state crackdown on fraudulent charities and charitable solicitors claiming to help police, firefighters, and veterans. Federal and state agencies will prosecute 60 law enforcement actions against fundraising companies, nonprofits, and individuals. The FTC and state agencies also released new education materials to help consumers recognize and avoid charitable solicitation fraud.

FTC Enforcement Actions

The FTC cases announced today include actions against defendants who allegedly tricked consumers into giving by claiming they were affiliated with law enforcement or veterans groups or misleading consumers about how much of the money would go to those groups. According to the FTC, the defendants used legitimate-sounding names to give their sham organizations a veneer of credibility. Their real goal, however, was to trick consumers into contributing money that the defendants used overwhelmingly to support themselves and their fundraisers.

Participating States

State officials participating in the sweep include the Attorneys General of Alabama, Alaska, Arkansas, Arizona, California, Colorado, Connecticut, Delaware, the District of Columbia, Florida, Hawaii, Idaho, Illinois, Indiana, Iowa, Kansas, Kentucky, Louisiana, Maine, Massachusetts, Michigan, Minnesota, Missouri, Montana, Nevada, New Jersey, New Mexico, North Carolina, North Dakota, Ohio, Oklahoma, Oregon, Pennsylvania, South Dakota, Texas, Vermont, Washington, West Virginia, and Wisconsin.

Also participating were other state agencies that register and sometimes regulate charities, including the Secretaries of State of Colorado, Georgia, Mississippi, North Carolina, Pennsylvania, South Carolina, West Virginia, and Washington, as well as the Georgia Governor's Office of Consumer Affairs, the Rhode Island Department of Business Regulation, and the Virginia Department of Agriculture and Consumer Services.

Consumer Education

The FTC today issued a consumer alert providing tips about charities that solicit donations on behalf of veterans and military families. According to the alert, which can be found on the FTC Web site at http://www.ftc.gov/charityfraud/, while many legitimate charities are soliciting donations to support the nation's military veterans, not all "charities" are legitimate. Some are operators whose only purpose is to make money for themselves. Others are paid fundraisers whose fees can use up most of the consumer's donation.

The new alert, "Supporting the Troops: When Charities Solicit Donations on Behalf of Vets and Military Families," offers the following tips to help consumers ensure that their donations go to a legitimate charity. Many of these tips apply to other charitable giving as well.

- Recognize that the words "veterans" or "military families" in an organization's name do not necessarily mean that veterans or the families of active-duty personnel will benefit from your donation.

- Donate to charities with a track record and a history. Charities that spring up overnight may disappear just as quickly.

- If you have any doubt about whether you have made a pledge or a contribution, check your records. If you do not remember making the donation or pledge, resist the pressure to give.

- Check out an organization before donating. Some phony charities use names, seals and logos that look or sound like those of respected, legitimate organizations.

- Call the office that regulates charitable organizations in your state to see whether the charity or fundraising organization is required to register in your state. In Alaska, the information is available at www.law.state.ak.us/consumer.

- Do not send or give cash donations. For security and tax record purposes, it is best to pay by check made payable to the charity.

- Ask for a receipt showing the amount of your contribution.

- Be wary of promises of guaranteed sweepstakes winnings in exchange for a contribution. You never have to give a donation to be eligible to win a sweepstakes.

  Some of the sites where consumers can check out a charity include:

- www.law.state.ak.us/consumer – for Alaska's charity registry

- www.guidestar.org - Guidestar

- www.bbb.org/us/charity/ - Better Business Bureau Wise Giving Alliance

- www.charitynavigator.org - CharityNavigator

- www.charitywatch.org – American Institute of Philanthropy
- www.ftc.gov/charityfraud - Federal Trade Commission

For additional consumer protection information go to www.law.state.ak.us/consumer
Brenda Mahlatini, Manager
550 W. Eighth Ave.
Anchorage, Alaska 99501
Phone: (907) 269-3666 or (800) 478-9996
Fax: (907) 269-3648

Arizona

Family Health/ Senior Citizen Resources:

http://az.gov/services_famhealth_sencitserv.html

Aging and Adult Services:

https://www.azdes.gov/common.aspx?menu=36&menuc=28&id=190

(The State of Arizona seems to offer little if any actual financial support towards in-home caregiving situations. I would be happy to be proved wrong.)

Division of Aging and Adult Services: https://www.azdes.gov/daas/aging/

Independent Living Supports (ILS) is a collection of programs that serve to protect the rights of older adults, prevent fraud and abuse, provide information and assistance on rights, benefits and options, while providing Home and Community-Based services to ensure many aspects of Independent Living.

Programs Include:

- Arizona State Health Insurance Assistance Program (SHIP) is a free health-benefits counseling service for Medicare beneficiaries and their families or caregivers. Our mission is to educate, advocate, counsel and empower people to make informed benefit decisions. SHIP also administers the "**SMP**" and "**Ferret Out Fraud**" medical fraud awareness and reporting programs for Arizona.
- AZ Links - Arizona's Aging & Disability Resource Center!
- The Family Caregiver Support Program provides services to family caregivers who are caring for an individual who is 60 years or older. The program also serves family caregivers who are 55 years or older and are the primary caretakers for a child, related by blood, marriage, or adoption, who is under 19 years of age and resides with the caregivers. The program provides information and assistance with obtaining community resources, counseling, training, and support groups; respite care; and supplemental services to complement care provided by a caregiver.

- <u>Home and Community Living Supports</u> is a comprehensive case-managed system of care, which offers an array of services designed to help aging and vulnerable individuals remain and live independently in their own home and community with the appropriate level of support. In-home services include personal care, home health aid, respite care, housekeeping, home-delivered meals, and home nursing. Community services include congregate meals, adult day care, health promotion, disease prevention, and transportation.
- <u>Legal Services Assistance</u> is available to older persons who may be unable to appropriately manage their own affairs. Some legal issues may include power of attorney, guardianship/conservatorship, wills, living wills, trusts, and tenant/landlord concerns.
- The <u>Long Term Care Ombudsman Program</u> - provides assistance to (and advocacy for) residents of long term care and assisted living facilities in understanding and maintaining their human and civil rights; and ensuring quality of life and quality of care.
- The <u>Mature Workers Program</u> empowers the economically disadvantaged person age 55 or older with job opportunities in training programs in order to enhance the quality of life of the participants.
- ILS, through contracts with the local Area Agencies on Aging, provides a <u>Nutrition Program</u> to older adults and eligible persons with disabilities. The program provides a range of related services through the aging network's nutrition service providers. Included are nutrition screening, assessment, education and counseling on health and nutrition needs, special health assessments for such diseases as hypertension and diabetes, instruction in shopping, planning and preparing economical and nutritious meals that optimize health and well-being.

Arkansas

Adult and Aging Services:

http://www.healthy.arkansas.gov/Pages/googleSearch.aspx?q=adult services

Resources and Reference Guides

Local Aging Resources

AARP Arkansas

1701 Centerview Drive, Suite 205

Little Rock, AR 72211

Telephone: (501) 217-1626

Email: araarp@aarp.org

Arkansas Geriatric Education Center (AGEC)

UAMS – Slot 798

4301 W. Markham St.

Little Rock, AR 72205

Email: AGEC@uams.edu

Arkansas Minority Health Commission

1123 S. University Ave., Suite 312

Little Rock, AR 72204

Telephone: (501) 686-2720 or 1-877-264-2826

Fax: (501) 686-2722

Email: arkmin@mail.state.ar.us

Arkansas Alzheimer's

10411 West Markham Street, Suite 130

Little Rock, AR 72205

501-224-0021 or 1800-689-6090

501-913-1878 after hours "Care Phone"

Alzheimer's Association –Oklahoma/Arkansas Chapter

411 S. Victory, Suite 202

Little Rock, AR 72201

501-265-0017

Community Health Centers of Arkansas, Inc. (CHC-AR)

420 W. 4th Street, Suite A

North Little Rock, AR 72114

Telephone: (501) 374-8225

Fax: (501) 374-9734

Division of Aging and Adult Services

Department of Human Services (DAAS)

PO Box 1437

Slot S-530

Little Rock AR 72203

Telephone: (501) 682-2441

Fax: (501) 682-8155

Donald W. Reynolds Center on Aging

4301 West Markham, Slot 748

Little Rock, AR 72205

Telephone: (501) 296-1000 or 1-800-942-8267

Fall Prevention (at Arkansas Department of Health) **{this goes to injury prevention}**

Geriatric Research, Education and Clinical Center (GRECC)

Little Rock GRECC (182/LR)

VA Medical Center

Little Rock, AR 72205

Telephone: (501) 257-5542

Fax: (501) 257-4531

University of Arkansas Cooperative Extension Service

Division of Agriculture

2301 S. University Ave.

Little Rock, AR 72204

Telephone: (501) 671-2000

Fax: (501) 671-2209

http://www.ar-ican.org/

Increasing Capabilities Access Network
ICAN AT4ALL

Welcome to Our Website!

ICAN AT4ALL is Arkansas' statewide assistive technology program designed to make technology available and accessible for everyone who needs it. **Assistive technology (AT)** is any kind of device or tool that helps people learn, work, communicate and live more independently. AT can be very simple and inexpensive, like a modified knife and fork, or it can be very sophisticated and costly, like a computerized speech device.

ICAN stands for **Increasing Capabilities Access Network** and **AT4ALL** is our philosophy—assistive technology for everyone! ICAN AT4ALL offers a number of services to help Arkansans of all ages find the AT they need for home, school, work and getting around in the community. Our services include:

- Information and Referral;
- Equipment Loans;
- Equipment Recycling;
- Equipment Exchange;
- Equipment Demonstrations;
- Training on devices and issues related to accessibility and AT;
- Presentations about ICAN and the benefits of technology;
- Exhibits of AT;
- Tours of the ICAN AT4ALL Clearinghouse;
- Information resources like this website and our newsletter; and
- Technical Assistance to employers, service providers, educators, and others.

The services offered by ICAN AT4ALL are available to all Arkansans, regardless of age, geographic area, disability, income or eligibility for any other service. Click here or visit the About ICAN page for more information about ICAN's services. To contact ICAN or visit the Location & Map page.

If you would like to call us, the number is 501-666-8868 in Little Rock or 1-800-828-2799 outside of the Little Rock area. We hope you'll enjoy this website!

http://www.livingandworkingwell.org/

http://www.ddcouncil.org/

California

Health and Safety: http://www.ca.gov/HealthSafety/HealthCare/

Services for Californians With Disabilities:
http://www.ca.gov/HealthSafety/HealthCare/Disabled.html

Independent Living : http://www.dds.ca.gov/LivingArrang/IndLiving.cfm

Independent Living is a service provided to adults with developmental disabilities that offers functional skills training necessary to secure a self-sustaining, independent living situation in the community and/or may provide the support necessary to maintain those skills. Individuals typically live alone or with roommates in their own homes or apartments. These homes are not licensed.

Independent living programs, which are vendored and monitored by regional centers, provide or coordinate support services for individuals in independent living settings. They focus on functional skills training for adults who generally have acquired basic self-help skills or who, because of their physical disabilities, do not possess basic self-help skills, but who employ and supervise aides to assist them in meeting their personal needs.

For more information about Independent Living Services, contact your local regional center or the:

California Department of Developmental Services
Residential Services Branch
P.O. Box 944202
Sacramento, CA 94244-2020

Services Provided By Regional Centers: http://www.dds.ca.gov/RC/RCSvs.cfm

Regional centers provide diagnosis and assessment of eligibility and help plan, access, coordinate and monitor the services and supports that are needed because of a developmental disability. There is no charge for the diagnosis and eligibility assessment.

Once eligibility is determined, a case manager or service coordinator is assigned to help develop a plan for services, tell you where services are available, and help you get the services. Most services and supports are free regardless of age or income.

There is a requirement for parents to share the cost of 24-hour out-of-home placements for children under age 18. This share depends on the parents' ability to pay. For further information, see Parental Fee Program. There may also be a co-payment requirement for other selected services. For further information, see Family Cost Participation Program.

Some of the services and supports provided by the regional centers include:

- Information and referral
- Assessment and diagnosis
- Counseling
- Lifelong individualized planning and service coordination
- Purchase of necessary services included in the individual program plan
- Resource development
- Outreach
- Assistance in finding and using community and other resources
- Advocacy for the protection of legal, civil and service rights
- Early intervention services for at risk infants and their families
- Genetic counseling
- Family support
- Planning, placement, and monitoring for 24-hour out-of-home care
- Training and educational opportunities for individuals and families
- Community education about developmental disabilities

For additional information about these services and supports, see:

- <u>Information About Programs and Services</u>

Info: (916) 654-1690

TTY: (916) 654-2054

Quick Links

- Laws & Regulations
- Budget Information
- Facts & Stats
- CDER
- DDS Forms
- Publications & Other Resources
- Employment Opportunities
- Public Records Requests
- Appeals, Complaints & Comments
- Small Business and Disabled Veterans Advocates
- Disabilities Advisory Committee
- Español
- Newsroom
- Links
- Contact Us

Information About Programs and Services:
http://www.dds.ca.gov/RC/ProgramSvcs.cfm

The Department of Developmental Services is responsible for designing and coordinating a wide array of services for California residents with developmental disabilities. <u>Regional centers</u> help plan, access, coordinate and monitor these services and supports.

A Person-Centered Planning approach is used in making decisions regarding where a person with developmental disabilities will live and the kinds of services and supports that may be needed. In person-centered planning, everyone who uses regional center services has a planning team that includes the person utilizing the services, family members, regional center staff and anyone else who is asked to be there by the individual. The team joins together to make sure that the services that people are getting are supporting their choices in where they want to live, how and with whom they choose to spend the day, and hopes and dreams for the future.

The following is a partial list of supportive services and living arrangements available for persons with developmental disabilities:

- Day Program Services
- Education Services
- Work Services Program *(formerly Habilitation)*
- Supported Employment
- Work Activity Programs
- Support Services
- Supported Living Services
- Affordable Housing
- Family Home Agency
- Foster Family Agency
- Independent Living
- In-Home Supportive Services
- Respite (In-Home) Services
- Transportation Services
- Community Care Facilities (CCFs)
- Intermediate Care Facilities (ICFs)

Services for Seniors: http://www.ca.gov/HealthSafety/HealthCare/Seniors.html

Health & Safety

Services for Seniors

- <u>California Department of Aging</u> - California Department of Aging
  Home- and community-based services throughout California.
- <u>Caregiver Resource Centers</u> - California Department of Managed Health
- <u>Area Agencies on Aging (listing by county)</u> - California Department of Aging
  Services to seniors in communities.
- <u>Medicare</u> - U.S. Department of Health and Human Services
  Find information on health plans, nursing homes, Medicare and more.
- <u>Choosing a Nursing Home</u> - U.S. Department of Health and Human Services
  Find information about Medicare and Medicaid certified

Department of Aging: http://www.aging.ca.gov/

The California Department of Aging (CDA) administers programs that serve older adults, adults with disabilities, family caregivers, and residents in long-term care facilities throughout the State. The Department administers funds allocated under the federal <u>Older Americans Act</u>, the <u>Older Californians Act</u>, and through the Medi-Cal program.

The Department contracts with the network of Area Agencies on Aging, who directly manage a wide array of federal and state-funded services that help older adults find employment; support older and disabled individuals to live as independently as possible in the community; promote healthy aging and community involvement; and assist family members in their vital care giving role. CDA also contracts directly with agencies that operate the Multipurpose Senior Services Program through the Medi-Cal home and community-based waiver for the elderly, and certifies Adult Day Health Care centers for the Medl-Cal program.

The Department's mission is to promote the independence and well-being of older adults, adults with disabilities, and families through

- ▪ Access to information and services to improve the quality of their lives;
- ▪ Opportunities for community involvement; and

- Support from family members providing care.

• WHERE TO CALL FOR LOCAL SERVICES

911

- 1-800-510-2020 (Senior Information Line)

- Mental Health Services

  - ○ 24 Hour Suicide Prevention Hotline 1-800-273-TALK (1-800-273-8255)

  - ○ 24 Hour Local Crisis Hotlines

  - ○ Mental Health Departments by County

- Adult Protective Services

- Area Agencies on Aging (AAA) by County

- Directory of Legal Service Providers in California (pdf)

- HICAP Number (Medicare Beneficiares and Long-Term

Care
Information)

- Long-Term Care
  Ombudsman
  CRISISline
  (For Resident
  complaints
  Ombudsman)

MORE

**I NEED INFORMATION
ON...**

- Alcohol/Substan
  ce Abuse

- Alzheimer's
  Disease

- Depression

- Medication
  Management

- Memory Loss

- Elder Abuse

- Employment

- Finding A
  Facility

- Health
  Insurance
  Counseling and
  Advocacy
  Program
  (HICAP)

- Home Safety
  and Housing

- In-Home
  Supportive
  Services (IHSS)

- Long-Term Care

- Long-Term Care
  Ombudsman
  Program

- Medicare &
  Other Insurance
- Medi-Cal

MORE

**TOOLS & TIPS
FOR CONSUMERS & CAREGIVERS**

- Advance
  Directives for
  Health Care and
  Other Issues
- Benefits Check
  Up
- Disaster
  Preparedness
  - Tip Sheets
    for Seniors
- Long-Term Care
  Guide
- Resident Rights
- Resources for
  Seniors
- Scam Alerts
- Senior
  Community
  Service
  Employment
  Program
  Eligibility
  Calculator
- Seniors and the
  Law: A Guide
  for Maturing
  Californians
  (State Bar of
  California)
- Wellness Fact
  Sheets
  - Health Tip
    Sheets

<u>MORE</u>

PROGRAMS & SERVICES FOR SENIORS, CAREGIVERS & ADULTS WITH DISABILITIES

- <u>ElderCare Locator</u>
- <u>Employment Links</u>
- <u>Information & Assistance</u>
- <u>Program List</u>

In Home Supportive Services: http://www.cdss.ca.gov/cdssweb/PG139.htm *If your loved one is a resident of California, disabled and/or over sixty-five, then this is the best place to start for in-home care. (From what I've heard, it is probably the best program in the country for in-home care.)*

IHSS: http://www.dss.cahwnet.gov/cdssweb/PG139.htm

In-Home Supportive Services

The IHSS Program will help pay for services provided to you so that you can remain safely in your own home. To be eligible, you must be over 65 years of age, or disabled, or blind. Disabled children are also eligible for IHSS. IHSS is considered an alternative to out-of-home care, such as nursing homes or board and care facilities. Click here for more information on IHSS eligibility.

The types of services which can be authorized through IHSS are housecleaning, meal preparation, laundry, grocery shopping, personal care services (such as bowel and bladder care, bathing, grooming and paramedical services), accompaniment to medical appointments, and protective supervision for the mentally impaired.

Important Notice For IHSS Providers About Changes to the Federal Medi-Cal In-Home Supportive Services (IHSS) Program

For Whom

You may be eligible for IHSS if you:

- Are a current recipient of Supplemental Security Income/State Supplementary Payment (SSI/SSP); or

- You meet all the eligibility criteria for SSI/SSP except that your income is in excess of the SSI/SSP income levels; or

- You meet all the eligibility criteria for SSI/SSP, including income, but do not receive SSI/SSP; or

- You are a Medi-Cal recipient who meets SSI/SSP disability criteria.

Where To Get Help

To apply for IHSS, complete an application and submit it to the local IHSS office at the county welfare department. To find your local office, look for the closest county welfare department office listed under the County Government Section in the telephone book.

Links:

- Adult Protective Services

- Disability Benefits

- SSI - SSP

County Information

- County Offices

Quality Assurance

- SB 1104 IHSS/PCSP QA Initiative Overview

Other Programs

- Residential Care

- Blind Services

- Office of Deaf Access

- Continuing Care

- Cash Assistance Program for Immigrants (CAPI)

Other Related Information

- DHS Web Site

- DHS Toll-Free Numbers

- Help Stop Medi-Cal and IHSS Fraud

Adults: Caregiver Resource Centers:
http://www.dmh.ca.gov/Services_and_Programs/Adults/Caregiver_Resource_Centers.asp

Services | Links | Reports

Caring for a loved one with cognitive disorder or another disabling condition forever changes the lives of families and caregivers. There can be devastating effects on those providing long-term care: financial pressures, legal quandaries, health problems, and emotional turmoil.

Fortunately, in California, there is help. **Eleven Caregiver Resource Centers** (CRCs), throughout the state serve thousands of families and caregivers of those with Alzheimer's disease, stroke, Parkinson's disease and other disorders. California was the first state in the nation to establish a statewide network of support organizations for caregivers; every resident has access to a CRC in their area (see below for services).

You can keep up with the latest news, training opportunities, and support strategies that you can use every month by subscribing to the <u>California Caregiver</u> e-newsletter.

REGIONAL CAREGIVER RESOURCE CENTER SERVICES

Each CRC provides the following core services to families and caregivers at low or no cost:

- **Specialized Information and Referral** - Referrals and advice related to caregiver stress, diagnoses and community resources.

- **Family Consultation and Care Planning** - Trained staff consultations to assess needs of persons with cognitive impairment and their families, explore care options, and develop a course of action.

- **Respite Care** - Financial assistance for temporary in-home support, adult day care services, short-term or weekend care and transportation.

- **Short-Term Counseling** - Individual, family and group sessions with licensed counselors to offer emotional support to caregivers

- **Support Groups** - Online or in-person meetings to share experiences and ideas to ease the stress of caregiving.

- **Professional Training** - Workshops on long-term care, patient management, public policy, legal and financial issues for health and service providers.

- **Legal and Financial Consultation** - Experienced attorneys consult on Powers of Attorney, Advance Directives, estate and financial planning, conservatorships and other matters.

- **Education** - Special workshops on topics such as cognitive disorders, dealing with dementia, long-term care planning and stress management to help caregivers cope with day-to-day concerns.

ADDITIONAL HELPFUL LINKS

- **FCA Web Resource** guide: A comprehensive directory for all aspects of caregiving, medical information, foundations, and support groups.

- Administration on Aging **National Family Caregiver Support:** Web resources for elders, caregivers, professionals and providers.

- **National Respite Locator Service:** Helps parents, caregivers, and professionals find respite services in their state and local area to match their specific needs.

Department of Healthcare Services: http://www.dhcs.ca.gov/Pages/default.aspx

CACareNET: http://calcarenet.ca.gov/?Page=Services

Frankly folks, as states go, California has a great number of programs available, and also frankly, too many to list in this book. However, the previous links should go a long way to getting you the information you will need.

Colorado

Colorado Department of Human Services: http://www.colorado.gov/cs/Satellite/CDHS-Main/CBON/1251575083520

Aging and Adult Services: http://www.colorado.gov/cs/Satellite/CDHS-SelfSuff/CBON/1251579250975

Homecare Allowance and Adult Foster Care: http://www.colorado.gov/cs/Satellite/CDHS-SelfSuff/CBON/1251579250975

Home Care Allowance (HCA) and Adult Foster Care (AFC)

Home Care Allowance (HCA) provides a financial allowance that must be used to purchase specific chore, personal care, and support services.

Adult Foster Care (AFC) provides a financial allowance to pay for residential care to an approved facility for eligible applicants.

What are the Benefits of HCA & AFC?

The HCA provides cash assistance to elderly and disabled individuals for unskilled care services paid directly to a home care provider of the client's choice. The home care provider assists the client with activities of daily living such as bathing, dressing, and transfers, and with supportive service such as money management, and appointment management.

The AFC program provides financial assistance to pay for residential care to an approved facility for eligible applicants.

Application for any services is made through the local County Offices, at:

Adams – Department of Human Services

Phone: (303) 287-8831

24/7 Hotline: (303) 412-5212

Dr. Donald M. Cassata, Director

7190 Colorado Boulevard

Commerce City, CO 80022

Alamosa – Department of Human Services

Phone: (719) 589-2581

Fax: (719) 589-9794

After Hours: Colorado State Patrol Dispatch (719) 589-5807

Larry Henderson, Director

P.O. Box 1310 (mail)

8900 Independence Way Bldg. C

Alamosa, CO 81101

Arapahoe – Department of Human Services

Phone: (303) 636-1130

24/7 Hotline: (303) 636-1750

Cheryl Ternes, Director

14980 East Alameda Drive

Aurora, CO 80012

Archuleta – Department of Human Services

Phone: (970) 264-2182

Fax: (970) 264-2186

After Hours: Police Dispatch (970) 264-2131

Erlinda Gonzales, Director

P.O. Box 240 (mail)

551 Hot Springs Boulevard

Pagosa Springs, CO 81147

Baca – Department of Public Welfare

Phone: (719) 523-4131

After Hours: Baca Sheriff Dispatch (719) 523-4511

Ruth Wallace-Porter, Director

772 Colorado Street

Springfield, CO 81073

Bent – Department of Social Services

Phone: (719) 456-2620

Fax: (719) 456-2945

William G. Schultz, Director

215 2nd Street

Las Animas, CO 81054

Boulder – Department of Housing and Human Services

Phone: (303) 441-1000

24/7 Hotline: (303) 441-1000

Frank Alexander, Director

3400 Broadway

Boulder, CO 80304

Broomfield – Department of Health and Human Services

Phone: (720) 887-2200

Fax: (720) 469-2110 (fax)

24/7 Hotline: (720) 887-2271

Debbie Oldenettel, Director

#6 Garden Center

Broomfield, CO 80020

Chaffee – Department of Health and Human Services

Phone: (719) 539-6627

Phone: (719) 530-2500

Fax: (719) 539-6430

After Hours: Police Dispatch (719) 539-2596

Philip Maes, Director

P.O. Box 1007 (mail)

448 East First Street, Room 166

Salida, CO 81201

Cheyenne – Department of Health and Human Services

Phone: (719) 767-5629

Fax: (719) 767-5101

After Hours: Law Enforcement Dispatch (719) 767-5633

Kindra Mulch, RN, Director

P.O. Box 146 (mail)

51 South 1st

Cheyenne Wells, CO 80810

Clear Creek – Department of Health and Human Services

Phone: (303) 679-2365

Fax: (303) 679-2443

After Hours: Clear Creek Sheriff's Office (303) 679 2393

Cindy Dicken, Director

P.O. Box 2000

405 Argentine Street

Georgetown, CO 80444

Conejos – Department of Social Services

Phone: (719) 376-5455

Fax: (719) 376-2389

After Hours: On-Call Phone (719) 588-1817 or State Patrol (719) 589-5807

Maria Garcia, Director

P.O. Box 68

Conejos, CO 81129

Costilla – Department of Social Services

Phone: (719) 672-4131

After Hours: Sheriff's Office Dispatch: (719) 672-0673

Tommy Vigil, Interim Director

P.O. Box 249

123 Gasper Street

San Luis, CO 81152

Crowley – Department of Human Services

Phone: (719) 267-3546

After Hours: Sheriff's Office Dispatch (719) 267-5235

Tonia Burnett, Director

631 Main Street, Suite 100 (physical)

Ordway, CO 81063

Custer – Department of Social Services

Phone: (719) 783-2371

Fax: (719) 783-2885

After Hours: Sheriff's Office (719) 783-2270

Laura Lockhart, Director

P.O. Box 929 (mail)

205 South 6th Street

Westcliffe, CO 81252

Delta – Department of Health and Human Services

Phone: (970) 874-2030

Fax: (970) 874-2068

After Hours: Delta County Dispatch (970) 874-2015

Chuck Lemoine, Director

560 Dodge Street

Delta, CO 81416

Denver – Department of Human Services

Phone: (720) 944-3666

Fax: (720) 944-3019

24/7 Hotline: (720) 944-3000

Patricia Wilson Pheanious, Director

1200 Federal Boulevard

Denver, CO 80204

Dolores – Department of Social Services

Phone: (970) 677-2250

Fax: (970) 677-2859

24/7 Hotline: (970) 565-8441

Dennis A. Story, Director

P.O. Box 485

409 North Main Street

Dove Creek, CO 81324

Douglas – Department of Human Services

Phone: (303) 688-4825

Fax: (303) 814-0923

After Hours: Douglas Sheriff's Office (303) 660-7500

Barbara Drake, Director

4400 Castleton Court

Castle Rock, CO 80109

Eagle – Department of Health and Human Services

Phone: (970) 328-8840

Fax: (970) 328-8829

After Hours: Vail Police Dispatch (970) 479-2200

Rachel Oys, Director

P.O. Box 660

551 Broadway

Eagle, CO 81631

Elbert – Department of Human Services

Phone: (303) 621-3149

Fax: (303) 621-0122

After Hours: Douglas County (303) 660-7500

Cathy Robinson, Director

P.O. Box 544 (mail)

214 Comanche Street

Kiowa, CO 80107

El Paso – Department of Human Services

Phone: (719) 636-0000

24/7 Hotline for reports of Child Abuse or Neglect ONLY: (719) 444-5700

Richard Bengtsson, Director

1675 Garden of the Gods Rd

Colorado Springs, CO 80907

Fremont – Department of Human Services

Phone: (719) 275-2318

Fax: (719) 275-5206

After Hours: Fremont Sheriff's Office: (719) 276- 5555 or 911

Steven A. Clifton, Director

172 Justice Center Road

Canon City, CO 81212

Garfield – Department of Human Services

Phone: (970) 945-9191

Fax: (970) 928-0465

After Hours: 911

Mary Baydarian, Director

108 8th Street, Suite 300

Glenwood Springs, CO 81601

Gilpin – Department of Human Services

Phone: (303) 582-5444

Fax: (303) 582-5798

After Hours: 911

Black Hawk Police Dispatch (303) 582-5878

Elizabeth Donovan, Director

2960 Dory Hill Road, Suite 100

Black Hawk, CO 80422

Grand – Department of Health and Human Services

Phone: (970) 725-3331

Fax: (970) 725-3696

After Hours: Grand County Sheriff's Office (970) 725-3347

Glen Chambers, Director

P.O. Box 204 (mail)

620 Hemlock

Hot Sulphur Springs, CO 80451

Gunnison – Department of Health and Human Services

Phone: (970) 641-3244

Fax: (970) 641-3738

After Hours: Gunnison County Dispatch (970) 641-8200

Renee Brown, Director

225 North Pine Street, Suite A

Gunnison, CO 81230

Hinsdale – Department of Public Health

Phone: (970) 944-2225

After Hours: Gunnison County Dispatch (970) 641-8200

Main County Office

311 North Henson Street

Lake City, CO 81235

Huerfano – Department of Social Services

Phone: (719) 738-2810

After Hours: Walsenburg Dispatch (719) 738-1044

Sheila Hudson, Director

121 West 6th Street

Walsenburg, CO 81089

Jackson – Department of Social Services

Phone: (970) 723-4750

Fax: (970) 723-4619

After Hours: Jackson County Sheriff (970) 723-4242

Glen Chambers, Director

PO Box 338 (main)

350 McKinley Street

Walden, CO 80480

Jefferson – Department of Human Services

Phone: (303) 271-1388

Child Protection Hot line:(303) 271-4131

Lynn A. Johnson, Executive Director

900 Jefferson County Parkway

Golden, CO 80401

Kiowa – Department of Social Services

Phone: (719) 438-5541

Fax: (719) 438-5370

After Hours: 911 or Bent Sheriff's Office (719) 456-1363

Dennis Pearson, Director

P.O. Box 187 (mail)

1307 Maine Street

Eads, CO 81036

Kit Carson – Department of Health and Human Services

Phone: (719) 346-8732

Fax: (719) 346-8066

After Hours: Law Enforcement Dispatch (719) 346-9325

Kindra Mulch, RN, Director

252 South 14th Street

Burlington, CO 80807

Lake – Department of Human Services

Phone: (719) 486-2088

Fax: (719) 486-4164

Hotline Number: (719) 486-2088

After Hours: Law Enforcement (719) 486-1249

Jeri M. Lee, Director

P.O. Box 884 (mail)

112 West 5th Street

Leadville, CO 80461

La Plata – Department of Human Services

Phone: (970) 382-6150

Fax: (970) 274-2208

After Hours: Answering Service (866) 382-9721

Lezlie Mayer, Director

1060 East Second Avenue

Durango, CO 81301

Larimer – Department of Human Services

Phone: (970) 498-6300

Fax: (970) 498-7987 (fax)

24/7 Hotline: (970) 498-6990

Ginny Riley, Director

1501 Blue Spruce Drive

Fort Collins, CO 80524

Las Animas – Department of Human Services

Phone: (719) 846-2276

After Hours: Trinidad Police (719) 846-4444

Las Animas Sheriff's Office (719) 846-2211

Catherine Salazar, Director

204 South Chestnut Street

Trinidad, CO 81082

Lincoln – Department of Human Services

Phone: (719) 743-2404

Fax: (719) 743-2879

After Hours: Lincoln Sheriff's Office at (719) 743-2426 (ask for the On-Call worker for DSS)

Colette Barksdale, Director

P.O. Box 37 (mail)

103 3rd Avenue

Hugo, CO 80821

Logan – Department of Social Services

Phone: (970) 522-2194

Fax: (970) 521-0853

After Hours: Sterling Police Dispatch (970) 522-3512

Fredrick J. Crawford, Director

P.O. Box 1746 (mail)

508 South 10th Ave., Suite 2

Sterling, CO 80751

Mesa – Department of Human Services

Phone: (970) 241-8480

Fax: (970) 248-2849

24/7 Hotline: (970) 242-1211

Tracey Garchar, Director

510 29-1/2 Road

Grand Junction, CO 81502

Mineral – Department of Social Services

Phone: (719) 657-3381, ext. 100

Fax: (719) 657-4013

After Hours: Law Enforcement (719) 658-2600

Jody Kern, Director

P.O. Box 40 (mail)

1015 6th Street

Del Norte, CO 81132

Moffat – Department of Social Services

Phone: (970) 824-8282

Fax: (970) 824-9552

After Hours: Law Enforcement Dispatch (970) 824-8111 (on-call worker will be paged)

Marie Peer, Director

595 Breeze Street

Craig, CO 81625

Montezuma – Department of Social Services

Phone: (970) 565-3769

After Hours: Sheriff Office (970) 565-8441

Dennis A. Story, Director

109 West Main, Room 203

Cortez, CO 81321

Montrose – Department of Health and Human Services

Phone: (970) 252-5000

Fax: (970) 252-5060

After Hours: (970) 252-3939

Peg Mewes, Director

1845 South Townsend

Montrose, CO 81401

Morgan – Department of Human Services

Phone: (970) 542-3531

Fax: (970) 542-3415

After 4:00 p.m.: Call 911

Steve Romero, Director

P.O. Box 220 (mail)

800 East Beaver Avenue

Fort Morgan, CO 80701

Otero – Department of Social Services

Phone: (719) 383-3100

24/7 Hotline: (719) 267-5454

Donna Rohde, Director

P.O. Box 494 (mail)

Courthouse, 3rd & Colorado

La Junta, CO 81050

Ouray – Department of Social Services

Phone: (970) 626-2299

Fax: (970) 626-9911

After Hours: Sheriff's Office (970) 325-7272

Allan Gerstle, Director

P.O. Box 530 (mail)

Ridgway, CO 81432

177 Sherman Street, Unit 104 (physical)

Ridgway, CO 81432

Park – Department of Human Services

Phone: (303) 816-5939

Fax: (303) 816-5942

After Hours: Call dispatch at (719) 836-4121

Joe Homlar, Director

59865 US Highway 285

Bailey, CO 80421

Phillips – Department of Social Services

Phone: 970-854-2280

Fax: 970-854-3637

After Hours: Sheriff's Office (970) 854-3644

Judy McFadden, Director

127 East Denver, Suite A

Holyoke, CO 80734

Pitkin – Department of Health and Human Services

Phone: (970) 920-5209

Fax: (970) 544-1850

Nan Sundeen, Director

0405 Castle Creek Road, Suite 8

Aspen, CO 81611

Prowers – Department of Social Services

Phone: (719) 336-7486

Fax: (719) 336-7198

After Hours Pager: (719) 336-6269

Linda Fairbairn, Director

P.O. Box 1157 (mail)

1001 South Main (physical)

Lamar, CO 81052

Pueblo – Department of Social Services

Phone: (719) 583-6160

Fax: (719) 583-6748

After Hours: (719) 583-6699

Jose Mondragon, Director

212 West 12th Street

Pueblo, CO 81003

Rio Blanco – Department of Social Services

Phone: (970) 878-9640

Fax: (970) 878-4893

After Hours: (970) 878-9620 (ask for the on-call caseworker)

Bonnie Ruckman, Director

345 Market Street

Meeker, CO 81641

Rio Grande – Department of Social Services

Phone: (719) 657-3381, ext. 100

Fax: (719) 657-4013

After Hours: Del Norte Sheriff's Office (719) 657-4000

Monte Vista Police Department (719) 852-5111

Jody Kern, Director

P.O. Box 40 (mail)

1015 6th Street

Del Norte, CO 81132

Routt – Department of Human Services

Phone: (970) 879-1540

Fax: (970) 870-5260

After Hours: Routt Sheriff's Office (970) 879-1090

Vickie Clark, Director

P.O. Box 772790 (mail)

136 6th Street

Steamboat Springs, CO 80477

Saguache – Department of Social Services

Phone: (719) 655-2537

Fax: (719) 655-0206

After Hours: Sheriff's Office (719) 655-2445

Jeannie Norris, Director

P.O. Box 215 (mail)

605 Christy Avenue

Saguache, CO 81149

San Juan – Department of Social Services

Phone: (970) 387-5326

Fax: (970) 387-5236

After Hours: Answering Service (866) 382-9721

Lezlie Mayer, Director

P.O. Box 376 (mail)

1557 Greene Street

Silverton, CO 81433

San Miguel – Department of Social Services

Phone: (970) 728-4411

Fax: (970) 728-4412

After Hours: Law enforcement (970) 728-1911

Allan Gerstle, Director

P.O. Box 96

333 West Colorado Avenue

Telluride, CO 81435

Sedgwick – Department of Human Services

Phone: (970) 474-3397, ext.227

Fax: (970) 474-9881

After Hours: Sedgwick Sheriff's Office (970) 474-3355 (on-call worker will be paged)

Lisa Ault, Director

P.O. Box 27 (mail)

118 West 3rd

Julesburg, CO 80737

Summit – Department of Social Services

Phone: (970) 668-6198

Fax: (970) 668-4115

After Hours: Summit Sheriff Dispatch (970) 668-8600

Susan Gruber, Director

P.O. Box 869 (mail)

37 County Road 1005

Frisco, CO 80443

Teller – Department of Social Services

Phone: (719) 687-3335

Fax: (719) 687-0429

After Hours: Sheriff's Office (719) 687-9652

Kim Mauthe, Director

P.O. Box 9033 (mail)

740 Highway 24

Woodland Park, CO 80866

Washington – Department of Human Services

Phone: (970) 345-2238

Fax: (970) 345-2237

After Hours: (970) 345-2244

Rick Agan, Director

PO Box 395 (mail)

126 West 5th

Akron, CO 80720

Weld – Department of Human Services

Phone: (970) 352-1551

Fax: (970) 353-5215

After Hours: 911

Judy Griego, Director

P.O. Box A (mail)

315 North 11th Avenue

Greeley, CO 80631

<u>Yuma – Department of Social Services</u>

Phone: (970) 332-4877

Fax: (970) 332-4978

24/7 Hotline: (970) 848-0464

David K. Henson, Director

340 South Birch Street

Wray, CO 80758

Connecticut

Living:

http://www.ct.gov/ctportal/taxonomy/taxonomy.asp?DLN=27189&ctportalNav=|27189|&ctportalPNav Ctr=|27357|#27357

⊞ Arts and Culture

⊟ Disability Services

> ▸ Board of Education and Services for the Blind
> ▸ Bureau of Rehabilitation Services (Department of Social Services)
> ▸ Disability Resource Directory
> ▸ Library for the Blind and Physically Handicapped

⊞ Children and Family

⊞ Driving

⊞ Government

⊞ Health

⊞ Housing

▸ ConneCT Kids

⊞ Leisure Activities

▸ Relocating

⊞ Media and News

⊞ Schools

⊞ Cities and Towns

⊞ Travel and Transportation

▸ Voting and Elections

⊞ Weather

▸ Long-Term Care

Department of Social Services: http://www.ct.gov/dss/site/default.asp

Programs For Elders: http://www.ct.gov/dss/cwp/view.asp?a=2345&Q=304924&dssNav=|

Aging Services: http://www.ct.gov/agingservices/cwp/view.asp?a=2510&q=313020

State of Connecticut Department of Social Services

The Department of Social Services (DSS) provides a broad range of services to the elderly, persons with disabilities, families, and individuals who need assistance in maintaining or achieving their full potential for self-direction, self-reliance and independent living. It administers over 90 legislatively authorized programs and one-third of the state budget.

Mission

The Connecticut Department of Social Services provides a continuum of core services to:
• Meet basic needs of food, shelter, economic support and health care
• Promote and support the choice to live with dignity in one's own home and community
• Promote and support the achievement of economic viability in the workforce

We gain strength from our diverse environment to promote equal access to all DSS programs and services.

Vision

The Connecticut Department of Social Services is people working together to support individuals and families to reach their full potential and live better lives. We do this with humanity and integrity.

Follow this link to learn more about the CT Department of Social Services

DSS Aging Services Division

The Aging Services Division, Connecticut's State Unit on Aging, ensures that Connecticut's elders have access to the supportive services necessary to live with dignity, security, and independence. The Division is responsible for planning, developing, and administering a comprehensive and integrated service delivery system for older persons in Connecticut.

To accomplish this, the Division conducts needs assessments, surveys methods of service administration, evaluates and monitors such services, maintains information and referral services, and develops, coordinates, and/or collaborates with other appropriate agencies to provide services.

More specifically, the Division administers Older Americans Act programs for supportive services, in-home services, and congregate and home-delivered meals. It also administers programs that provide senior community employment, health insurance counseling, and respite care for caregivers.

We work closely with our aging network partners to provide these services. Our partners include Connecticut's five area agencies on aging, municipal agents for the elderly, senior centers, and many others who provide services to older adults.

The Connecticut Statewide Respite Care Program:
http://www.ct.gov/agingservices/cwp/view.asp?a=2513&q=313026

As of May 1, 2010 The Connecticut Statewide Respite Care Program has been re-opened for new intake.

New applicants on or after this date will be placed on a waitlist and served once all of the clients on the existing waitlist are served. If you were placed on the waitlist prior to May 1, 2010, please call 1-800-994-9422 and notify the Care Manager at your local Area Agency on Aging if you are still interested in receiving services. If you did not file an application prior to May 1, 2010, please apprise them of your interest in being placed on the current waitlist. You may also be screened for other programs for which you may be eligible at that time.

This program offers relief to stressed caregivers by providing information, support, the development of an appropriate plan of care, and services for the individual with Alzheimer's Disease or related dementias. There is a maximum of three thousand five hundred dollars in services available per year to each applicant, and a maximum of 30 days of out of home respite care services (excluding Adult Day Care) available per year to each applicant. This program is a joint partnership between the Alzheimer's Association Connecticut Chapter, the Area Agencies on Aging, and the State of Connecticut Department of Social Services, Aging Services Division.

The eligibility criteria are as follows:

1. An application must be completed which includes a Physician's statement certifying the condition of the individual with Alzheimer's disease or a related dementia.

2. Applicants (individuals with Alzheimer's or a related dementia) must have an income of $41,000 a year or less, liquid assets of $109,000 or less, and cannot be enrolled in the Connecticut Homecare Program for Elders. Income is considered to be Social Security (minus the Medicare Part B premiums), Supplemental Security Income, Railroad Retirement Income, veteran's benefits, and any other payments received on a one-time or recurring basis. Liquid assets include checking and savings accounts, stocks, bonds, IRAs, certificates of deposit, or other holdings that can be converted into cash.

3. A Co-payment of 20% of the cost of services is required unless waived by the Agency on Aging Care Manager due to financial hardship.

Governor M.Jodi Rell signs into law a bill expanding the Connecticut Statewide Respite Program's eligibility parameters to include individuals under 65 on the Medicaid program.

For more information on the CT Statewide Respite Program, call 1-800-994-9422 to be directed to your nearest Area Agency on Aging or contact the Care Manager directly:

Joan Marshall

Senior Resources (Eastern CT)

(860) 887-3561

Betsy Wieland

Agency on Aging of South Central CT

(203) 785-8533

Katie Halligan

Mary Ellen Girard

Southwestern CT Agency on Aging

Western CT Area Agency on Aging

(203) 333-9288

(203) 757-5449

Karen Asheh
North Central CT Area Agency on Aging
(860) 724-6443

Follow this link to the map of Connecticut to find the Area Agency on Aging serving your town.

For information on the CT Nursing Home Diversion Modernization Project and how it works with the CT Statewide Respite Care Program please follow this link.

Please follow this link to view "Choices At Home" a video on self-directed care and an on-line training tool for Caregivers and Consumers.

For more information on Alzheimer's Disease, as well as counseling and support groups, call the Connecticut Chapter of the Alzheimer's Association at 1-800-356-5502 or (860) 828-2828.

Additional links to Alzheimer's Disease and supports:

The Alzheimer's Association, Connecticut Chapter: www.alz.org/ct

The Alzheimer's Association, National Office: www.alz.org

The National Institute on Aging's Alzheimer's Disease Education and Referral Center: www.alzheimers.nia.nih.gov

The National Alzheimer's Contact Center is a free tool for caregivers available 24 hours/day, 365 days/year. It offers an integrated network of information specialists and clinicians who can provide you with free consultation and support by phone or online. A senior housing finder, group calendars, message boards and other free online tools are accessible at the website: http://www.alz.org/we_can_help_caresource.asp

Or call the 24-hour helpline toll free # at 1-800-272-3900.

For more information on caregiver supports, the following websites are available:

The National Alliance for Caregiving: www.caregiving.org

The National Family Caregiver Association: www.nfcacares.org

Administration on Aging Caregiver Resources: www.aoa.gov/prof/aoaprog/caregiver/caregiver.asp

If you have any questions concerning this program or related services, feel free to contact Cynthia Grant at (860) 424-5279 or Cynthia.grant@ct.gov.

DSS Programs for Elders: http://www.ct.gov/dss/cwp/view.asp?a=2345&Q=304924&dssNav=|

These programs are general Department of Social Services programs that you may be eligible for as an older individual. Further information about Caregiving, Employment, Health Insurance, Health & Wellness, Housing, Legal, Long Term Care Insurance, Nutrition, Volunteerism and other programs is available. Please click here to visit the Aging Services website if the information you are seeking is not on this page. Aging Services Division

The Long Term Care Ombudsman Program works to improve the quality of life and quality of care of Connecticut residents living in long term care facilities. Ombudsman activity is performed on behalf of, and at the direction of residents. The Ombudsman Program responds to, and investigates complaints brought forward by residents, family members, and/or other individuals acting on their behalf and all communication is held in strict confidence. The Program brings residents to the forefront to voice their concerns directly to public officials and supports residents in their quest to shape their own legislative agenda. The Ombudsman Program offers information and consultation to consumers and providers, monitors state and federal laws and regulations, and makes recommendations for improvements.

Caregiving

- Alzheimer's Respite Care Program
- Grandparents as Parents (GAPS)
- National Family Caregiver Support Program

Cash Assistance

- Adult Services Division

Employment Services

- Employment and Training
- Aging Services Division - Employment

Food Assistance

- SNAP (Formerly known as Food Stamps)
  - Programs and Services
  - Nutritional Assistance Programs
- Food Banks
  - Nutritional Assistance Programs
- Nutrition
  - Aging Services - Nutrition

Housing Assistance

- Locating Affordable Rental Housing
- Congregate Housing
  - Housing
- Emergency Homeless Shelters
  - Housing
- Eviction Prevention Program
  - Social Work
  - Social Work Services
  - Community Services
- Homeshare Program
  - Aging Services Division - Housing
- Home Care for Elders
  - Alternate Care Unit
- Rental Assistance Program
  - Housing
- Security Deposit Program
  - Housing - Security Deposit
  - Housing
- Shelters and Services for Victims of Domestic Violence
  - Housing - Security
  - Preventive Services to Families
- Transitional Living Program
  - Housing

Medical

- CHOICES Program (Health Insurance Assistance for Individuals with Medicare)
  - Aging Services Division - CHOICES
- ConnPACE
  - ConnPACE.com
- ConnTrans - Connecticut Organ Transplant Program
  - Adult Services Division
  - Brochures: ConnTRANS - Connecticut Program for Organ Transplant Recipients

- CHCPE - Connecticut Home Care for Elders
  - Alternate Care Unit
- Medicaid (Title XIX)
  - Adult Services Division
  - Community Medicaid
  - Money Follows the Person
- Medicare
  - Medicare Savings Programs

Bureau of Aging, Community, and Social Work Services

- Prevention Services
  - Social Work Services
- Protective Services for the Elderly
  - Social Work Services

Winter Heating Aid

- Connecticut Energy Assistance Program
- Refugee Assistance Services

CHCPE Alternate Care Unit: http://www.ct.gov/dss/cwp/view.asp?a=2353&q=305170

Alternate Care Unit - Connecticut Home Care Program for Elders (CHCPE)
This Web site explains the CT Home Care Program for Elders including who is eligible for the program, what services are available, how to apply for services, and how to contact the program.
To be eligible, applicants must be 65 years of age or older, be a CT resident, be at risk of nursing home placement and meet the program's financial eligibility criteria. To be at risk of nursing home placement means that the applicant needs assistance with critical needs such as bathing, dressing, eating, taking medications, toileting. The CHCPE helps eligible clients continue living at home instead of going to a nursing home. Each applicant's needs are reviewed to determine if the applicant may remain at home with the help of home care services. For more information on eligibility criteria, please see the link below.
Services may include:
Care Management Services
Adult Day Health Services
Companion Services
Home Delivered Meals
Homemaker Services
Assisted Living Services
*Personal Care Attendant Services - family members are NOT eligible to be paid for taking care of relatives with very rare exceptions.
*Chore Assistance - only available as part of a package of services to applicants who meet all other eligibility criteria.
Co-Pay Requirement

Public Act 10-179, Section 21 instituted a 6% copay amount for clients in the state funded home care program, effective 7/1/10. Effective 7/1/11, Public Act 11-6 increases the copay amount to 7%. The care manager assigned to you can explain the process in detail. Failure to pay the copay will result in the termination of services under the CT Home Care Program for Elders.

Assisted Living Demonstration Program residents (The Retreat), Hebert T. Clark, Smithfield Gardens and Luther Ridge) are excluded from copay requirements, per Section 17b-347e of the CT General Statutes. For more information, or to start the application process, please call 1-800-445-5394 (toll-free) or 860-424-4904 locally in the Hartford area.

PROGRAM INFORMATION: Click on the links below for more information:

General Program Information

Program Brochure

Program Brochure - Spanish

Contact Information

HOME AND COMMUNITY-BASED SERVICES WAIVER APPLICATION

CT Home Care Program for Elders Waiver Renewal 2010

Assisted Living

Assisted Living Options

Assisted Living Program Flyer - English

Assisted Living Flyer - Spanish

Participating Assisted Living Facilities in CT

For further information about Assisted Living Facilities in CT, see

www.ctassistedliving.com/providers.cfm

CT Adult Day Care Centers 5-2011

Eligibility

Spousal Assessments (revised 5/10)

Financial and Functional Eligibility

Transfer of Assets

Eligibility Information

Eligibility, Categories of Service and Cost Caps

PCA

Personal Care Attendant Guidelines (Rev. 7/10)

CT Home Care Prorgam for Disabled Adults

The CT Home Care Program for Disabled Adults (CHCPDA)

(see "Forms" below for application form)

CHCPE Annual Report

2009 Annual Report

2008 Annual Report

2007 Annual Report

2006 Annual Report

FORMS FOR POTENTIAL CLIENTS:

Program Application (Rev. 8/10)

Program Application (Spanish)

CHCPE Referral Form - to make a referral to the program

CT Home Care Program for Disabled Adults application form

FORMS FOR PROVIDERS ONLY

Health Screen Form - for health care professionals only

W-1510 Part II - for access agencies only (Rev. 2010)

Assessment Tool for Providers - for Access Agency/provider use only

Performing Provider Enrollment Form

Performing Provider Agreement

Programs for People With Disabilities:

http://www.ct.gov/dss/cwp/view.asp?a=2345&Q=304922&dssNav=|

Programs for People with Disabilities

Medical

- Connecticut Organ Transplant Program (ConnTRANS)
  - Adult Services Division
  - Brochures: ConnTRANS - Connecticut Program for Organ Transplant Recipients
- ConnPACE
  - ConnPACE.com
- Medicaid (Title XIX)
  - Acquired Brain Injury (ABI)
  - Medicaid for the Employees with Disabilities
  - Department of Mental Retardation (DMR) Waiver
  - Personal Care Attendant

- o   Money Follows the Person
- Medicare
  - o   Medicare Savings Programs

Food Assistance

- SNAP (Formerly known as Food Stamps)
  - o   Programs and Services
  - o   Nutritional Assistance Programs
- Food Banks
  - o   Nutritional Assistance Programs

Cash Assistance

- Temporary Family Assistance (TFA)
  - o   Welfare Reform - TFA
- Employment Services
  - o   Welfare Reform - Employment Services

Employment

- Bureau of Rehabilitation Services (BRS)
- Connect to Work Program
- Connect-Ability

Repatriation (U.S. Citizens abroad)

- No URL at this time

Social Work Services

- Preventive Services
  - o   Preventive Services to Families
  - o   Social Work
  - o   Social Work Services
  - o   Community Services
- Safety Net Services
  - o   Safety Net Program

Winter Heating Aid

- Connecticut Energy Assistance Program
- Refugee Assistance Services

Housing Assistance

- Locating Affordable Rental Housing

- Congregate Housing
  - Housing
  - Publications: Services for Seniors (181KB)
- Emergency Homeless Shelters
  - Housing
- Eviction Prevention Program
  - Social Work
  - Social Work Services
- Homeshare Program
  - Aging Services Division - Housing
- Rental Assistance Program
  - Housing
- Section 8 Housing
  - Housing
  - Housing - Section 8
- Section 8 Moderate Rehabilitation Program
  - Housing
- Security Deposit Program
  - Housing - Security Deposit
  - Housing
- Shelters and Services for Victims of Domestic Violence
  - Housing - Security
  - Preventive Services to Families
- Transitional Living Program
  - Housing

Affirmative Action

- ADA (Americans with Disabilities Act)

Housing: http://www.ct.gov/agingservices/cwp/view.asp?a=2513&q=313058

Homeshare

Housing Options

Reverse Annuity Mortgages

Homeshare: http://www.ct.gov/agingservices/cwp/view.asp?a=2513&q=313058

Home Share Program:

Single adults who are having difficulty maintaining their homes and/or don't want to live alone, may share a home with another single adult who needs affordable housing and is willing to either make a financial contribution or perform services.

Housing counseling and/or opportunities for single individuals, one of whom must be over age 60, to share a house are available through three home share programs in Connecticut. Applicants to the program are screened and interviewed by the program staff. The staff introduces individuals found to be compatible, helps them to develop a home sharing-agreement, and offers follow-up counseling if a match is made. If a home share arrangement is not appropriate, staff will counsel applicants, and/or refer them to other appropriate housing services. Interested parties should call the program closest to them or in the area they wish to live.

Connecticut's Home Share Programs

1. Agency on Aging of South Central Connecticut
One Long Wharf Drive, Suite 1L
New Haven, CT 06511
Phone: 203 785-8533
Fax: 203 785-8873
Website: www.aoapartnerships.org

2. North Central Area Agency on Aging
151 New Park Ave., Suite 15
Hartford, CT 06106
Phone: 860 724-6443
Fax: 860 251-6107
Website: www.ncaaact.org

Delaware

http://dhss.delaware.gov/dhss/main/aging.htm

Division and Services for Aging and Adults With Physical Disabilities:
http://dhss.delaware.gov/dhss/dsaapd/index.html

Services Overview Guide: http://dhss.delaware.gov/dhss/dsaapd/files/aging_and_disabilities_guide.pdf

Office Locations: http://dhss.delaware.gov/dhss/dsaapd/ofclocations.html

The Division of Services for Aging and Adults with Physical Disabilities has three office locations: in New Castle, Newark, and Milford. Hours of operation are 8:00 AM to 4:30 PM, Monday through Friday.

1901 N. Du Pont Highway, Main Bldg.
New Castle, DE 19720
DMS Fiscal Management: (302) 255-9265
DSAAPD: (302) 255-9390

256 Chapman Road
Oxford Building
Newark, DE 19702
DPH Cancer Registry: (302) 283-7200>
DPH HIV/AIDS: (302) 283-7210
DSAAPD: (302) 453-3820 or (800) 223-9074

18 N. Walnut Street
Milford, DE 19963
DPH Child Development Watch: (302) 424-7300 or (800) 752-9393
DSAAPD: (302) 424-7310 or (800) 223-9074

Assistance For Caregivers: http://dhss.delaware.gov/dhss/dsaapd/caregivers_assistance.html

Service Related Links: http://dhss.delaware.gov/dhss/dsaapd/links.html

Florida

(As far as I could determine, The Great State of Florida which has one of the largest senior populations in the country offers virtually no publicly funded services other than those of Adult Protective Services and some assisted living facilities both long term and residential. I could find nothing on the subject of in-home care, in some way assisted through Florida's auspices. I would however be pleased to be proven incorrect...).

http://www.myflorida.com/

Aging Resource Centers: http://www.agingresourcecentersofflorida.org/

About Florida's Aging Resource Centers

Florida's Aging Resource Centers are committed to helping persons age 60 and above and those who care about them understand and navigate the complex web of available services, agencies and other options. Our goal is to help you find the information, resources and services you need to make informed decisions.

Florida's eleven Aging Resource Centers help persons age 60 and above and their loved ones find agencies and individuals who can provide assistance on a variety of issues – from housing and home care to meals, transportation and other vital areas of concern.

We will help you find answers to the many questions you have as you or someone you love face the challenges of growing older. And let's face it: life gets a bit more complicated as we get older, so it's good to know where to turn for help.

At Florida's Aging Resource Centers, our primary job is to listen. We listen to your questions and concerns, and provide a list of resources – including names, addresses, telephone numbers and websites - where you will find the information you need to make sound decisions. It's that simple. You call, we respond. We're on your side and we're here to help. Give us a call or visit us online. Our goal is to help you find the information, resources and services you need to make informed decisions.

Growing older has its rewards. One of the finest is your Aging Resource Center. Florida's Aging Resource Centers are staffed by trusted, compassionate and professional people who will help find real answers to life's questions.

Senior Resource Alliance:
http://www.seniorresourcealliance.org/InfoByCateg/Caregiving.aspx?wadi=iOFaTT0z011hxlaMKHoW5l1sZnzNW5001anSGOzg2gmL%2bL2YMuyvKA%3d%3d

Caregiving

Becoming a Caregiver

It's 1:00 a.m. and the phone rings. The hospital is calling to tell you that your father has suffered a stroke. A neighbor found him and called 911. Come quickly, they say. You rush to your father's side, but the stroke has left him partially paralyzed and unable to speak. The doctor says a full recovery is unlikely; he begins telling you a whole list of things you need to do and arrangements you need to make. Looking back, it's all a blur. What happened? Life has called YOU to become a caregiver!

Most of us never think about who will care for our parents when they get older. Many times, middle-aged children don't even recognize their parents' aging. They may see them infrequently or may simply not recognize small changes that indicate a problem could be developing. What's more, many older adults cover up problems. In any case, few of us plan ahead for these changes; usually they take us by surprise—financially and emotionally.

Who is a caregiver? A caregiver is anyone who takes care of or provides assistance to an older or disabled person. Interestingly, few adults identify themselves as elder caregivers, but at least one in four American families are doing so. The National Alliance for Caregiving and AARP teamed up to produce a scale that measures the level of intensity for caregiving. "Intense" caregivers are those who perform personal care tasks (bathing, dressing, etc.) for an average of 12-87 hours per week. "Informal" caregivers provide, on average, fewer than 10 hours of care per week. This may include transportation, help with homemaking or yard maintenance, meals, and financial and emotional support.

Caregiver Support and Training

So what do you do if, as in the story above, you find yourself thrust into a caregiving role with no preparation or training? Currently, there's no easy answer, but some places to look for help are these online resources:

http://www.nfcacares.org/ This is the website of the National Family Caregivers Association. It can link you to a wide variety of training resources and service information. There are also ways to connect with other family caregivers for peer learning and support.

http://www.familycaregiving101.org/ This website has even more specific tips and training ideas for family caregivers.

http://www.caregiving.org/ This is the website of the National Alliance for Caregiving, and it is full of great information for family caregivers, including helpful explanations about the hospital discharge process.

http://www.redcross.org/ The American Red Cross offers caregiving classes at some of its local chapters, including the Central Florida Chapter on Bumby Ave. in Orlando. Contact them by calling (407) 894-4141 or see a complete list of courses on their website: www.centralflorida.redcross.org/courses.php . The Space Coast Chapter in Rockledge does not currently offer the caregiver training, but does offer CPR and Nurse Assistant training. Contact them at 321-890-1002.

Cooperative Caregiving

An approach to dividing caregiving tasks, according to the skills and abilities of each family member or friend, is called Cooperative Caregiving. This approach recognizes that no one person can or must do it all. Rather, caregiving is a team effort with the elder at the center of the action, calling the plays, whenever possible.

Whether you are the family elder, a family member or other caregiver, the following list of "job titles" might help you identify the specific type of assistance that you need or can provide.

Personal Care Assistant	Transportation Assistant
Cook and Nutritionist	Medical Manager
Mobility Assistant	Legal Assistant
Listener and Companion	Investment Advisor
Financial Assistant	Administrative Clerk
Emergency Responder	Home Care Assistant

Each family member or helper can commit to fill a specific role or roles, knowing that other roles can be filled by others. If no one in the family's network is willing or able to perform a specific role that must be filled, then outside resources can be explored, only to fill this specific need.

The Care Manager Role

Another key role is that of Care Manager. As the assembler of caregiving resources, the Care Manager's job may be compared to that of a general contractor in charge of building a house. It is the contractor's role to identify and secure willing and qualified resources to perform the many different types of construction tasks. Whether a family member fulfills this function or you contract with a professional depends on several factors. Being the "general contractor" for your own or your elder's care is a big job in itself and may be more than you can handle alone.

If the role seems too much for you, consider hiring a professional **Geriatric Care Manager**, a social worker or elder care professional who performs these general contracting tasks for a fee. To learn more about what geriatric care managers do and what they charge or to find one in your area, go to: www.caremanager.org. If your case is complicated, you live a considerable distance from your loved one, or if you lack family members to assist you, contracting with a Geriatric Care Manager may be well worth the cost.

Georgia

Disability and Mental Health: http://www.georgia.gov/00/channel_title/0,2094,4802_5001,00.html

Seniors: http://www.georgia.gov/00/channel_title/0,2094,4802_5007,00.html

Division of Aging Services: http://aging.dhr.georgia.gov/portal/site/DHS-DAS/

Help at Home: http://aging.dhr.georgia.gov/portal/site/DHS-DAS/menuitem.9e91405d0e424e248e738510da1010a0/?vgnextoid=5dc466ef2affff00VgnVCM100000bf01010aRCRD

    Caregiver Programs: http://aging.dhr.georgia.gov/portal/site/DHS-DAS/menuitem.9e91405d0e424e248e738510da1010a0/?vgnextoid=baf466ef2affff00VgnVCM100000bf01010aRCRD

Home & Community Based Services

Non-Medicaid Home and Community Based Services include a range of solutions to help older Georgians live safely, healthily, and independently in their homes and communities.
The Home and Community Based Services program is mandated through the Older Americans Act. It assists individuals age 60 and older and their caregivers. (Note that consumers may be eligible at 55 years old for some programs such as senior employment and kinship care.)
The Division of Aging Services administers, contracting with 12 Area Agencies on Aging, to regionally manage the program and consumer case management.
How to Get Local Help
For information & assistance, eligibility screening, and referral to community services/ resources, contact your regional Area Agency on Aging.

At this point you must choose a region and city from two drop down menus for further contact information

Available services in your community may include:
Nutrition and Wellness
- ♦ Congregate (group) Meals at Senior Centers
- ♦ Home-Delivered Meals
- ♦ Nutrition and Wellness Education
- ♦ Counseling
- ♦ Health Promotion and Disease Prevention
(See CDSMP under "Other Services.")
- ♦ Physical Fitness Classes
- ♦ Senior Recreation

In-Home Services
- ♦ Emergency Response Services
- ♦ Respite Care
(services that offer a brief period of rest for family caregivers)
- ♦ Friendly Visiting
(home visits to reduce isolation)

♦ Telephone Reassurance
(regular phone calls to reduce isolation and check on an elder's safety)
♦ Homemaker Services
(light housekeeping, meal preparation, etc.)

♦ Chore Services
♦ Personal Care Assistance
(stand-by prompting or hands-on help with bathing, dressing, and similar activities of daily living)

Caregiver Programs
♦ Respite

♦ Education and Support Groups

♦ Adult Day Services
(daytime care and meals in a supervised group community setting)
♦ Mobile Day Care (Click here.)

Kinship Care Programs
(Grandparents and Other Relatives Raising Children)
♦ Education and Support
♦ Case Management
♦ Counseling
♦ Access to Respite
(services to provide a brief period of relief for caregivers, exs: summer camps and child care)
♦ Information about Special Services
(Exs: Legal Assistance, Tutoring, Respite, etc.)

Other Services
♦ Home Modification and Repair
♦ Home Management Training
(training in self-help and self-care skills, training in daily living skills)
♦ Material Aid
(Limited Availability: payments to or on behalf of an elder for housing/shelter, transportation, utilities, food, etc.)

♦ Mental Health Counseling

♦ Community and Public Education

♦ Home Sharing

♦ Transportation
♦ **Senior Community Service Employment Program** (Click here)
(Adults who are 55 or older and who meet income eligibility requirements can receive training, on-the-job experience in community settings, and assistance with securing private employment through SCSEP services.)
♦ **Chronic Disease Self Management Program (CDSMP)**
CDSMP is an evidence-based, train-the-trainer program developed by Stanford University to help promote the empowerment of persons with chronic conditions or those caring for persons with chronic conditions to be able to live well and not be consumed by the condition. Participants of a

Live Well CDSMP Workshop meet for 2-1/2 hours, once a week, for six weeks and learn techniques to deal with the common symptoms shared across various conditions (pain, fatigue, shortness of breath, depression, difficult emotions, tense muscles, and stress/anxiety).

♦ **Livable Communities Initiatives**

Special initiatives help communities build their capacity to meet the needs of a growing aging population. Livable Communities efforts relate to housing, community mobility, environmental health, civic engagement, and more.

POLICIES

Online Directives Information System (ODIS)

RELATED LINKS

Live Well Age Well

Grandparents Raising Grandchildren

National Alliance for Caregiving

VIDEO

Mobile Day Care

PUBLICATIONS

Alzheimer's Disclosure Form (pdf)

Caregiving in Georgia: Role of Focus Groups (pdf)

Caregiving in Georgia - Focus Group Follow up (pdf)

Caregiving in Georgia Report, Summer 2003 (pdf)

Distance Caregiving - Final 3-09 (pdf)

Georgia Senior Homeowner's Resource Guide (Rev 2010) (pdf)

Mobile Day Care Fact Sheet (pdf)

Self Directed Care Guidebook (pdf)

Self Directed Care Fact Sheet

You may also click upon the "Contact Us" button on the left side of the above page to go to local AAA (Area Agencies on Aging), then pick the most pertinent

Hawaii

http://portal.ehawaii.gov/

Seniors: http://portal.ehawaii.gov/residents/seniors.html

General Resources

Executive Office on Aging (EOA)

The designated lead agency in the coordination of a statewide system of aging and caregiver support services in the State of Hawai'i.

Hawai'i Aging and Disability Resource Center

Your one-stop source for information, assistance, and access to community resources and services for older adults, people with disabilities, and family caregivers.

How To Obtain a Disabled Persons Parking Permit

Find instructions and application for applying for a disabled persons parking permit.

Department of Human Services Adult Services and Programs

Programs such as: adult and grandparent foster care, transportation assistance, chore services, and senior companionship.

Department of Health Useful Websites

Various links to useful websites, both Hawai'i and national.

Hawai'i AARP

Provides general information on aging and sometimes acts as an advocate concerning fraud and abuse, age discrimination, prescription-drug issues and economic security; also, refers members to local attorneys who handle issues related to the elderly.

SeniorNet

Provides older adults education and access to computer technology.

Kokua Mau: Hawai'i's Hospice and Palliative Care Organization

Find support groups, information on advance directives, and other resources for improving quality of life by promoting excellence in hospice, end-of-life care, palliative care, and early advance care planning.

Staying Active

Retired and Senior Volunteer Program (RSVP)

Provides volunteer opportunities for persons 55 and older to remain as active, contributing members of the community through volunteer involvement.

Department of Parks & Recreation, Senior Citizens Section, O'ahu

City-sponsored clubs at recreation centers, classes and events for seniors.

Lanakila Multi-Purpose Senior Center (Catholic Charities), O'ahu

Kaunoa Senior Services, Maui

Activities for Seniors, Kaua'i

Elderly Recreation Services, County of Hawai'i

Medical

Hawai'i QUEST, Medical assistance to qualified persons (Medicaid)

SagePlus, Health insurance and Medicare counseling.

United States Government Websites

- Medicare Insurance
- Social Security Administration
- Administration on Aging

Executive Office on Aging (EOA): http://hawaii.gov/health/eoa/index.html

EXECUTIVE OFFICE ON AGING (EOA)

The Executive Office on Aging (EOA) is the designated lead agency in the coordination of a statewide system of aging and caregiver support services in the State of Hawaii, as authorized by federal and state laws.

The federal Older Americans Act establishes an Aging Network and provides federal funding for elderly support services, nutrition services, preventive health services, elder rights protection, and family caregiver support services. Chapter 349 of the Hawaii Revised Statutes establishes the Executive Office on Aging as the focal point for all matters relating to older adults' needs and the coordination and development of caregiver support services within the State of Hawaii.

To learn about EOA's efforts to develop comprehensive and coordinated systems to serve older adults and family caregivers in the State of Hawaii, please read the Hawaii State Plan on Aging: 2008-2011.

Programs & Services

Healthy Aging Partnership
A statewide public-private partnership committed to improving the health and well-being of residents. The partnership offers evidence-based health promotion and disease prevention programs: the EnhancedFitness (EF) Program on Kauai and the Ke Ola Pono Disease Self-Management Programs-Chronic Disease Self-Management (CDSMP), Arthritis Self-Management (ASMP) and Diabetes Self-Management (DSMP). Ke Ola Pono classes are open to adults 18 and older.

For information on accessing these services in your local area, please contact your county office on aging:
Honolulu: (808)768-7705 • Hawaii: (808)961-8600 • Maui/Molokai/Lanai: (808)270-7774 • Kauai: (808)241-4470

Senior Medicare Patrol Hawaii (SMP Hawaii)
A volunteer-based program to ensure Medicare is not billed for health care services, medical supplies, and equipment not received. If you suspect fraud or errors when reviewing your Medicare statement, please contact SMP Hawaii at 586-7281 on Oahu and toll-free at 1-800-296-9422 from the neighbor islands.

Hawaii's Fraud Prevention & Resource Guide is designed to help residents protect themselves against fraud.
The 134-page guide provides information about different types of fraud, including identity theft, securities fraud, marketing fraud, and healthcare fraud.

Sage PLUS Program
This program provides free health insurance information, education, counseling, and a referral service for people with Medicare. Volunteers are trained and certified to assist members and their families with questions about Medicare benefits, Medicare Advantage Program, Long-Term Care financing, and Medicare Part D - the prescription drug benefit. For assistance, please contact Sage PLUS at 586-7299 on Oahu and toll-free at 1-888-875-9229 or 1-866-810-4379 (TTY).

The Long-Term Care Ombudsman Program (LTCOP)

This program provides information, outreach, and advocacy for residents of long-term care facilities. If you have a problem, complaint, or question regarding services provided at a long-term care facility, please call the LTC Ombudsman at 586-7268(Oahu).

To ensure that all long-term care residents are aware of the services provided by the Long-Term Care Ombudsman, volunteers are trained and certified by the LTC Ombudsman Volunteer Program to regularly visit licensed LTC settings. To become a certified volunteer, please complete the LTCOP Volunteer Application and mail it to the LTCO Volunteer Coordinator at Executive Office on Aging, 250 South Hotel Street, #406, Honolulu, HI 96813.

In-Home and Community-Based Services

Services are available to assist older adults in remaining independent and active. Types of services provided: adult day care, assisted transportation, attendant care, case management, chore services, congregate meals, home delivered meals, homemaker/housekeeper, information and assistance, legal assistance, nutrition education, personal care, and transportation.

For information on accessing services in your local area, please contact your county office on aging:
Honolulu: (808)768-7705 • Hawaii: (808)961-8600 • Maui/Molokai/Lanai: (808)270-7774 • Kauai: (808)241-4470

Family Caregiver Support Program

Support services are available to family caregivers such as: information, assistance, individual counseling, support groups and training, respite, and supplemental services.

For information on accessing these services in your local area, please contact your county office on aging:
Honolulu: (808)768-7705 • Hawaii: (808)961-8600 • Maui/Molokai/Lanai: (808)270-7774 • Kauai: (808)241-4470

Resources for Older Adults and Family Caregivers

Useful Websites • Reports/Publications • Family Caregiver Newsletter • Advance Health Care Directive Form •

Physician Orders for Life Sustaining Treatment Form

Contact Information

Executive Office on Aging
No. 1 Capitol District
250 South Hotel Street, Suite 406
Honolulu, Hawaii 96813-2831
email: eoa@doh.hawaii.gov

Phone: (808) 586-0100 • FAX: (808) 586-0185

If you are calling from a neighbor island, use the toll-free State of Hawaii access numbers (when prompted, enter 60100)
Kauai - 274-3141
Maui - 984-2400
Hawaii - 974-4000
Molokai, Lanai - 1-800-468-4644

Family Caregiver Support Program: http://hawaii.gov/health/eoa/CG.html

The Family Caregiver Support program provides caregiver support services to enable care recipients to remain in their familiar environment. These caregiver support services are available to adult family members, or other individuals who are informal, unpaid providers of in-home and community care to older adults age 60 and older.

Caregiver support services are also available to grandparents or relatives (not parents) age 55 or older who are taking care of a child, age 18 and younger and/or a relative 18 and older with a disability.

Please contact your county office on aging for more information about accessing these services.

Caregiver Support Services

- **Access Assistance** - A service that assists caregivers in obtaining access to the services and resources that are available within their communities.

- **Counseling** - Counseling to caregivers to assist them in making decisions and solving problems relating to their caregiving roles. This includes counseling to individuals, support groups, and caregiving training.

- **Information Services** - A service for caregivers that provides the public and individuals with information on resources and services available to the individual within their communities.

- **Supplemental Services** - Services provided on a limited basis to complement the care provided by caregivers. Examples of supplemental services include, but are not limited to, home modifications, assistive technologies, emergency response systems, and incontinence supplies.

- **Respite Care** - Services which offer temporary, substitute supports or living arrangements for care recipients in order to provide a brief period of relief or rest for caregivers.

Contact Information

For caregiver services in your local area, please contact your county office on aging.

Elderly Affairs Division (Honolulu)
phone:(808)768-7705 • website: www.elderlyaffairs.com

Hawaii County Office of Aging
phone: (808)961-8600 • website: www.hcoahawaii.org

Maui County Office on Aging
phone: (808)270-7755 • website: http://www.co.maui.hi.us/departments/Housing/aging.htm

Kauai Agency on Elderly Affairs
phone: (808)241-4470 • website: www.kauai.gov/elderly

Aging and Disabled Resource Center: http://www.hawaiiadrc.org/site/439/resources.aspx

Resources

Policy Advisory Board for Elderly Affairs Orientation Trainings

The first time you access the trainings below, the WebEx server will automatically download and install WebEx player. If you are having difficulties viewing the trainings, please contact Tania Kuriki at 808-586-0100 or tania.kuriki@doh.hawaii.gov

Module 1: PABEA Orientation

Speakers: Wes Lum, EOA Director

Recorded on 7/26/2011, 37 minutes

Module 2: Older Americans Act and Hawaii State Plan on Aging

Speakers: John Grant, Grants Supervisor and David Kanno, Planner

Recorded on 7/28/2011, 1 hour and 11 minutes

Module 3: EOA Program Presentations

Speakers: John McDermott, LTC Ombudsman; Brenda Lau, Sage PLUS Assistant Coordinator; Laurie Paleka, SMP Assistant Coordinator; John Grant, Grants Supervisor; Tania Kuriki, Statistician; and Trina Adaro, Secretary/Office Manager

Recorded on 7/29/2011, 1 hour

Module 4: ADRC, Kupuna Care, and Special Projects

Speakers: Nancy Moser, Grants Manager; Caroline Cadirao, Grants Manager; and Wes Lum, EOA Director

Recorded on 8/4/2011, 1 hour and 13 minutes

Executive Office on Aging Publications

Hawaii ADRC 5-Year Operational Plan

Hawaii State Plan on Aging (2007-2011)

Business Plan on Sustainability and Marketing for Evidence-Based Programs (November 2010)

Hawaii's Fraud Prevention and Resource Guide (May 2008)

Advance Health Care Directive Form

Physician Orders for Life Sustaining Treatment (POLST)

Senior Medicare Patrol Hawaii Program Materials

SMP Volunteer Recruitment Handout

Other Informational Website Links

State of Hawaii

Hawaii State Department of Health

Hawaii State Department of Human Services

Hawaii Disability and Long-Term Care Information and Resources

AARP Hawaii

Hawaii Medical Library (The Queen's Medical Center)

Kokua Mau Program (Resources on end-of-life care)

Hilopa'a Family to Family Health Information Center (QUEST Expanded Access (QExA)

Kapiolani Community College-Kupuna Education Center

Listing of Hawaii Adult Residential Care Homes and Assisted Living Facilities

United States Government Websites

Medicare Insurance

Social Security Administration

Administration on Aging

Home and Community Services: http://hawaii.gov/health/eoa/KC.html

HOME AND COMMUNITY SERVICES

Home and community services help older adults, age 60 and older, remain active and independent. Please contact your county office on aging for more information about accessing these services.

DESCRIPTION OF SERVICES

Adult Day Care/Adult Day Health - Personal care for dependent older adults in a supervised, protective, and group setting during some portion of the day.

Assisted Transportation - Door-to-door transit service, including escort, for those who have difficulties (physical or cognitive).

Attendant Care - Companion assistance/oversight of older adults who are frail or have one or more disabling conditions.

Case Management - Assistance to identify needs, explore options, and develop a care plan to achieve greater independence.

Chore Services - Assistance for those unable to perform yard and heavy housework.

Congregate Meals - A meal provided to an older adult in a group setting.

Home Delivered Meals - Meals delivered to frail and vulnerable older adults at their place of residence.

Homemaker/Housekeeper - Help in preparing meals, grocery shopping, managing money, using the telephone, doing housework, and taking medication.

Information and Assistance - A service that provides older adults information on services available within their communities and links them to these services.

Legal Assistance - Legal advice, counseling, and representation by an attorney or legal assistant.

Nutrition Education - Culturally sensitive health information and instruction on maintaining good nutrition.

Personal Care - Assistance to older adults who are unable to bathe, eat, dress, toilet, and/or transfer from bed to chair by themselves.

Transportation - Transportation from one location to another.

Contact Information

For more information about services in your local area, please contact your county office on aging.

Elderly Affairs Division (Honolulu)
phone: (808)768-7705 • website: www.elderlyaffairs.com

Hawaii County Office of Aging
phone: (808)961-8600 • website: www.hcoahawaii.org

Maui County Office on Aging
phone: (808)270-7755 • website: http://www.co.maui.hi.us/departments/Housing/aging.htm

Kauai Agency on Elderly Affairs
phone: (808)241-4470 • website: www.kauai.gov/elderly

While most disabled specific services seem to be covered in the previous material, here is one more link:

Disability and Communication Access Board: http://hawaii.gov/health/dcab/home/index.htm

Idaho

Citizen Services: http://www.idaho.gov/online_services/citizen.html

Idaho Commission on the Aging: http://www.idahoaging.com/

Welcome! The Idaho Commission on Aging is designated by the Governor as Idaho's State Unit on Aging. The Commission administers and ensures compliance of federally funded programs under the Federal Older Americans Act and state funded programs under the Idaho Senior Services Act. We plan, coordinate, fund, and monitor a variety of services, in conjunction with the Area Agency on Aging, to address the present and future needs of older Idahoans, and serve as a catalyst for improvement in the organization, coordination, and delivery of aging services in Idaho.

Idaho Adult Protection Services Public Comment Opportunity:

The Idaho Commission on Aging (ICOA) announces a statewide public comment opportunity regarding Idaho's Adult Protection Services (APS). As the state designated agency responsible for the oversight of the APS Program, ICOA seeks community stakeholder input in an effort to identify opportunities for program improvements as a component of an overall program review.

Your comments and viewpoints are important to this process; therefore ICOA welcomes your participation. The public comment period is scheduled from 2:00 p.m. to 6:00 p.m. to allow for an open house format. It is not required to stay for the entire four hour period. Public comments made in person will be limited to three (3) minutes; however written comments may be submitted at the public meeting or directly to ICOA via the following options:

Mail: Fax: Email:

Idaho Commission on Aging (208) 334-3033 ICOA@aging.idaho.gov

341 W. Washington Street

Boise, ID 83702

August 2 – Idaho Falls
Idaho Falls Public Library
2:00 p.m. to 6:00 p.m.
457 West Broadway, Idaho Falls

August 3 – Pocatello
SICOG Area Agency on Aging
2:00 p.m. to 6:00 p.m.

214 E. Center, Pocatello

August 4 – Twin Falls
Office on Aging, College of Southern Idaho

2:00 p.m. to 6:00 p.m.

Room 248, CSI Student Union Building, Twin Falls

August 22 – Boise

Sage Community Resources

2:00 p.m. to 6:00 p.m.

125 E. 50th Street, Garden City

August 30 – Coeur d'Alene

Area Agency on Aging of North Idaho

2:00 p.m. to 6:00 p.m.

2120 Lakewood Drive, Suite B, Coeur d'Alene

August 31 – Lewiston

Community Action Partnership conference room

2:00 p.m. to 6:00 p.m.

124 New 6th Street, Lewiston

Please contact Sharon Duncan, ICOA Deputy Administrator, at (208)334-3833 with any questions.

ICOA Programs and Services:

http://www.idahoaging.com/IdahoCommissиononAging/ICOAProgramsandServices/tabid/153/Default.aspx

ICOA Programs and Services

The Idaho Commission on Aging is the agency of state government responsible for carrying out the mandates of the <u>Older Americans Act</u> (OAA), as amended, and to distribute federal funds appropriated under the Act for a range of services addressing the needs of Idaho's 60 population. We also administer state monies appropriated under the Senior Services Act. We fund and oversee such services as congregate and home delivered meals, transportation, homemaker and other supportive services. ICOA also provides access to information on work opportunities for seniors, fulfilling both seniors' and business owners' needs.

ICOA has designated six regional offices called <u>"Area Agencies on Aging"</u> to provide tax-supported services to seniors. The AAAs provide some services directly and contract with local providers for other services. This allows easy access to services based on geographical areas and close proximity to those being served. Further information on each program or service, and contact information, both state-wide and regional, can be found on each program page (listed to the left) within this website. Your regional Area

Agency on Aging is the first and best place to start to obtain services and information.

The National Council on the Aging has created two websites, BenefitsCheckUp and BenefitsCheckUpRx, to help older adults to quickly identify services and prescription drug programs that may improve the quality of their lives. A simple questionnaire explains what benefit programs you may be eligible for and how to apply for them. The questionnaire does not ask your name, address or any information that could be used to identify you, and is completely confidential.

These programs and services assist individuals to live independently in a home environment based on their medical needs. Contact your local Area Agency on Aging for information about In-Home Services or to search for services and service providers in your area 211 Idaho CareLine.

In Home Supportive Services:

http://www.idahoaging.com/IdahoCommissiononAging/ICOAProgramsandServices/InHomeSupportServices/tabid/137/Default.aspx

These programs and services assist older individuals to live independently in a home environment. Contact your local Area Agency on Aging for information about receiving In-Home Services. For Information on line, please click on the link to the Idaho ADRC website.

Case Management

Case Management is the gateway to In-Home services. This program primarily serves frail individuals who have multiple needs and who require assistance to access available programs and services. The purpose of the program is to reduce the risk of institutionalization for people who can no longer adequately attend to their own affairs without some degree of guidance or active intervention.

Home-Delivered Meals

Home-bound seniors are able to remain in their homes in part because of the delivery of hot, cold or frozen meals, often by a volunteer. Volunteers delivering meals decrease social isolation for these vulnerable seniors. Area Agency on Aging Case Managers develop individualized plans for this and other In-Home services and assistance for participants.

Homemaker

Essentially a housekeeping service, the Homemaker Program provides assistance with laundry, meal preparation, and other essential activities around the home which frail individuals can no longer manage alone.

Chore

Chore workers assist frail older individuals with minor home repair and maintenance necessary to protect their health and safety. Typical Chore services include shoveling snow off walkways, clearing trash out of a yard, replacing locks and minor plumbing repairs such as unclogging drains.

Respite

This program provides full-time caregivers of homebound persons much needed occasional breaks from their caregiving responsibilities.

Benefit Check up: http://www.benefitscheckup.org/ This appears to be a National Council on the Aging website.

Idaho Council on Developmental Disabilities: http://www.icdd.idaho.gov/

Disability Rights Idaho: http://www.disabilityrightsidaho.org/

DisAbility Rights Idaho is a statewide non-profit agency which provides advocacy and legal services for people with disabilities in Idaho. We have offices in Boise, Pocatello and Moscow.

Anyone may call DisAbility Rights Idaho for information or referrals. Direct representation is available to Idahoans whose issues are directly related to their disability. Available resources may affect the kind of assistance we are able to provide.

Disability Rights Idaho Services: http://www.disabilityrightsidaho.org/services/

Services Overview

DisAbility Rights Idaho provides advocacy and legal services to people with disabilities. We do this in many ways, such as:

- Informing people with disabilities of their rights under the law
- Providing information, tools and referrals that empower people to advocate for themselves
- Assisting people in cases where an advocate or legal help may be needed
- Pursuing policy changes that benefit many people with disabilities
- Monitoring conditions in public and private facilities

DisAbility Rights Idaho receives more requests for services than we can provide. DisAbility Rights Idaho must also follow the requirements of the grants it receives to provide services. To meet both the demand for services and ensure we are in compliance with our mandates, priorities and objectives are approved by the Board of Directors on an annual basis. Click here to read more.

Please note that we cannot provide direct assistance in the following areas:

- Any issue or problem not directly related to your disability
- Any issue for a person who already has an attorney working on the same issue
- Criminal law
- Divorce
- Out-of-state issues

☐ Worker's compensation
☐ General medical malpractice and personal injury
☐ General consumer bankruptcy issues
☐ Assistance finding employment, housing or financial assistance
☐ Assistance filling out forms and Social Security applications
☐ Anything that is not the wish of the person with the disability

Disability Resources: http://www.disabilityrightsidaho.org/resources/links.aspx

Idaho Resources

Brain Injury Association of Idaho

Center on Disability and Human Development

Court Assistance Offices Project

Directory of Idaho Legal Services

Epilepsy Foundation of Idaho

Family Support 360

Idaho Assistive Technology Project

Idaho Commission on Human Rights

Idaho Department of Education: Special Education

Idaho Department of Health & Welfare

Idaho Division of Vocational Rehabilitation

Idaho Infant Toddler Program

Idaho Legal Aid Services

Idaho Parents Unlimited, Inc. (IPUL)

Idaho State Council on Developmental Disabilities

Idaho State Independent Living Council (SILC)

Idaho System of Care

Idaho Volunteer Lawyers Program

Life, Inc.

Living Independence Network Corporation (LINC)

National Alliance for the Mentally Ill (NAMI) - Idaho Chapter

United Cerebral Palsy of Idaho

Senior Resources: http://www3.irissoft.com/tow1/search.asp

Illinois

Senior and Retirees: http://www2.illinois.gov/family-home/Pages/SeniorsAndRetirees.aspx

1. **State of Illinois Home**

2. **Family & Home**

3. Seniors & Retirees

Seniors & Retirees

- Senior Help Line
- Illinois Supportive Living Program
- Grandparents Raising Grandchildren
- Legal Assistance for Seniors
- Elder Abuse & Prevention
- Home & Community Assistance
- Caregivers
- Long-term Care Facilities Information
- Agencies & Organizations Serving Seniors
- Intergenerational & Volunteer Programs
- Illinois Cares Rx, Medicare Part D, & Other Pharmaceutical Drug Programs (Illinois Benefits)
- Circuit Breaker
- Senior Illinoisans Hall of Fame

Retirement

- State Employees' Retirement System
- Teachers' Retirement System for Illinois Educators
- State Universities Retirement System of Illinois
- Legal Assistance for Seniors

Illinois Department on Aging, Family Caregiver Support Program:
http://www.state.il.us/aging/1caregivers/caregivers-main.htm

There is a Caregiver Resource Center near you.

Each center can help you locate such services as...

- Adult day service for the senior citizen and respite services for the caregiver
- Individual counseling and support groups
- Services that help senior citizens remain in their homes:
  - Home-delivered meals
  - Assistance in housekeeping
  - Home modification
  - Assistance finding assistive devices
  - Training, counseling and emotional support
  - Transportation services
- Financial information and services
- Legal services
- Caregiver training
- Case management assistance
- Employment programs

Illinois has an amazing number of counties listed on this page with their respective Caregiver Resource Center contact information, and the pertinent services as listed above:
http://www.state.il.us/aging/1caregivers/crc.htm

Illinois Disability Information Home Page: http://www2.illinois.gov/family-home/Pages/Disabilities.aspx

Supportive Living Program: http://www.slfillinois.com/ This is not in-home.

DHS Home Services Program: http://www.dhs.state.il.us/page.aspx?item=29738

What is the purpose of this service?

We provide services to individuals with severe disabilities so they can remain in their homes and be as independent as possible.

What services are offered?

Our program offers numerous options for independence:

- **Personal Assistant (PA):** Provides assistance with household tasks, personal care and, with permission of a doctor, certain health care procedures. PAs are selected, employed, and supervised by individual customers.

- **Homemaker Services:** Personal care provided by trained and professionally supervised personnel for customers who are unable to direct the services of a PA. Instruction and assistance in household management and self-care are also available.

- **Maintenance Home Health:** Services provided through a treatment plan prescribed by a physician or other health care professional. Other services include nursing care and physical, occupational, and speech therapy.

- **Electronic Home Response**: Emergency response system offered by hospitals and community service organizations. This rented signaling device provides 24-hour emergency coverage, permitting the individual to alert trained professionals at hospitals, fire departments, or police departments.

- **Home Delivered Meals**: Provided to individuals who can feed themselves but are unable to prepare food.

- **Adult Day Care**: The direct care and supervision of customers in a community-based setting to promote their social, physical, and emotional well-being.

- **Assistive Equipment**: Devices or equipment either purchased or rented to increase an individual's independence and capability to perform household and personal care tasks at home.

- **Environmental Modification**: Modifications in the home that help compensate for loss of ability, strength, mobility or sensation; increase safety in the home, and decrease dependence on direct assistance from others.

- **Respite Services**: Temporary care for adults and children with disabilities aimed at relieving stress to families. Respite services may be provided for vacation, rest, errands, family crisis or emergency. Services may include personal assistant, homemaker or home health.

We also provide specialized services for people (who may be over age 60) with:

- HIV/AIDS
- Traumatic brain injuries

Our Community Reintegration Program helps individuals with disabilities who live in nursing homes move into community with the supports they need to live as independently as possible.

Who can receive these services?

We serve people with severe disabilities under age 60 who need help with daily living activities in their homes. Many of these people are at risk of moving into a nursing home or other facility.

How are services provided?

Customers may hire their own PAs to assist in their home, based on the service plan they have jointly developed with their DRS rehabilitation counselor.

Homemaker agencies may supply workers for persons who need someone to supervise their PA in the home.

How to apply?

Use the online Rehabilitation Services Web Referral to refer yourself or someone else for services.

We provide services in 48 local offices located in communities throughout the state. Use the DHS Office Locator and search for Rehabilitation Services to find the nearest local office or call toll-free: (800) 843-6154 (Voice, English or Español) or (800) 447-6404 (TTY).

Indiana

Family and Health: http://www.in.gov/core/family.html

Older Adults

- Assisted Living Facilities Directory
- Hoosier Rx
- Indiana Long Term Care Insurance Program
- Medicare Assistance
- Senior Health Insurance Information Program - SHIIP
- Other Older Adult Assistance Services

Resources for Citizens with Disabilities

- Blind & Visually Impaired Services
- Deaf & Hard of Hearing Services
- Indiana Centers for Independent Living
- Library for the Blind & Physically Handicapped
- Vocational Rehabilitation Services

Division of Aging: http://www.in.gov/fssa/2329.htm

CHOICE

The Community and Home Options to Institutional Care for the Elderly and Disabled (CHOICE) provides case management services, assessment, and in-home and community services to individuals who are at least 60 years of age or persons of any age who have a disability due to a mental or physical impairment and who are found to be at risk of losing their independence.

CHOICE funds may only be utilized after an applicant has been determined and documented ineligible for Medicaid or If currently eligible for Medicaid, after a determination that the requested service(s) is not available from Medicaid.

The following are services available under CHOICE:

Adult Day Service - Adult Day Service are community-based group programs designed to meet the needs of adults with impairments through individual plans of care. These structured, comprehensive, non-residential programs provide health, social, recreational, and therapeutic activities, supervision, support services, and personal care.

Attendant Care - Attendant Care is hands on assistance for older adults and persons with disabilities who have physical needs and is provided to allow the client to remain in their own home and carry out functions of daily living, self-care, and mobility. Assistance can include help with bathing, oral hygiene, hair care, shaving, dressing, applying cosmetics, transfer between bed and chair, meal planning, preparation and cleanup, toileting assistance, escorting client to medical appointments and other day-to-day activities. It should be noted that an attendant has to be a hired third party and can not be a loved one.

Behavior Management - Behavior Management is training, supervision or assistance in appropriate expression of the emotions and desires, compliance, assertiveness, acquisition of socially appropriate behaviors, and the reduction of inappropriate behaviors.

Congregate Meals - Congregate meals are meals which comply with the Dietary Guidelines for Americans published by the Secretaries of the Department of Health and Human Services and the United States Department of Agriculture and are available to eligible clients or other eligible participants at a nutrition site, senior center or another congregate setting.

Counseling Support Groups - Counseling Support Groups are services or activities that assist the caregiver in the areas of health, nutrition, financial literacy, decision making and problem solving. This includes counseling provided by a licensed professional or support groups that allow caregivers to discuss their attitudes, feelings, and problems with other individual(s) to achieve a greater understanding of their situation, role, and problems that arise with care giving. This also includes training and education for the caregiver to assist them in acquiring knowledge and skills that allow them to provide care.

Environmental Modifications - Environmental modifications are minor physical adaptations to the individual's own home or family owned home, as required by the individual's Plan of Care/Cost Comparison Budget. Rented homes or apartments are allowed to be modified only when a signed agreement from the landlord is obtained. The modifications must be necessary to ensure the health, welfare and safety of the individual and enable them to function with greater independence in the home, and without which the individual would require institutionalization.

Gerontology Counseling - Gerontology Counseling is the process of helping older individuals to overcome losses, to establish new goals while in the process of discovering that living may be limited in years but not necessarily in quality, and to reach decisions based on the importance of being in the present as well as looking for future opportunities.

Habilitation Day Group - Habilitation Day Group is assistance with acquisition, retention, or improvement in self-help, socialization and adaptive skills which takes place in a non residential setting that is separate from the home or facility in which the individual resides. Services are normally furnished four (4) or more hours per day on a regularly scheduled basis for one (1) or more days per week unless provided as an adjunct to other day activities included in an individual's care plan.

Handy Chore - Handy Chore are minor home maintenance activities, that are planned and monitored, that are essential to an individual's health and safety. They can include plumbing, heating, storm door, window, and screen repairs; gutter and roof patching; heavy cleaning; broken step repair; installation of health and safety equipment such as handrails, ramps, deadbolts, fire extinguishers, smoke detectors, locks. Ground maintenance is also included and can be lawn moving, snow removal, and minimal hard cleanup to assure safe entrance and departure from premises.

Homemaker - Homemaker is direct and practical assistance with household tasks and related activities. Services assist clients who have lost ability to perform instrumental activities of daily living that allow them to live in a clean, safe, healthy home environment. The service is available when the client is unable to meet daily needs and there is no informal caregiver who could meet those needs. Activities can include dusting, vacuuming, cleaning the kitchen and bathroom, doing dishes, laundry, making beds, disposing of trash, yard clean up and mowing, snow removal, grocery shopping, preparing meals, running errands and several others.

Home Delivered Meals - Home Delivered Meals are meals brought to the client's home which comply with the Dietary Guidelines for Americans and published by the Secretaries of the Department of Health and Human Services and the United States Department of Agriculture.

Home Health Aide - Home Health Aide duties include the provision of hands-on personal care, performance of simple procedures as an extension of therapy or nursing services, assistance in ambulation or exercises, and assistance in administering medications that are ordinarily self-administered. Any home health aide services offered by a Home Health Agency and must be provided by a qualified home health aide.

Individual Counseling - Individual Counseling services are provided by a licensed psychologist with an endorsement as a health service provider in psychology, a licensed marriage and family therapist, a licensed clinical social worker, or a licensed mental health counselor.

Information Assistance - Information Assistance ensures that adults and disabled individuals have access to all available benefits and services. This includes providing answers to questions, assisting clients to receive needed service, and follow up to make sure that referred services are appropriate.

Legal Assistance - Legal Assistance assists older adults understand and maintain their rights, exercise their choices, help them benefit from available services and resolve disputes. The program also promotes the need for lifetime planning through the understanding and the use of advance directives.

Licensed Practical Nurse - A Licensed Practical Nurse furnishes services in accordance with agency policies, prepares clinical and progress notes, assists the physician and registered nurse in performing specialized procedures, prepares equipment and materials for treatments observing aseptic technique as required, and assists the patient in learning appropriate self-care.

Nutrition Counseling - Nutrition Counseling helps individuals who are at nutritional risk, because of their health or nutritional history, dietary intake, medication use or chronic illnesses, with options and methods for improving their nutritional status. The service is performed by a health professional in accordance with state law and policy.

Nutrition Education - Nutrition Education is a program that promotes better health by providing accurate and culturally sensitive nutrition, physical fitness, or health (as it relates to nutrition) information and instruction to participants and caregivers in a group or individual setting. The program is overseen by a dietitian or individual of comparable expertise.

Occupational Therapy - Occupational Therapy provides evaluation, treatment, and training programs such as gross and fine motor function, self-care, sensory and perceptual motor function. It also includes remedial techniques that include the design, fabrication, and adaptation of materials and equipment to an individual's needs.

Outreach - Outreach assists with identifying potential clients or their caregivers and encouraging their use of existing services and benefits.

Pest Control - Pest Control services are designed to prevent, suppress, or eradicate anything that competes with humans for food and water, injures humans, spreads disease and/or annoys humans and is causing or is expected to cause more harm than is reasonable to accept. Pests include insects such as roaches, mosquitoes, and fleas; insect-like organisms, such as mites and ticks; and vertebrates, such as rats and mice.

Physical Therapy - Physical Therapy provides treatment and training programs designed to preserve and improve abilities for independent functioning, such as gross and fine motor skills, range of motion, strength and muscle tone, activates of daily living, and mobility to prevent progressive disability through such means as the use of purposeful activities, orthopedic and prosthetic devices, assistive and adaptive equipment, positioning, behavior adaptation, and sensory stimulation.

Private Duty Nurse - Private Duty Nursing are nursing services for recipients who require more individual and continuous care than is available from a visiting nurse or routinely provided by the nursing staff of the hospital or skilled nursing facility.

Personal Emergency Response Systems (PERS) - PERS is an electronic device which enables certain individuals at high risk of institutionalization to secure help in an emergency. The individual may also wear a portable help button to allow for mobility. The system is connected to the person's phone and programmed to signal a response center once a "help" button is activated. The response center is staffed by trained professionals. PERS is limited to those individuals who live alone, or who are alone for significant parts of the day, and have no regular caregiver for extended periods of time, and who would otherwise require extensive supervision, professionals.

Private Hire Attendant Care - Attendant Care is hands on assistance for older adults and persons with disabilities who have physical needs and is provided in order to allow the client to remain in their own home and carry out functions of daily living, self-care, and mobility. Assistance can include help with bathing, oral hygiene, hair care, shaving, dressing, applying cosmetics, transfer between bed and chair, meal planning, preparation and cleanup, toileting assistance, escorting client to medical appointments and other day-to-day activities.

Residential Based Habilitation - Residential Based Habilitation is assistance with the acquisition, retention or improvement in skills related to activities of daily living, such as personal grooming and cleanliness, bed making and household chores, eating and the preparation of food, and the social and adaptive skills necessary to enable the individual to live in a non-institutional setting.

Respite Care - Respite Care are temporary substitute supports or living arrangements for care recipients in order to provide a brief period of relief or rest for caregivers. This can include in-home respite (personal care, homemaker, and others), respite provided by attendance of the client at a senior center or other non-residential program and institutional respite which is provided by placing the resident in a non-institutional setting such as a nursing facility for a short period of time as a respite service for the caregiver, or a summer camp in the case grandparents caring for children.

Registered Nurse - The registered nurse makes the initial evaluation visit, regularly reevaluates the patient's nursing needs, and initiates the plan of care and necessary revisions. They also furnish those services requiring substantial and specialized nursing skills, initiate appropriate preventive and rehabilitative nursing procedures, prepare clinical and progress notes, coordinate services, and other related needs, participate in in-service programs, and supervise and teach other nursing personnel.

Speech Therapy - Speech Therapy is provided by a licensed speech pathologist and includes screening, assessment, direct therapeutic intervention and treatment for speech and hearing disabilities such as delayed speech, stuttering, spastic speech, aphasic disorders, injuries, lip reading or signing, or the use of hearing aids.

Vehicle Modification - Vehicle Modifications are the addition of adaptive equipment or structural changes to a motor vehicle that permit an individual with a disability to be safely transported in a motor vehicle. Vehicle modifications, as specified in the Plan of Care/Cost Comparison Budget, may be authorized when necessary to increase an individual's ability to function in a home and community based setting to ensure accessibility of the individual with mobility impairments. These services must be necessary to prevent or delay institutionalization. The necessity of such items must be documented in the plan of care by a physician's order. Vehicles necessary for an individual to attend post secondary education or job related services should be referred to Vocational Rehabilitation Services.

Specialized Medical Equipment and Supplies - Specialized Medical Equipment and Supplies are medically prescribed items required by the individual's Plan of Care/Cost Comparison Budget which is necessary to assure the health, welfare and safety of the individual, and allow an individual to function with greater independence in the home, and without which the individual would require institutionalization. Items include but are not limited to direct selection communicators, alphanumeric communicators, scanning communicators, speech amplifier, electronic speech aids/devices, standing boards/frames, adaptive switches/devices, specially adaptive locks.

Transportation - Transportation services allow individuals to gain access to community services, activities and resources, specified by the plan of care. There are two levels of transportation: Level 1 in which the individual does not need medical assistance to travel and Level 2 in which the individual does need medical assistance to travel.

Money Follows the Person: http://www.in.gov/fssa/da/3475.htm

What is the Money Follows the Person Demonstration Program?

The Money Follows the Person Demonstration (MFP Program) is a special project developed by the federal government to assist Hoosiers moving from a nursing facility or hospital to a residential setting in the community, such as:

- A home owned or leased by the individual or the individual's family
- An apartment with a personal lease that includes living, sleeping, bathing, and cooking areas
- Adult Foster Care - A residence in which no more than four unrelated individuals reside
- Assisted Living

Who is eligible to participate in the MFP Program in Indiana?

To participate in the MFP Program, the individual must:

- Have lived in a nursing facility and approved for long-term placement or hospital for at least three (3) months
- Be Medicaid eligible for one (1) day prior to discharge
- Have health needs that can be met through services available in the community
- Voluntarily consent to participation by signing a consent form
- Be eligible for either the Aged & Disabled (A/D), Traumatic Brain Injury (TBI), or Developmental Disabilities (DD) waiver

How does the MFP Program Work?

The MFP Program will assist Hoosiers transitioning from a nursing facility or hospital by providing:

- Information to help participants make informed choices regarding transition and participation in the MFP Program and waivers
- Assessment by a nurse indicating that the individual can safely move and live independently
- Access to transition services and assistance from a transition nurse and transition specialist (Case Manager)
- Post-discharge follow-up by a transition nurse and transition specialist to ensure the move is satisfactory and the individual's community-based needs are being met

The MFP Program will help participants locate a place to live and will arrange for medical, rehabilitative, home health, and other services in the community, as needed. MFP participants will be covered by the program for 365 days, after which time, the A/D or TBI, or DD waiver will provide ongoing services specific to the waiver to which they will be transitioning.

In what areas of the state will the MFP Program Operate?

The MFP Program will operate throughout the state from fall 2008 through September 30, 2016.

What services are available through the MFP Program?

In addition to services provided by regular Medicaid and the A/D, TBI, and DD waivers, MFP participants will also receive:

- *Personal Emergency Response System (PERS),* a 24-hour emergency response service for increased health and safety
- *Enhanced transportation* to provide transportation above what is available through the waiver. For example, MFP will provide transportation to the grocery store, to the beauty/barber shop, and to leisure activities, such as dining out or to the movie theater
- *Targeted Case Management* – screening to determine the eligibility of an individual and transition activities into the MFP program.

What are Home and Community-Based Waiver Services (HCBS)?

HCBS are services that are available to individuals who move from nursing facilities or hospitals into the community. These services are provided in addition to medical services that may be needed, to help recipients live independently in the community.

For participation in the MFP demonstration grant, individuals must be eligible for either the A/D, TBI, or DD waiver.

Who is eligible for the A/D, TBI, and DD Waivers?

Applicants may choose the waiver that will best serve their individual needs, as long as the following eligibility requirements are met:

- *A/D Waiver*: Individuals who meet nursing facility level of care and Medicaid eligibility requirements and who are aged (age 65 or older) or disabled may be eligible for the A/D waiver.
- *TBI Waiver*: Individuals who meet nursing facility level of care and Medicaid eligibility requirements and who are disabled and have traumatic brain injuries may be eligible for the TBI waiver.
- *DD Waiver*: Individuals who meet level of care for an Intermediate Care Facility for the Mentally Retarded (ICF/MR) and Medicaid eligibility requirements may be eligible for the DD waiver.

How do I participate or get more information?

If an individual is eligible to participate in the MFP Program based on the criteria on this page, willingness to assist in the development of the plan of care is all that is needed to become a participant.

Social Security or other income will cover rent and other basic necessities and the MFP Program will cover the costs of services listed on the Medicaid Waivers page on this website for the first, transitional year. If you would like more information about the MFP Program or Medicaid Waivers, please call the Division of Aging at 1-888-673-0002.

Indiana Council on Independent Living: http://www.in.gov/fssa/ddrs/2762.htm

Independent Living Centers This page seems primarily for those with disabilities.

Independent Living Centers In Indiana

accessABILITY Center for Independent Living, Inc.
5302 E. Washington Street
Indianapolis, IN 46218
317-926-1660
info@abilityindiana.org
http://www.abilityindiana.org/

ATTIC
Patricia Stewart, Executive Director
1721 Washington Avenue
Vincennes, IN 47591
(812) 886-0575 office
(812) 886-1128 fax
(877) 962-8842 Toll Free
inattic1@aol.com

Community Options for Independent Living (or also known as Future Choices)
Beth Quarles, Executive Director
309 N. High Street
Muncie, IN 47305
765-741-8332 office
765-741-8333 fax
bquarles@futurechoices.org

Everybody Counts Center for Independent Living (ECCIL) Teresa Torres, Executive Director
9111 Broadway Suite A
Broadfield Center
Merrillville, IN 46410
219-769-5055 office
219-769-5325 fax
219-756-3323 TTY
888-769-3636 Toll free
ecounts@netnitco.net

Independent Living Center of Eastern Indiana (ILCEIN)
Jim McCormick, Executive Director
1818 W. Main Street
Richmond, IN 47374
765-939-9226 office
765-935-2215 Fax/TTY
877-939-9226 Toll Free
jimm@ilcein.org

League for the Blind & Disabled (The League)
David Nelson, Executive Director
5821 South Anthony Blvd.
Fort Wayne, IN 46816
260-441-0551 office V/TTY
260-441-7760 fax
800-889-3443 (toll free)
The.League@verizon.net

Southern Indiana Center for Independent Living (SICIL)
Al Tolbert, Executive Director
Stone City Plaza

651 X Street
Bedford, IN 47421
812-277-9626 office V/TTY
812-277-9628 fax
800-845-6914 Toll free
sicildir@msn.com

Wabash Independent Living and Learning Center
The WILL Center
Peter Ciancone, Executive Director
4312 S. Seventh Street
Terre Haute, IN 47802
812-298-9455 office
812-299-9061 Fax
info@thewillcenter.org

HoosierRX: http://www.in.gov/fssa/ompp/2669.htm For Medicare Part D assistance

HoosierRx Helps Pay for your Medicare Part D Plan

Indiana's State Pharmaceutical Assistance Program, HoosierRx, can help pay the monthly Part D premium, up to $70 per month, for members enrolled in a Medicare Part D Plan working with HoosierRx.

To be eligible for HoosierRx you must:

1. Be an Indiana resident, 65 years old or older.
2. Have a yearly income of $16,485 or less for a single person, or $22,095 or less for a married couple living together.
3. Have applied for the "Medicare Extra Help" through Social Security to pay for your Medicare Part D plan, and received either a "Notice of Award" or "Notice of Denial" from Social Security.
   - Your Social Security "Notice of Denial" must be because your **resources are above the limit established by law.**
   - Your Social Security "Notice of Award" must state that you are receiving **partial extra help** subsidy to help pay for your Medicare Part D premium.

If you think you meet these eligibility requirements please call a HoosierRx representative at 1-866-267-4679 or visit the HoosierRx website at www.IN.gov/HoosierRx.

Companies offering Prescription Drug Plans working with HoosierRx: AARP/United Healthcare, CIGNA Healthcare, Clarian Health Plans (with Part D coverage), Community Care Rx, Coventry AdvantraRx, EnvisionRx, First Health, PrescribaRx, SilverScript, and WellCare.

Iowa

Iowa Department on Aging: http://www.aging.iowa.gov/

Iowa's Area Agencies on Aging: http://www.aging.iowa.gov/aaa/index.html

Click the links to jump down to information on:

Services Provided by Area Agencies | Locate Your Area Agency

About Area Agencies

Area Agencies on Aging (AAAs) were established under the Older Americans Act (OAA) in 1973 to respond to the needs of Americans aged 60 and over in every local community. Iowa has thirteen AAAs, covering all 99 counties.

Iowa's 13 Area Agencies on Aging strive to meet the needs of the rapidly-growing number of older Iowans. Iowa's Area Agencies:

- Assess current needs of older Iowans;
- Assess available services, programs, and institutions;
- Develop plans to help address service gaps via the Senior Living Program;
- Assure access to services, programs, and institutions;
- Advocate for the needs of older Iowans;
- Finance and administer contracts to direct providers of services;
- Provide a central leadership role for older Iowans; and
- Provide information and assistance services for older Iowans and their caregivers

Area Agencies are funded by approximately 50% in federal funds, 10% state funds, and 40% local contributions. Collaboration with local human service networks leads to more effective use of tax dollars.

Back to Top

Services Provided by Area Agencies

Area Agencies in Iowa provide resources to older Iowans, including, but not limited to: adult day services, chore services, companion & respite care, congregate meals, consultations about other problems, employment assistance, health-care aides, home-delivered meals, home repairs, legal assistance, meal sites, modifying the home for disabilities, nursing & homemaker services, senior centers, and transportation.

Locate Your Local AAA

To identify the contact information for the AAA nearest you, please click your home county on the map below, or click here for a full listing of Iowa Area Agencies on Aging.

Area Agency on Aging Contact Information: http://www.aging.iowa.gov/aaa/aaacontact.html

If you wish to select the area agency by county, use our Interactive Map.

NORTHLAND AGENCY ON AGING

Serving: Allamakee, Clayton, Fayette, Howard and Winneshiek Counties

Director:	Bruce Butters
Address:	808 River Street
	Decorah, IA 52101
Phone:	563-382-2941 or 1-800-233-4603
Fax:	563-382-6248

Email Address: mail@northlandaging.com

Web site: www.northlandaging.com

Back to Top

ELDERBRIDGE AREA AGENCY ON AGING

Offices located in Mason City, Fort Dodge and Carroll, IA.

Serving: Audubon, Calhoun, Carroll, Cerro Gordo, Crawford, Floyd, Franklin, Greene, Guthrie, Hamilton, Hancock, Humboldt, Kossuth, Mitchell, Pocahontas, Sac, Webster, Winnebago, Worth, and Wright Counties

Director:	Beth Bahnson
Address:	22 North Georgia, Suite 216
	Mason City, IA 50401
Phone:	641-424-0678 or 1-800-243-0678
Fax:	641-424-2927
Address:	308 Central Ave
	Fort Dodge, IA 50501-3736
Phone:	515-955-5244 or 1-800-543-3280
Address:	603 N West
	Carroll, IA 51401-2346

Phone: 712-792-3512 or 1-800-543-3265

Email Address: Elderbridge@elderbridge.org

Web site: www.elderbridge.org

Back to Top

NORTHWEST AGING ASSOCIATION

Serving: Buena Vista, Clay, Dickinson, Emmett, Lyon, O'Brien, Osceola, Palo Alto, and Sioux Counties

Director: Tresa Knoff
Address: 714 10th Avenue East
             Spencer, IA 51301
Phone: 712-262-1775 or 1-800-242-5033
Fax: 712-262-7520

Email Address: tknoff@nwaging.org

Web site: www.nwaging.org

Back to Top

SIOUXLAND AGING SERVICES

Serving: Cherokee, Ida, Monona, Plymouth, and Woodbury Counties

Director: Kim Keleher
Address: 2301 Pierce Street
             Sioux City, IA 51104
Phone: 712-279-6900 or 1-800-798-6916
Fax: 712-233-3415

Email Address: siouxlandaging@siouxlandaging.org

Web site: www.SiouxlandAging.org

Back to Top

HAWKEYE VALLEY AREA AGENCY ON AGING

Serving: Black Hawk, Bremer, Buchanan, Butler, Chickasaw, Grundy, Hardin, Marshall, Poweshiek, and Tama Counties

Director:	Mike Isaacson
Address:	2101 Kimball Avenue
	Suite 320
	Waterloo, IA 50702
Phone:	319-272-2244 or 1-800-779-8707
Fax:	319-272-2455

Email Address: hvaaa@hvaaa.org

Web Site: www.hvaaa.org

Back to Top

SCENIC VALLEY AREA VIII AGENCY ON AGING

Serving: Delaware, Dubuque, and Jackson Counties

Director:	Linda McDonald
Address:	Fountain Park Springs Bldg
	2728 Asbury Road
	Dubuque, IA 52001
Phone:	563-588-3970
Fax:	563-588-1952

Email Address: scenicaaa@aol.com

Web Site: www.scenicvalley.org

Back to Top

GENERATIONS AREA AGENCY ON AGING

Serving: Clinton, Muscatine, and Scott Counties

Director:	Christa Merritt
Address:	935 E 53rd Street
	Davenport, IA 52808-3788
Phone:	563-324-9085
Fax:	563-324-9384

Email Address: cmerritt@genage.org

Web Site: www.genage.org

Back to Top

HERITAGE AREA AGENCY ON AGING

Serving: Benton, Cedar, Iowa, Johnson, Jones, Linn and Washington Counties

Director:	Ingrid Wensel
Address:	6301 Kirkwood Blvd., SW
	PO Box 2068
	Cedar Rapids, IA 52406
Phone:	319-398-5559 or 1-800-332-5934
Fax:	319-398-5533

Email Address: ingrid.wensel@kirkwood.edu

Website: www.heritageaaa.org

Back to Top

AGING RESOURCES OF CENTRAL IOWA

Serving: Boone, Dallas, Jasper, Madison, Marion, Polk, Story and Warren Counties

Director:	Joel Olah
Address:	5835 Grand Avenue
	Suite 106
	Des Moines, IA 50312-1437
Phone:	515-255-1310 or 1-800-747-5352
Fax:	515-255-9442

Email Address: agingres@aol.com

Website: www.agingresources.com

Back to Top

SOUTHWEST 8 SENIOR SERVICES, INC.

Serving: Cass, Fremont, Harrison, Mills, Montgomery, Page, Pottawattamie, and Shelby Counties

Director:	Barbara Morrison
Address:	300 West Broadway, Suite 240
	Council Bluffs, IA 51503
Phone:	712-328-2540 or 1-800-432-9290
Fax:	712-328-6899

Email Address: bmorrison@southwest8.org

Web Site: www.southwest8.org

Back to Top

AREA XIV AGENCY ON AGING

Serving: Adair, Adams, Clarke, Decatur, Ringgold, Taylor, and Union Counties

Director:	Steve Bolie
Address:	215 East Montgomery
	Creston, IA 50801
Phone:	641-782-4040
Fax:	641-782-4519

Email Address: areaxiv@iowatelecom.net

Web Site: www.areaxivaaa.org

Back to Top

SENECA AREA AGENCY ON AGING

Serving: Appanoose, Davis, Jefferson, Keokuk, Lucas, Mahaska, Monroe, Van Buren, Wapello and Wayne Counties

Director:	Connie Holland
Address:	117 North Cooper Street
	Suite 2
	Ottumwa, IA 52501
Phone:	641-682-2270 or 1-800-642-6522
Fax:	641-682-2445

Email Address: seneca@seneca-aaa.org

Web Site: www.seneca-aaa.org

Back to Top

SOUTHEAST IOWA AREA AGENCY ON AGING, INC.

Serving: Des Moines, Henry, Lee and Louisa Counties

Director:	Dennis Zegarac
Address:	509 Jefferson Street
	Burlington, IA 52601-5427
Phone:	319-752-5433 or 1-800-292-1268
Fax:	319-754-7030

Email Address: zegarac.dennis@mchsi.com

Web Site: www.southeastiowaaaa.org

Housing and Service Programs: http://www.aging.iowa.gov/services/index.html

Housing & Services Programs

Click the links below to jump to:

Assisted Living | Iowa Able Foundation Loan Program | CNA Recruitment & Retention | Performance Outcome Measures Grant | Seamless Project | Iowa NAPIS | Family Caregiver Support | Legal Assistance Program | Additional Resources | IDA Commission Presentation: Policy Changes in Assisted Living, Elder Group Homes, and Adult Day Service Programs

Senior Living Program- Funded by the Senior Living Trust, the goal of this program improve upon the current system of long-term care. Follow the link above for more information on this program.

Assisted Living and Elder Group Homes - The Iowa Department on Aging (IDA) no longer possesses statutory authority for the regulation of assisted living, elder group homes and adult day service programs due to the Eighty-second General Assembly passage of House File 909 which transfers full responsibility for the oversight of assisted living programs, adult day service programs, and elder group homes from the Iowa Department on Aging to the department of inspections and appeals effective July 1, 2007.

Back to Top

Iowa Able Foundation Loan Program- The Iowa Able Foundation helps Iowans with disabilities, their families, and older Iowans access adaptive devices / equipment, and home modifications through its loan programs. The Iowa Able Foundation offers an alternative financial solution by providing low interest loans with flexible terms to help individuals increase their independence. This statewide 501(c)(3) nonprofit program will loan funds for any item, piece of equipment, product, or home modification that is used to improve an individual's functional capabilities, mobility, and quality of life.

Loans for Assistive Technology and Home Modifications- In an effort to counter the lack of financial resources many individuals with disabilities and older Iowans face, Iowa Able offers low interest loans for the purchase of assistive technology and home modifications.

Assistive technology is defined as any item, piece of equipment or device that enables an individual to improve individual independence and quality of life. There must be a demonstrable connection between the end user's disability and the need for the equipment.

Allowable equipment includes but is not limited to: wheelchairs, motorized scooters, Braille equipment, voice simulation systems, scanners, assistive listening devices, telecommunications devices for the IDAf, augmentative communication systems, environmental control units, computers and adaptive peripherals, building modifications for accessibility, and motor vehicles and vehicle modifications.

Loans for Telework- The Telework Program seeks to increase home-based employment and self-employment opportunities for individuals with disabilities across the State of Iowa. Telework has proven to be a viable solution for assisting individuals with disabilities to integrate into the workplace due to its elimination of transportation barriers and barriers to accessibility.

The purpose of the Telework Program is to assist individuals to earn an income through the use of the technology or home modifications purchased with program funds.

Allowable equipment for the Iowa Able Telework Program includes but is not limited to: the purchase of computer and peripheral equipment; Internet services; assistive technology hardware, software and equipment; equipment deemed by the employer as necessary for telecommuting; equipment deemed by the entrepreneur as necessary for home-based employment; modifications to home-based work site to facilitate increased productivity.

For more information or to apply for a loan, please visit the Iowa Able Foundation web site at http://www.iowaable.org.

Back to Top

Performance Outcome Measures Grant- IDA and the Hawkeye Valley Area Agency on Aging collaborate on this project, funded by the Administration on Aging. The goal of this initiative is to develop survey tools, field test these surveys and evaluate performance outcome measures of selected services offered through the aging network to Iowa's elderly population. This grant will enable IDA and Hawkeye Valley AAA to continue present field testing of survey tools in Caregiving, Case Management, Home Delivered Meals, Physical Functioning, Transportation, and Barriers to Service and Capacity Building, and carry on data collection, base line development, and evaluate how community services used benefited Iowa's frail elders.

<u>Back to Top</u>

Seamless Project- IDA administers the $1.5 million Seamless Project, developed in collaboration with Senator Tom Harkin and his staff. The project seeks to begin the planning process to streamline Iowa's home and community based long-term care delivery infrastructure to better meet the needs of Iowa's seniors. IDA will collaborate with the Iowa Department of Human Services, the Iowa Department of Public Health, the Iowa Information Technology Department, the Area Agencies on Aging, the Iowa Research Council, and the American Association of Retired Persons (AARP) on this project.

Currently, funding for elderly services comes from as many as 17 sources. Older Iowans are left to complete separate applications to these sources, each of which has different eligibility requirements. Conversely, intake personnel in each agency spend valuable time and resources inputting data in an effort that is duplicated by other agencies. This translates into lost time and resources, which could be better used to provide services to elderly clients. The Seamless Project attempts to correct these inefficiencies by streamlining systems, to the benefit of consumers of services, caregivers, providers, the Area Agencies on Aging, and the State of Iowa.

The proposed system will include clear access points for frail seniors and their caregivers, accessibility to the right services at the right time, and efficiency in the delivery of services for seniors, professional caregivers, and for those who pay the cost of services. It is proposed that the total project will cover a three-year period (years 2 & 3 would be funded at $1.5 million each as well, but it should be noted that funding is not guaranteed). Year one, currently underway, will focus on assessing existing systems and will implement a new streamlined approach to the Case Management Program for the Frail Elderly (CMPFE). CMPFE will serve as the model for the transformation of the state's service delivery infrastructure. Year two focuses on implementation and streamlining of additional services, and training and receiving input from those services. In year three, additional training will be provided and the system will be evaluated.

Family Caregiver Support Program (Title III-E) - The Administration on Aging (AoA) has determined that for Title III-E, the actual family caregiver is the client, not the older person receiving the services. Iowa NAPIS (National Aging Program Information System) collects and reports Title III-E service/performance data and related program management information to the federal and state government in a format like the other Title III services. The major shift in reporting relates to who is the client. As a result, this Title III-E Client/Service Unit Report shows the number of caregivers who receive services and the number of units by service category from the Title III-E funding of the Older Americans Act, the AoA, and limited state general fund dollars. Additionally, it shows the number of persons served by individual services and total "unduplicated" client count across all services. In other words, if you add the total number of clients (caregivers) from all services, it is higher than the actual number of persons served across all services because some people need and receive more than one service. *(Please note: this is preliminary data, and may be subject to change.)*

Legal Assistance Program - The SFY legal assistance activity report that follows is based on data compiled from the Legal Assistance Program quarterly reports submitted to the Department by Area Agencies on Aging (AAA) and their legal providers.

For additional resources on Housing & Services programs, consult the <u>Housing Resources for Seniors</u> section on our Related Links page.

Family Caregiver Support Program: http://www.aging.iowa.gov/living/caregiver.html

Family Caregiver Resources

Most family members who help older people don't see themselves as caregivers. Yet a caregiver is anyone who helps an older person with household chores, errands, personal care, or finances. You are a caregiver if you do any of these things. You are a family caregiver if you help someone who cannot do or is limited from doing any of these things for him/herself.
The goal of all caregivers is to help older adults maintain the highest level of independence that they can and remain safe. Like anyone else, older adults need to be self-reliant, in control of their own lives, feel safe, be understood, and be respected.

Common issues facing older adults include adequate income, physical and mental health, suitable housing, a variety of community services, retirement in health, honor and dignity, opportunity for meaningful activity, access to transportation, and protection from abuse, neglect and exploitation.

Caregivers may be related to older persons as spouses, children, in-laws, or other family members. Sometimes, caregivers are not related but assist as friends or neighbors. The caregiver role is complex and differs for everyone depending on the needs of the person who is aging.

Family and informal caregivers are the backbone of our long-term care system. The vast majority of long-term care in Iowa and the nation is provided informally and privately at no public cost. Often at great sacrifice, families keep a loved one at home, avoiding more costly institutional care. Most caregivers are reluctant to use formal help. They often provide care with little support, experience adverse consequences to their own physical and emotional well-being, and use formal services only when faced with a crisis. But, even the most self-sufficient people may need information and direct services to best meet the needs of both aging family members and themselves. This Family Caregiver section will provide links to information and resources that can help you and your loved one on your caregiving journey.

Below are some web sites that can help you to manage the practical day-to-day process of Caregiving as well as the emotional highs and lows that you as caregiver are sure to experience. By clicking on the links, you can find a wealth of information that will help you to work through your questions and concerns.

Back to Top

Iowa Family Caregiver Program: What do they do?

1. Plan and develop services and programs for older Iowans to help them maintain independence and quality of life as long as possible.
2. Advocate for federal and state policies which affect the quality of life for older Iowans.
3. Serve as the coordinating entity with other governmental and community based organizations involved in area development efforts affecting older Iowans.
4. Increase public awareness, including that of government and community leaders, of the help available to older Iowans through the Area Agencies on Aging and other community entities.

Ensure that older Iowans and family caregivers have accurate and easily accessible information about what help is available to them and their older loved ones.

The Iowa Association of Area Agencies on Aging (I4A) offers a searchable website for services. For example, your loved one lives in Monona County and you live in Polk County and you need to find a person or agency that can provide home-delivered meals once a day. On the I4A website, you can conduct a search by county and by service from drop down lists - easy! It is an excellent resource even if your loved one lives with you so that you can find the resources/services that you need for any occasion. If you can't find the resources, or have questions that cannot be answered, you can also find the local area agency on aging and their contact information on the same site. www.I4A.org

Back to Top

Family Caregiving - It's Not All Up to You: If you're caring for a loved one who is ill or disabled, this site was created for you. It's a great place to find assistance, answers, new iIDAs and helpful advice - for you and your loved one.

- www.familycaregiving101.org

Back to Top

Family Caregiver Support: If you are caring for a grandchild or a relative's child, you are not alone. More than six million children in the United States - about 1 in 12 children - are living in households headed by grandparents or other relatives. In many of these households, grandparents or other relatives are primary caregivers for children whose parents are unwilling or unable to care for them because of many different reasons including substance abuse, mental health problems, unemployment, family violence, divorce, incarceration and others.

Kinship caregivers come from all walks of life and their numbers are increasing every year. Kinship caregivers are grandparents, aunts, uncles, other siblings, and even great grandparents.

The Iowa Foster and Adoptive Parents Association (IFAPA) supports kinship caregivers in a variety of ways including peer support, training and resources. Additional information can be found on their website by clicking here: www.ifapa.org

Back to Top

Housing - Ensuring a Safe Living Environment: Comfort and a place for self-expression are vital for everyone's well-being. Being able to stay in their own home gives our loved one feelings of their treasured independence. But their home should also be a place in which he/she can be safe from accidents and injuries. Listed below are resources for assessing the safety of a home, making changes in design to include the needed safety elements, and, when staying alone in their own home is no longer possible, what other housing options are available.

- A Housing Safety Checklist for Older Adults
- Removing Barriers in a Home
- Universal Design for Homes
- A Safe Home is in Your Hands

If the person for whom you care has dementia or Alzheimer's Disease, there is a website that has been created to provide information on best strategies and home safety for dementia care.

It also provides social networking so caregivers can share information, ask questions and find support from the online community. This new resource will help caregivers learn new strategies that enhance the safety and well-being of their loved ones. The website also provides information to help the person they care for lice a healthier, more meaningful life.

A unique and beneficial part of this website is its Home Safety-0Virtual Care Section that allows visitors to explore research-based solutions to home safely and daily care issues by a simple mouse click over a room. Visit the Caring Home webstie at: www.thiscaringhome.org

If you and your loved one make the decision that living in her/his own home is not the best housing option, there are others such as elder group homes, assisted living and long-term care facilities. These options provide a continuum of care and are suited to the individual's care needs. More information can be found on this website by clicking on this link: Help Me Stay Home.

There may be home modifications that you would like to make either to your loved one's home, or your own home if you decide to move your loved one in to live with you. The Iowa Able Foundation offers low interest loans for many types of home modifications and purchase of assistive devices to those who qualify. You can access more information about this program through the Iowa Able Foundation website.

Back to Top

Iowa's Aging and Disability Resources: Many people do not think about what it takes to live well with a disability or age-related concerns until they need help or a crisis occurs. You can prepare for the many transitions that occur in one's lifetime by planning. Whether you are responding to a current need or planning for the future LifeLong Links can help you find the way through an array of choices, information, and options. You can make decisions about the services you or your loved one need using the information on this site. A broad range of services and supports are available when a person's independence is limited. In the aging community, these are sometimes called "long-term care" or "aging in place." In the disability community, these are "community supports" or "supports for independent living."

- LifeLongLinks.org (provides links for both populations)

Back to Top

Caring for You, the Caregiver: Caregiving for an older adult is rewarding, but let's face it, caregiving can also be stressful - physically, emotionally, and financially. It is vital that you take good care of yourself so that you can remain in good health and thrive - not merely survive your caregiving experience. We do that by managing our self-care - that means we:

- Take responsibility for our personal well-being;
- Have realistic expectations about what our loved one can and cannot do;
- Focus on what we can do - be clear about what you can and cannot change and "let go" of the ones you can't change;
- Communicate effectively with others including family members, friends, health care professionals and your loved one;
- Learn from your emotions - realize there will be ups and downs and learn how to manage your emotions appropriately
- Get help when needed - an important part of self-care is knowing when you need help and how to find it; and finally;
- Set goals and work toward them. Be realistic in the goals that you set and take steps toward reaching those goals. Changes do not need to be major to make a significant difference.

One problem that caregivers frequently experience is trying to do it all and do it all alone. Ask yourself - is it possible to do it all? The answer to the question can be both "yes" and "no". It really depends on you. What is critical is how you define what it means to "do it all" and whether or not your definition of "doing it all" includes taking care of yourself.

Regular breaks from the tasks of caregiving are essential. Decide on the time, date, and activity - then follow through. Breaks don't have to be long to make a positive difference. It's important to plan some time for yourself in every day, even if that time is only for 15 minutes or half an hour. Most important is to do something that fulfills you and helps you to feel better. If you have difficulty taking breaks for yourself, consider taking them for your loved one. Care receivers also benefit from caregivers getting breaks.

For additional information on family caregiving visit http://www.iowafamilycaregiver.org.

Family Caregiving: It's Not All Up to You: http://www.familycaregiving101.org/

Welcome to the Family Caregiving 101 Web site. If you're caring for a loved one who is ill or disabled, this site was created for you. It's a great place to find assistance, answers, new ideas and helpful advice — for you and your loved one.

Where do you start? Try clicking on the Top 10 Questions.:
http://www.familycaregiving101.org/top_10/

Respite: http://www.familycaregiving101.org/manage/respite.cfm

Respite

It isn't possible to talk about self-care for family caregivers without talking about respite. More than any other service respite is what family caregivers want most. The primary purpose of respite care is to provide relief from the extraordinary and intensive demands of ongoing care to someone with special needs, thereby strengthening the family's ability to provide care. Respite care is planned and proactive. Respite means taking a break before extreme stress and crisis occurs.

A respite doesn't have to mean a week on the French Riviera, although that sounds pretty nice. It doesn't even have to be a weekend visiting friends, at least not at first. A respite can be as simple as lying on the couch with the lights dimmed listening to your favorite music, especially if you do it on a regular basis. It can be going to the movies or having a manicure every other week. You might even think of your three times a week exercise routine as a respite, if you enjoy it, rather than thinking of it as something you do because it is good for you.

What you do on a respite break, regardless of its length, is up to you. It has to meet your needs, break your tensions, and renew your spirit. It needs to be the right medicine to cure, or at least ameliorate your current stress. It needs to be for you, precisely because you do so much for others and because you deserve it.

Next time you feel guilty for even thinking about taking a break, remember it is only partially for your benefit. Your loved one will reap a great deal of the benefit as well. Respites are guaranteed to take the edge off your tension, renew your energy and give you a fresh dollop of patience with which to pick up your caregiving duties once again. Respite is the primary mechanism you have as a family caregiver to refill your tank and thereby keep on going.

> The following is excerpted from Love, Honor, & Value by Suzanne Mintz, President/Co-founder of the National Family Caregivers Association
>
> "I've come to think of respite as coming in three sizes..." MORE

Two family members volunteered to give us relief [from caring for my mom] for a week's family vacation. We had a wonderful time with our sons and came back refreshed.
- Ruthann S. McDonough, Carmel, Indiana

A number of studies have proven the value of respite to caregivers and their loved ones. A paper published in fall, 2001 in Focal Point, a journal of the Regional Research Institute for Human Services at Portland State University explored the benefits of respite for parents of children with emotional and behavioral disorders, showed that respite enhanced the capacity to cope with stress, lessened the number of institutionalizations, and created greater optimism about the caregiver's ability to continue to provide care.

A study of caregivers of Alzheimer's patients published in the Journal of the American Medical Association in 1996 showed that respite and counseling lessens depression and helps caregivers avoid nursing home placement for their loved one for as much as a year.

Click here for a list of Respite Resources

Respite Resources: http://www.familycaregiving101.org/help/respite.cfm

National Organizations, Programs and Referral Sources

Easter Seals
230 West Monroe Street, Suite 1800
Chicago, IL 60606
800-221-6827
Web site: www.easter-seals.org

Easter Seals provides a variety of services at 400 sites nationwide for children and adults with disabilities, including adult day care, in-home care, camps for special needs children and more. Services vary by site.

Faith in Action
Wake Forest University School of Medicine
Medical Center Boulevard
Winston-Salem, NC 27157
877-324-8411
Web site: www.fiavolunteers.org
e-mail: info@fiavolunteers.org

Faith in Action is an interfaith volunteer caregiving program of The Robert Wood Johnson Foundation. Faith in Action makes grants to local groups representing many faiths who volunteer to work together to care for their neighbors who have long-term health needs. There are nearly 1,000 interfaith volunteer caregiving programs across the country.

Family Friends
National Council on the Aging, Inc.
409 Third Street, SW
Washington, DC 20024
202-479-6672
Web site: www.family-friends.org

This group provides respite (and other services) by matching men and women volunteers over the age of 50 with families of children who have disabilities or chronic illness. Programs are located throughout the country.

National Adult Day Services Association, Inc.
8201 Greensboro Drive, Suite 300
McLean, VA 22102

866-890-7357
Web site: www.nadsa.org

This association provides information about locating adult day care centers in your local area.

National Respite Coalition
4016 Oxford Street
Annandale, VA 22003
703-256-9578
Web site: www.archrespite.org/NRC.htm

NRC provides a list of states that have respite coalitions. These state coalitions then list respite services available in their state. The majority of the information is focused on helping families of children with special needs, but lately there has been an effort to enlarge their referral base to include lifespan respite information. The NRC is working to gain passage of national lifespan respite legislation.

National Respite Locator Service
800 Eastowne Drive, Suite 105
Chapel Hill, NC 27514
800-473-1727, ext. 222
Web site: http://www.respitelocator.org/index.htm

Access a list of sites nationwide. While the vast majority focus on respite care for families of special needs children, the service now assists programs that provide respite for caregivers of adults and the elderly.

Shepherd's Centers of America
One West Armour Boulevard, Suite 201
Kansas City, MO 64111
800-547-7073
Web site: www.shepherdcenters.org
e-mail: staff@shepherdcenters.org

The organization provides respite care, telephone visitors, in-home visitors, nursing home visitors, home health aides, support groups, adult day care, and information and referrals for accessing other services available in the community. Services vary by center.

Home Care Resources: http://www.familycaregiving101.org/help/home_care.cfm

Finding Home Care

Home Care Agencies, Assisted Living and Nursing Homes Watchdog Agencies

Homecare is a general term that represents a wide range of community-based services to support someone that is recuperating from an acute situation, such as a hip fracture, or services needed by persons with on-going chronic conditions, such as stroke or cerebral palsy. The skills and duties of home care personnel vary, but all have one thing in commonÑthey make it possible for care recipients to remain at home in a safe, environment and in some cases have more independence than they did before. In the process, they also provide family caregivers with a chance to replenish their depleted physical and emotional reserves.

Most people with chronic or disabling conditions live in the community, on their own or with family.. For those who live in the community and their family caregivers, knowing agencies that can help provide help at home is important. If you think your loved one will need to move to an assisted living facility or a nursing home, youÕll need information on how to do that as well.

Consumer Consortium on Assisted Living
2342 Oak Street
Falls Church, VA 22046
703-533-8121
Web site: www.ccal.org

CCAL is a national consumer-focused organization that is dedicated to representing the needs of residents in assisted living facilities and educating consumers, professionals, and the general public about assisted living issues. Family caregivers can request the publication "Choosing an Assisted Living Facility: Strategies for Making the Right Decision," which provides helpful information and a concise checklist for those contemplating this next step.

National Citizens' Coalition for Nursing Home Reform
1424 16th Street, NW, Suite 202
Washington, DC 20036
202-332-2275
Web site: www.nccnhr.org

This organization serves as an information clearinghouse and offers referrals nationwide for help with concerns about long-term care facilities.

National Association for Home Care and Hospice
228 7th Street, SE
Washington, DC 20003
202-547-7424
Web site: www.nahc.org

This organization for home health care agency providers allows family caregivers to use the Internet to access a list of member agencies across the country.

New LifeStyles
4144 N. Central Expressway, Suite 1000
Dallas, TX 75204
800-869-9549
Web site: www.NewLifeStyles.com

New LifeStyles publishes regional directories of nursing homes, assisted living and retirement communities. Call for a free copy or visit them on the Web.

Support Groups: http://www.familycaregiving101.org/help/support_groups.cfm

Support Groups for Family Caregivers

Choosing a Support Group that you are comfortable with is a difficult task. Click here for guidance and questions to ask before you join a Support Group.

Children of Aging Parents (CAPS)
1609 Woodbourne Road, Suite 302A
Levittown, PA 19057
800-227-7294
Web site: www.caps4caregivers.org

CAPS assists caregivers of the elderly with information and referrals, a network of support groups, and publications and programs that promote public awareness of the value and the needs of family caregivers.

Family Caregiver Alliance (FCA)
690 Market Street, Suite 600
San Francisco, CA 94104
415-434-3388
800-445-8106
Web site: www.caregiver.org
e-mail: info@caregiver.org

FCA is the lead agency in California's system of Caregiver Resource Centers. FCA provides support and help to family caregivers and champions their cause through education, services, research and advocacy. Services are specific to California, although information can be accessed nationally.

Family Voices, Inc.
3411 Candelaria NE, Suite M
Albuquerque, NM 87107
888-835-5669
Web site: www.familyvoices.org

Family Voices offers information on healthcare policies relevant to children with special needs in every state.

Friends' Health Connection
PO Box 114
New Brunswick, NJ 08903
800-483-7436
Web site: www.48friend.org

Friends' Health Connection links persons with illness or disability and their family caregivers with others experiencing the same challenges.

Well Spouse Foundation
63 West Main Street, Suite H
Freehold, NJ 07728
800-838-0879
Web site: www.wellspouse.org
e-mail: info@wellspouse.org

Well Spouse is a national membership organization that gives support to husbands, wives and partners of the chronically ill and/or disabled. Well Spouse has a network of support groups and also a newsletter for spouses.

Financial Help and Advice: http://www.familycaregiving101.org/help/financial.cfm

Health Insurance, Prescription Drug, Medical Care Support and Information Programs

Family caregivers can contact their county or state Department of Health and Human Services, or area social service agencies such as Catholic Charities or the Association of Jewish Family and Children's Agencies, as well as local chapters of voluntary health agencies to find out if they offer any financial support programs and how to apply for them. Don't forget the Medicare and Medicaid websites: www.medicare.gov and www.medicaid.gov. Also, The Center for Medicare and Medicaid Services (CMS), which is the government agency that administers the Medicare Program and works in partnership with the states to administer the Medicaid Program, has a Web site that provides information about the Medicare and Medicaid Programs (www.cms.hhs.gov).

Benefits Check-Up and Benefits Check-Up RX
Web sites: www.benefitscheckup.org

A service of the National Council on the Aging, Benefits Check-Up and Benefits Check-Up RX help people over the age of 55 find federal, state, and local public and private programs that may pay for some of their medical care and/or prescription costs.

HealthInsurance.com
800-942-9019
Web site: www.healthinsurance.com

This fairly new Web site provides consumers and small businesses with quotes for health insurance, and may help those who have lost their health insurance find an affordable alternative.

Hill-Burton Free and Reduced Cost Health Care Program
800-638-0742
Web site: www.hrsa.gov/hillburton/default.htm

Hospitals and other health care facilities that receive federal funds for construction or modernization under this program must provide a specific amount of free or below-cost health care services to eligible people. The program will provide a list of participating facilities as well as information on eligibility.

Medicare Rights Center
1460 Broadway, 11th Floor
New York, NY 10036
888-HMO-9050
Web site: www.medicarerights.org

The Center provides hotlines for direct services, education/training, policy briefs, and a list of discount drug programs. The Web site also has a list of phone numbers for each state's "State Health Insurance Assistance Program and information on the new Medicare law Prescription Drug Cards."

Medicine Program
PO Box 515
Doniphan, MO 63935
573-996-7300
Web site: www.themedicineprogram.com

This program is for persons who do not have coverage either through insurance or government subsidies for outpatient prescription drugs, and who cannot afford to purchase medications at retail prices.

MetDesk
Division of Estate Planning for Special Kids
Web site: http://www.metlife.com/desk/

This service links MetLife agents who have special needs children with other parents of special needs children and provides advice on financial planning for the long-term care of special needs children. Visit the Web site for information on workshops, free assistance, and other services.

Patient Advocate Foundation
700 Thimble Shoals Boulevard, Suite 200
Newport News, VA 23606
800-532-5274
Web site: www.patientadvocate.org

The Patient Advocate Foundation serves as a liaison between patients and their insurer, employer and/or creditors to resolve insurance, job retention and/or debt crisis matters relating to a patient's condition.

Partnership for Prescription Assistance
Web site: www.helpingpatients.org/

This is the site of the Pharmaceutical Manufacturers Association and has all the information related to the companies' discount and free programs.

Together Rx Access
1-800-444-4106
Web sites: http://www.togetherrxaccess.com

A FREE prescription-savings card for eligible residents of the United States and Puerto Rico who have no prescription drug coverage. Plus information Medicare Part D

Kansas

I would note here that I could find no specific information on the subject of "Disabled", Disabled Care", or "Disabled Resources" on the Kansas State's government website...

Health and Social Welfare: http://www.kansas.gov/community/health-social-welfare/

Senior Health Insurance Counseling For Kansas (SHICK):
http://www.agingkansas.org/SHICK/shick_index.html

Senior Health Insurance Counseling for Kansas (SHICK) is a free program offering older Kansans an opportunity to talk with trained, community volunteers and get answers to questions about Medicare and other insurance issues. SHICK provides you with many resources that will help you with your struggle through the Medicare maze.

Our volunteers at SHICK know their stuff! The role of the volunteer counselor is to help people stay informed on changing conditions in health care insurance and to cut through the confusion.

Our volunteer counselors receive training on Medicare, Medicare Supplement Insurance, Long-Term Care and other health insurance subjects that concern older Kansans.

Our volunteer counselors do not work for any insurance company. The goal is to educate and assist the public to make informed decisions on what's best for them.

Click here to view Upcoming SHICK events

Medicare Prescription Drug Coverage Information

The Center for Medicare and Medicaid Services (CMS) has developed a **Medicare Prescription Drug Coverage Personal Information Worksheet** to help Medicare-eligible persons make informed choices about the Medicare prescription drug coverage.

Also, the **Medicare Prescription Drug Plan Finder** provides a way to make specific plan comparisons. It is available electronically at www.medicare.gov or by calling a customer service representative at 1-800-633-4227. The Drug Plan Finder allows you to personalize your search for a drug plan that most closely fits your needs.

For more information call the KDOA Senior Health Insurance Counseling for Kansas (SHICK) at 1-800-860-5260.

SHICK offers you:

- Free, Confidential Counseling: An opportunity to speak with real people, not telephone machines
- Employment and Medicare Information
- Disability and Medicare Information
- Supplemental Rate Comparisons via the Kansas Insurance Department Website

- Help with the Prescription Drug Program

Publications from the Kansas Insurance Department:

- Long-Term Care Insurance Shopper's Guide
- Medicare Supplemental Insurance Shopper's Guide

These Kansas Insurance Department publications may be mailed directly to you by visiting its website.

Still need more information? Visit our links page for more useful websites.

Who Benefits from SHICK?

Everyone who calls:
Toll Free: 1-800-860-5260
Wichita, Kansas 67202-3850
Fax: 316-337-6731

The following page was under construction...

Prescription Drug Information: http://www.agingkansas.org/SHICK/pdp_home.html

This page is a map one clicks upon for agency location...

Coordinator and Volunteer Info: http://www.agingkansas.org/SHICK/psa_map.html

This is a generalized information page for seniors...

Healthy Aging: http://www.agingkansas.org/HealthyAging/HealthyAging_Index.html

Caregivers information: http://www.agingkansas.org/Caregivers/Caregivers.html

Senior Support Resources: A generalized page under the generalized page
http://www.agingkansas.org/SeniorSupport/SeniorSupport_Index.html

Kentucky

For Seniors: http://kentucky.gov/residents/Pages/seniors.aspx

Information, services, and resources for seniors of the Commonwealth.

Aging Adults Services

Links to programs available through the Office of Aging Services such as Aging Network, Adult Day Care and Alzheimer's Disease support

Aging News

News articles from the Office of Aging Services

Aging Senior Centers by Area

Aging Network Organization, the Kentucky Area Agencies on Aging with contact numbers.

Alzheimer's Disease and Related Disorders Council

A community group that assists the Office of Aging Services with identifying issues that will help with the treatment of persons with memory loss and their families.

Application for Exemption under Homestead/Disability Amendment

Application for Exemption under Homestead/Disability Amendment.

Assisted Living Communities

Assisted Living Communities in Kentucky are certified by the Kentucky Office of Aging Services.

Caregiver Support Project

KinCare, the caregiver Support Services. Includes

Consumer Protection for Seniors

Protecting Kentucky's seniors through crime prevention education

Energy Saving Ideas

Find quick, easy ideas that will help save energy.

Energy Watch

A snapshot of state and national energy issues

Gas Mileage Tips

Here are some tips to help you reduce the amount of gas you use.

Homecare Program

The Homecare Program helps adults who are unable to perform some activities of daily living and are at risk of institutional care to remain in their own homes by providing supporte services and coordinating the help of family, friends and provider agencies.

Kentucky Insurance Program for Seniors (KIPS)

The Kentucky Department of Insurance has addressed the challenge of a steadily increasing aging population by creating this special unit.

Legislative Process

Learn about the Legislative Branch of Kentucky government.

Long-Term Care Ombudsman Program

Serves as an advocate and resource for individuals (and their families) who are living in or need the services of a long-term care facility, which includes nursing homes, personal care homes and family care homes. LTC Ombudsmen are trained to resolve problems in long-term care settings and are a public voice advocating for improvements needed by residents of long-term care facilities.

Low Income Energy Assistance Program

This vital program helps approximately 150,000 Kentucky families pay their utility bills each winter.

Medicaid Covered Services and Information

Medicaid covered services and service information.

Medicaid Eligibility Guidelines

Medicaid is a program for families and individuals who have income and resources within the established guidelines. The guidelines and income standards are not the same in every state and this website explains the Kentucky medicaid requirements.

Medicare Prescription Drug Assistance

Medicare is now offering a prescription drug discount card as the first step toward a drug benefit that will begin in 2006. The discount card provides Medicare beneficiaries price reduction of 10 - 20 percent on their pharmaceutical medications. Visit this website to learn more.

Problems with Utility Service?

The Public Service Commission can answer your questions about your utility service and help you resolve your utility complaints.

Quick Tips on Saving Energy

Tips on saving energy and money at home from the Department of Energy.

Renewable Energy in Kentucky

Renewable and alternative energy in Kentucky helps prevent pollution and reduces America's dependence on foreign energy sources.

Report Elder Abuse

Learn about and report possible elder abuse

Seniors Crime College

Seniors Crime College is a program offered by the Attorney General's Office in conjunction with other law enforcement agencies to help senior citizens better protect themselves from physical and financial crimes.

Social Security

Retirement, Medicare, disability, widows, and other survivors resources

USA.Gov for Seniors

USA.Gov for Seniors will empower citizens to obtain valuable health and security information and services at one location via the Internet.

Utility Rate Intervention

The Office of Rate Intervention serves as a watchdog for consumers in matters relating to health insurance, natural gas, water, sewer, electric and telephone rates.

Weatherization Assistance Help

The Weatherization Assistance Program enables low-income families to reduce their energy bills by making their home more energy efficient. Check here for eligibility and to find the agency

Aging and Adult Care: http://chfs.ky.gov/dail/Programs.htm

Department for Aging and Independent Living

Program Services:

Aging and Disability Resource Center Program (ADRC) - streamline access to long-term care. ADRCs serve as highly visible and trusted places available in every community across the commonwealth where people of all ages, incomes and disabilities go to get information on the full range of long-term support options.

Aging Network - provides services through the fifteen Kentucky Area Agencies on Aging and Independent Living.

Adult Day Care and Alzheimer's Disease Respite - provides services for physically disabled or frail people 60 and older in need of supervision for part of the day. Alzheimer's respite includes services provided at adult day centers or in the home for people of any age with Alzheimer's disease or other dementia disorders

Alzheimer's Disease and Related Disorders Council - Alzheimer's Disease and Related Disorders Council - is a governor appointed council that helps the Department for Aging and Independent Living identify issues to advance the treatment of people with memory loss and provide support and assistance to their families.

Assisted Living Community information and certification - Assisted living is a private-pay living alternative between total independence and higher levels of residential care. Assisted living communities in Kentucky are certified by the Kentucky Department for Aging and Independent Living.

Caregiver Support Services - include the National Family Caregiver Support Program that helps families with their roles as caregivers, and the Kentucky Family Caregiver Program that helps Kentucky grandparents care for grandchildren.

Chronic Disease Self Management Program - empowers individuals with chronic diseases such as diabetes, high blood pressure, heart disease and others to better manage their conditions to live longer, healthier lives.

Consumer Directed Option (CDO) - allows eligible Medicaid waiver members to choose their own providers for non-medical and non-residential services. This choice gives members greater flexibility in the delivery of services that are needed to stay in their homes. Members may also purchase goods and finance minor home adaptations through CDO.

Elder Abuse Prevention - Elder abuse is often a silent crime, rarely noticed behind closed doors and rarely reported by those who think "it's none of my business." The law says it is our business to report elder abuse when we witness or suspect it. Visit the CHFS Elder Abuse Prevention site to learn more about the signs of elder abuse, what you can do to prevent it and how to report it.

Guardianship - is a program with offices in each Kentucky region. Guardianship is a legal relationship between a court appointed party that assumes the responsibility of guardian and a ward, a person declared "legally disabled" by the court who cannot manage their own well-being.

Hart-Supported Living - provides flexible funding to disabled Kentuckians for supports that promote independence to live at home and function within the community. Types of supports typical for this program include: supported living community resource developers; home modifications for accessibility; homemaker services; personal care services; transportation; adaptive and therapeutic equipment; and in-home training and home management assistance. Other supports not listed may also be considered. Applications for funding are accepted once a year and are due on or before April 1.

Health Promotion and Disease Prevention - includes routine health screening, nutrition counseling and education services, health promotion programs, home injury prevention, mental health screenings, benefits counseling, medication management screening education, and rehabilitation information through the area agencies on aging and independent living.

Homecare - provides in-home services for individuals 60 and older with functional disabilities who are at-risk for requiring long-term, institutional care. Services include personal care, home management, home health aide, home-delivered meals, home repair, help with household chores, respite, escort and case management and assessment.

Institute for Aging - advises the Secretary of the Cabinet for Health and Family Services and other officials of the Commonwealth on policy matters related to the development and delivery of services to the aged. The Institute operates in partnership with the Department for Aging and Independent Living.

Long-Term Care Ombudsman - established under the Older Americans Act, the Kentucky Long-Term Care Ombudsman Program operates out of the 15 Area Development Districts through their Area Agencies on Aging and Independent Living. The LTCO works to improve the lives of people living in long-term care by enhancing their quality of life, improving their quality of care, protecting individual rights and promoting the dignity of each resident.

Nutrition Program for the Elderly - includes home delivered meals (meals on wheels) and congregate meals at senior centers. The program helps improve the eating habits of participants, offers social networking opportunities and helps the participants remain healthy and independent by reducing hunger and food insecurity.

Personal Care Attendant Program - has one purpose: to enable eligible, severely physically disabled adults who otherwise may be at risk for institutional care to live where one wishes and how one wants to live. The program provides a subsidy to eligible participants. The eligible participant must have the ability to hire, supervise and pay an attendant.

Senior Citizen Centers - are located throughout Kentucky. There are more than 200 senior centers with at least one located in each of Kentucky's 120 counties. The centers provide information and assistance, wellness opportunities, citizenship, volunteer opportunities, and social activities and services related to people 60 and older.

Senior Community Service Employment Program - provides training and part-time employment opportunities to low-income people age 55 and older. Participant benefits include: earned income; training and experience to develop employment skills; annual physical exams; the chance to obtain unsubsidized employment; social and physical activities; and engagement in activities that support independence.

State Health Insurance Assistance Program (SHIP) - is a statewide program that provides free and objective counseling and assistance to people with questions or problems regarding Medicare and other related health insurances. SHIP operates through the state's 15 Area Agencies on Aging and Independent Living (AAAIL's).

Traumatic Brain Injury Trust Fund - was established to provide assistance to children and adults with brain injuries. The TBI Trust Fund Program is administered by a Board of Directors to assure that individuals with a brain injury and their families are provided effective services and supports to promote independence and personal productivity.

The Traumatic Brain Injury Behavioral Program - establishes identification of those affected by Traumatic Brain Injury who are in need of behavioral services. The TBI Behavioral Program will provide services through crisis intervention, residential, targeted case management and wrap-around services.

Area Agencies on Aging and Independent Living/Disability Resource Markets:
http://chfs.ky.gov/dail/AreaAgenciesonAging.htm

To find a senior center in your area, you would click on one of the following Area Agencies on Aging (AAA) on this webpage.

Barren River Area
Allen, Barren, Butler, Edmonson, Hart, Logan, Metcalfe, Monroe, Simpson, Warren
Big Sandy Area
Floyd, Johnson, Magoffin, Martin, Pike
Bluegrass Area
Anderson, Boyle, Bourbon, Clark, Estill, Fayette, Franklin, Garrard, Harrison, Jessamine, Lincoln, Madison, Mercer, Nicholas, Powell, Scott, Woodford
Buffalo Trace Area
Bracken, Fleming, Lewis, Mason, Robertson
Cumberland Valley Area
Bell, Clay, Harlan, Jackson, Knox, Laurel, Rockcastle, Whitley

FIVCO Area
Boyd, Carter, Greenup, Elliott, Lawrence

Gateway Area
Bath, Menifee, Montgomery, Morgan, Rowan
Green River Area
Daviess, Hancock, Henderson, McLean, Ohio, Union, Webster

KIPDA Area
Bullitt, Henry, Jefferson, Oldham, Shelby, Spencer, Trimble

Kentucky River Area
Breathitt, Knott, Lee, Leslie, Letcher, Owsley, Perry, Wolfe

Lake Cumberland Area
Adair, Casey, Clinton, Cumberland, Green, McCreary, Pulaski, Russell, Taylor, Wayne
Lincoln Trail Area
Breckinridge, Grayson, Hardin, Larue, Marion, Meade, Nelson, Washington
Northern Kentucky Area
Boone, Campbell, Carroll, Gallatin, Grant, Kenton, Owen, Pendleton

Pennyrile Area
Caldwell, Christian, Crittenden, Hopkins, Livingston, Lyon, Muhlenberg, Todd, Trigg
Purchase Area
Ballard, Calloway, Carlisle, Fulton, Hickman, Graves, Marshall, McCracken

Louisiana

Department of Health and Hospitals: http://new.dhh.louisiana.gov/

Office of Aging and Adult Services: http://new.dhh.louisiana.gov/index.cfm/subhome/12/n/7

COMMUNITY AND FAMILY SUPPORTS PROGRAM: The Community and Family Supports Program provides goods and/or services in a flexible manner to help eligible people with severe physical and/or cognitive disabilities live independently.

LOUISIANA DEPARTMENT OF HEALTH AND HOSPITALS/ OFFICE OF AGING AND ADULT SERVICES

Community and Family Supports Program:
http://new.dhh.louisiana.gov/assets/docs/OAAS/publications/CommunityFamily_Supports_Fact_Sheet.pdf

What is the purpose of the Community and Family Supports Program?

The Community and Family Support Program is intended to provide goods and/or services in a flexible manner to eligible people with severe physical and/or cognitive disabilities in order to help them live independently.

If I qualify, what services can be paid for by this program?

Communication services such as Braille devices, interpreters, etc.
Community supports such as dental and medical care not covered by Medicare
Companion or roommate services
Crisis intervention
Equipment and supplies such as prosthetics, mobility and sensory aids, etc.
Home and vehicle modifications needed for accessibility
Personal assistance services such as assistance with going to the bathroom, dressing, bathing, etc.
Counseling services

Home health Services
Homemaker services
Recreation services to improve access to community recreation and to educate service providers
Service coordination
Specialized diagnosis and evaluation
Specialized nutrition
Specialized utility costs
Therapeutic services, such as occupational and physical therapy, speech and language therapy, etc.
Respite care
Rent subsidy

For more information about the Community and Family Supports program or to apply for services, please call the ARC of Louisiana at 225-383-1033 or 1-866-966-6260.

PROGRAM FOR ALL-INCLUSIVE CARE FOR THE ELDERLY (PACE):
http://new.dhh.louisiana.gov/assets/docs/OAAS/publications/CommunityFamily_Supports_Fact_Sheet.pdf

What is the purpose of PACE?

Program for All-Inclusive Care for the Elderly (PACE) coordinates and provides all needed preventive, primary, acute and long term care services so that older people can continue living in the community. The emphasis is on enabling you to remain in your community while enhancing your quality of life.

How does the PACE program work?
As a PACE enrollee, you will be transported to and from the PACE center from your residence to receive needed services.

PACE providers are responsible for providing all services which are currently available through Medicare and Medicaid insurances.

Once you voluntarily enroll in PACE, Medicare and/or Medicaid will no longer pay any other provider for services. All your care will be provided or coordinated by PACE.

What Are some of the Services Provided by PACE

Primary Care
Personal Care/Supportive Services
Nutritional Counseling
Transportation
Medical Specialty Services Procedures
Prescriptions and Biological
Nursing Facility Care
Acute Inpatient Care
Day Center Services

Prosthetics, Orthotics, DME Corrective Vision, Assistive Devices, Hearing Aids, Dentures (Repair and Maintenance of these items are also covered.)
Social Work
Restorative Therapies
Recreational Therapy
Meals
Lab Tests, x-rays, diagnostic
Other services determined necessary to improve or maintain your overall health status

How is PACE paid?
Both Medicare and Medicaid reimburse PACE a payment based on what would have been paid under the fee-for-service system.

Once you are enrolled in PACE, Medicare and/or Medicaid will no longer pay any other provider for services. All your care will be provided or coordinated by the PACE provider. The PACE provider is at full risk; this means your PACE provider is responsible for all care costs, even if it exceeds the monthly capitated payment they receive each month.

Am I eligible for PACE?
You must be 55 years of age or older

Live in a PACE provider service area

You must be certified by the State to need nursing home care

Meet the requirements for Medicaid eligibility,

Individual income of no more than $2,022 per month, total resources must be less than $2,000. The income limits are different when an individual is married and this can change.

Can I change my mind if I no longer want to be in PACE?
Yes, you can disenroll from PACE and return to your regular benefits in Medicare and Medicaid at any time.

Where are the current PACE providers in Louisiana?

PACE Greater New Orleans, sponsored by Catholic Charities, can be reached at 504-945-1531.
Pace Baton Rouge, sponsored by the Franciscan Ministries of Our Lady Health System (FMOLHS), can be reached at 225-490-0604
945-1531.

For more information on PACE, please call the PACE Greater New Orleans at 504-945-1531
PACE Baton Rouge at 225-490-0604

Maine

Department of Health and Human Services:

Office of Elder Services: http://www.maine.gov/dhhs/oes/

Aging and Disability Resource Center (ADRC): http://www.maine.gov/dhhs/oes/resource/adrc.html

Aging and Disability Resource Center (ADRC)

Cultural Considerations of Serving Veterans Conference - Monday, September 12, 2011

On this page:

- Answer any question about long-term support services
- What can I expect when I call an Aging & Disability Resource Center (ADRC)?
- Fun look at finding an Aging and Disability Resource Center

- To contact an Aging & Disability Resource Center in Maine
- More Background
- More Information

Answer any question about long-term support services:

The five Aging & Disability Resource Centers in Maine serve as "one-stop-shops" to answer questions from older adults, or from any individuals with disabilities, about a wide range of in-home, community-based, and institutional services.

Aging and Disability Resource Centers are expert at answering questions in-home care services and all kinds of *long-term support*. Maine's five Aging and Disability Resource Center sites:

- provide information and assistance to individuals needing either public or private long-term care resources,
- serve professionals seeking assistance on behalf of their clients' long-term care needs,
- serve individuals planning for their future long-term care needs, and
- serve as the entry point to publicly administered long-term supports including those funded under Medicaid, the Older Americans Act and state revenue programs.

Goal: Empowerment: The goal of these Aging & Disability Resource Centers is to empower callers to make informed choices about long-term support and to streamline peoples' access to long-term support.

People Served: Maine's Aging & Disability Resource Centers are designed to serve all older adults, people with disabilities and their caregivers, who have long-term care community or program needs.

What can I expect when I call an Aging & Disability Resource Center (ADRC)?

Anyone can call their local Aging and Disability Resource Center (often called the Area Agency on Aging) to receive help in many ways. There is no charge for the assistance you receive. First, you will speak with the ADRC's phone staff, who may collect basic information about you. Phone staff are trained to listen carefully, ask questions, and write down your need or request. The phone staff may be able to answer your question or send information to you immediately. However, to make sure that your question is fully answered the phone staff may transfer you to other staff in the ADRC who can spend more time answering your question in more depth.

Your conversation with the ADRC program staff will probably be more in-depth in order to figure out how best to meet your needs and see if you are interested in any other services that may be available.

Assistance or services from the ADRC:

- **Information and referrals:** you may just need information, simple or complicated. You also can receive referrals to services within your community such as transportation, housing, home care, and Meals on Wheels.
- **Services:** the ADRC can help you access services such as congregate or home-delivered meals, prevention of falls, managing chronic diseases, Alzheimer's respite services, adult day care, access to legal services, employment training, or health insurance counseling
- **Medicare/Health Insurance counseling:** help in choosing the best policy for your situation, understanding the different plans, and assisting you with applications
- **Educational Opportunities:** the ADRC can connect you with educational opportunities
- **Options Counseling:** If you are interested in learning more about services you may need over time, for yourself or someone you care for, the ADRC staff can help you figure out what "options" of services might work well for you.
- **Advocacy:** the ADRC works for you – feel free to ask for what you need – we'd like to try to help!
- Caregiver Support Services: may include respite, caregiver training, support groups, helpful information, and individual support

Below are some comments from people who have used the services of the Aging and Disability Resource Center in the past:

- "A great organization to help older people who have no one to help them..."
- "The staff person I spoke with was very kind and helpful. She was quite knowledgeable, will do additional research, and get back to me with information if necessary."
- "Everyone has been very helpful and considerate. As an RN I thought I could handle this alone and am so relieved now I don't have to. Thank you!"
- "A pleasant experience all around. Would highly recommend to anyone else!"

To contact an Aging & Disability Resource Center in Maine:

Aroostook Area Agency on Aging – Aging & Disability Resource Center	
County Served	Aroostook
ADRC Coordinator	Sharon Berz
Website:	http://www.aroostookaging.org
Phone:	207-764-3396
Fax:	207-764-6182
Address:	1 Edgemont Drive Suite 2 Presque Isle, Maine 04769
Hours of Business:	8:00 a.m. to 4:30 p.m. Monday-Friday

[Back to list]

Eastern Area Agency on Aging – Aging & Disability Resource Center	
Counties Served	Piscataquis, Penobscot, Washington, Hancock
ADRC Coordinators	Dyan M. Walsh, MSW
Website:	http://www.eaaa.org/dashnetwork.shtml www.eaaa.org www.easternagencyonaging.org
Phone:	(207) 941-2865 1-800-432-7812
Fax:	(207) 941-2869
TTY:	(207) 992-0150
Address:	Eastern Agency on Aging 450 Essex Street Bangor, ME 04401
Hours of Business:	8:00 a.m. to 4:30 p.m. Monday-Friday

[Back to list]

Spectrum Generations - Aging & Disability Resource Center	
Counties Served	Knox, Lincoln, Waldo, Somerset, Sagadahoc, & Kennebec
ADRC Coordinators	Leslie Bray
Website:	http://www.seniorspectrum.com/
Phone:	1-800-639-1553
Fax:	207-622-7857
TTY:	1-800-464-8703
Address:	One Weston Court Suite 203 Augusta, ME 04330
Hours of Business:	8:00 a.m. to 4:30 p.m. Monday-Friday

[Back to list]

SeniorsPlus – Aging & Disability Resource Center	
Counties Served	Franklin, Oxford, Androscoggin
ADRC Coordinator	Connie Jones – Director, SeniorsPlus - Aging and Disability Connections
Website:	http://www.seniorsplus.org/aaoa/index.html
Phone:	1-800-427-1241 207-795-4010
Fax:	207-795-4009
TTY:	207-795-7232
Address:	8 Falcon Road P.O. Box 659 Lewiston, ME 04243-0659
Hours of Business:	8:00 a.m. to 5:00 p.m. Monday - Friday

[Back to list]

Southern Maine Area Agency on Aging – Aging & Disability Resource Center	
Counties Served	Cumberland and York
ADRC Coordinators	Katlyn Blackstone MS, LSW Director, Information & Advocacy Program
Website:	http://www.smaaa.org/
Phone:	207-396-6503
Fax:	207-764-6182
Address:	136 US Rt. 1 Scarborough, Maine 04074
Hours of Business:	8:00 a.m. to 4:30 p.m. Monday-Friday

[Back to list]

More Background:

The Aging and Disability Resource Center national initiative is funded by means of a collaboration between the U.S. Administration on Aging (AoA) and the federal Centers for Medicare & Medicaid Services (CMS).

AoA and CMS envision ADRCs as highly visible and trusted places available in every community across the country where people of all ages, incomes and disabilities go to get information on the full range of long-term support options. Nationally, ADRC programs have taken important steps towards meeting AoA and CMS's vision by

- creating a person-centered, community-based environment that promotes independence and dignity for individuals;

- providing easy access to information to assist consumers in exploring a full range of long-term support options; and

- providing resources and services that support the range of needs for family caregivers.

ADRCs target services to the elderly and individuals with physical disabilities, serious mental illness, and/or developmental/intellectual disabilities. The ultimate goal of the ADRCs is to serve all individuals with long-term care needs regardless of their age or disability.

Maine has received three grants to develop Aging & Disability Resource Centers in Maine, in 2003, 2006, and 2009. With these grants, we have been able to provide Aging & Disability Resource Center services for the entire state.

National perspective on "Why Transform Long Term Supports and Services?"

The U.S. Administration on Aging supports states' efforts in developing and sustaining a person-centered, self-directed national long term care system. This system should effectively assist consumers with identifying and accessing a range of home and community based resources which maintain independence of older citizens and persons with disabilities and slow the rate of growth and expenditures in the states' Medicaid programs.

1. The national long term care system has already begun to evolve with programs such as CMS's Real Choice Systems Change Grants, Cash and Counseling, and other consumer-centered and consumer-directed programs.

2. There is an opportunity to build upon this recent innovation and creatively resolve inefficiencies in the nation's long term care system using identified best practices and programmatic strategies developed by the Aging Network and its partners.

3. State budgets will not be able to support the current system of Medicaid long-term care and spend-down without creating a plan to slow the rate of its growth and expenditures.

4. The "Silver Wave" is coming and many states are not prepared.

5. States' fiscal crises must be resolved to effectively build service capacity and infrastructure for the growing numbers of elderly people and individuals with disabilities.

Consumer Satisfaction and Lessons Learned in Maine

The evaluation of the ADRCs was conducted in 2008 through the use of consumer satisfaction surveys and interviews with key stakeholders. The Muskie School of Public Service designed and administered the surveys, monitored the data collection protocols and analyzed the results.

The consumer satisfaction survey was mailed to individuals who had accessed the ADRCs for information or services. Staff at each ADRC sent names and addresses of "first time" contacts to the evaluation team at the Muskie School approximately every two weeks. Surveys were mailed to contacts immediately so that the interaction with the ADRCs would be fresh and accurately recalled. Over 1,900 surveys were mailed from the Muskie School along with a cover letter and a postage-paid business reply envelope to facilitate return of the completed surveys. Overall, there was a 28% response rate.

The Lewin Group has provided technical assistance to ADRCs and to the evaluators. The following Maine ADRC satisfaction survey results have been organized and reported under the key domains outlined by the Lewin Group: Visibility/Trust; Efficiency; Responsiveness; and Effectiveness.

The survey shows that consumers are pleased with the service and information they receive from the ADRCs.

Caregivers: http://www.maine.gov/dhhs/oes/caregivers.htm

Caregivers Information

As a person providing care for a loved one, you are faced with an enormous amount of responsibility and work. Often there are no others there to help you, and you have little time to take care of your own needs.
Below are some resources which may be helpful. If you are aware of any support groups, programs or other resources which you feel may be helpful to others, please contact the Office of Elder Services at OES.Info@maine.gov or call us at 1-800-262-2232

Family Caregiver Support Program

If you are interested in a home and community care assessment to help learn what services are available, visit our Maine Home & Community Care page.

Respite/alternative care

- Respite care - Alzheimers
- Early Memory Loss Family Support Group
- Adult Day Care Programs

Support Groups

- SeniorsPlus / Western Area Agency on Aging (Word | PDF) (*free viewer)
- The Brain Injury Association of Maine 🗗
- Seacoast Online group Listing 🗗
- The Aroostook Medical Center listing 🗗
- Southern Maine Agency on Aging 🗗
- Central Maine Medical Center 🗗

Miscellaneous

- **2009 National Family Caregiving Awards Program - Applications Are Now Being Accepted**

The National Alliance for Caregiving and MetLife Foundation are pleased to announce that applications are being accepted for the 2009 National Family Caregiving Awards Program.

- <u>Connections</u> - A Guide for Family Caregivers in Maine
  This guide includes information about home care, assisted living and nursing facility care, end of life care, kinship parents, legal issues, health insurance, dementias, and long-term care as well as other services that people caring for older adults might want to know about.

- Maine SAVVY CAREGIVER Training, sponsored by the Office of Elder Services, Department of Health and Human Services and funded by the Administration on Aging, provides family caregivers of people with dementia the knowledge, skills and attitude essential for successful caregiving. The 12-hour training is provided in 6 sessions.

Maryland

Living: http://www.maryland.gov/Living/Pages/Living.aspx

Sections on this page and under Disabilities:

- Adult Care Services
- American Council of the Blind of Maryland
- Americans with Disabilities Act
- Deaf and Hard of Hearing
- Developmental Disabilities Administration
- Disability Entitlement Advocacy Program (DEAP)
- DisabilityInfo.gov
- In Home-Aide Services
- Maryland Relay
- Maryland Relay - Video Relay Service (VRS)
- Motorists with Disabilities
- National Federation of the Blind
- Park Accessibility For All
- Project HOME
- Special Olympics
- Technology Assistance Program
- Transportation For People With Disabilities

Sections on this page and under Senior Citizens:

- Adult Evaluation and Review Services
- American Geriatrics Society
- Assisted Living
- Falls Among Older Adults: An Overview
- Flu Information
- Guide to Assisted Living Facilities
- Healthy Aging
- Housing Information
- Local Agencies on Aging
- Maryland Senior Olympics
- Maryland Tax Information for Seniors
- Medicaid Long Term Care Services
- Medicaid Waiver Program
- Medicare Part D Pharmacy

- MTA for Senior Citizens
- National Association of Retired Federal Employees (NARFE)
- National Institute on Aging (NIA)
- Nursing Home Guide
- Nursing Homes - Locate A Facility In Your Area
- Nursing Homes - What You Need To Know
- Older Adult Drivers
- Social Security

Under Independent Living/ Housing information is this pertinent section:

Continuing Care At Home

The Maryland Department of Aging is authorized to regulate Continuing Care At Home (CCAH), a new concept in delivering services to the elderly. Similar to the Continuing Care Retirement Community (CCRC) structure, subscribers to CCAH will pay a one-time entrance fee and monthly premiums to access comprehensive, managed long term care services in their own homes. This housing option is designed for persons 60 years of age and older with moderate to higher incomes and who are living independently in the community.

CCAH services include: care coordination, home inspections by occupational therapist, assistance with activities of daily living in subscriber's home, skilled nursing services in subscriber's home, routine services of an assisted living facility, routine services of a comprehensive care facility, and assistance with the maintenance of the subscriber's dwelling.

CCAH providers must meet the same requirements as CCRCs, including approval of a feasibility study, and review and approval of the language contained in the CCAH contract. A copy of the regulations for Continuing Care at Home is available by individual request. The Maryland Department of Aging urges anyone who is considering entering into a Continuing Care At Home agreement to consult with an attorney and financial advisor before signing any documents. Although the Department of Aging regulates CCAH providers, it does not rate, endorse, or guarantee a CCAH provider.

The Maryland Department of Aging provides a comprehensive information packet for consumers and developers interested in learning more about these communities, the law and the regulations. Interested persons may use the mail response form to request a Consumer or Developer CCAH packet.

Continuing Care at Home became available to consumers in December 2002; however, it is not currently available to new consumers. There is currently one provider registered with the Maryland Department of Aging:

MESH Life Care at Home, Inc.
7600 Georgia Avenue, NW, Suite 402
Washington, DC 20012-1616

It is not, however, specifically for family caregivers. The following page did seem more useful, at least for support purposes...

Senior Information & Assistance: http://www.aging.maryland.gov/senior.html#SeniorLocalOffices

Senior Information & Assistance

Senior Information and Assistance Local Offices

Eldercare Locator web site

Home and Community-Based Services

Medicaid Waiver for Older Adults

Senior Health Insurance Assistance Program

Helpful links for Legal Assistance

Senior Legal Assistance

Making Health Care Decisions for Others

Public Guardianship

In lieu of a suitable guardian, the Secretary of the Department of Aging or the Director of a local Area Agency on Aging may be appointed as a public guardian for persons ages 65 and older who have been declared by the Courts to be incapable of making their own decisions.

Guardians may be required to determine appropriate living arrangements, oversee the provision of services or consent to medical treatment for persons under their guardianship.

For more information or to speak with a Public Guardian in your area, you may contact any of the Local Area Agencies on Aging throughout Maryland.

How may we help you? Click on any of the links below.

"A Guide to Adult Guardianship and Guardianship Alternatives in Maryland " Handbook

Report Elder Abuse

1-800-91-**PREVENT**
1-800-917-**7383**

Visit the **Department of Human Resources** website at:

http://www.dhr.state.md.us/oas/protect.htm

Long Term Care Ombudsman/Elder Abuse Prevention

The Maryland Long Term Care Ombudsman Program helps residents in long term care facilities maintain their legal rights, control over their own lives, and personal dignity. Long term care facilities include nursing homes and assisted living communities.

Major Responsibilities of the Ombudsman Program

- **Receives** and resolves complaints made by or for residents of long term care facilities.
- **Educates** consumers and long term care providers about residents' rights and good care practices.
- **Promotes** community involvement through volunteer opportunities.
- **Provides** information to the public on nursing homes and other long term care facilities and services, residents' rights, and legislative and policy issues.

The Ombudsman Program is authorized by the Older Americans Act and Maryland law. In Maryland, Federal, State and local governments fund program operations in 19 regional offices covering all of Maryland's 23 counties and Baltimore City. Ombudsman Program Coordinators act as advocates for residents. In many jurisdictions, they also recruit, train and supervise volunteers who carry out the goals of the program.

Anyone may contact the Ombudsman

The Ombudsman is required to keep any information provided confidential.

There is absolutely no charge for the services of the Ombudsman program.

The State and local Ombudsman's office can be reached Monday through Friday during normal business hours.

- Allegany 301-777-5970
- Anne Arundel 410-222-4464
- Baltimore City 410-396-3144
- Baltimore County 410-887-4200
- Calvert 410-535-4606
- Carroll 410-386-3800
- Cecil 410-996-5295
- Charles 301-934-0133
- Frederick 301-600-1605
- Garrett 301-334-9431
- Harford 410-638-3025
- Howard 410-313-6423
- Montgomery 240-777-3369
- Prince George's 301-265-8458
- Queen Anne's 410-758-0848

- St. Mary's 301-475-4200 ext. 1050
- Washington 301-790-0275
- For Dorchester, Somerset, Wicomico, Worcester Counties, contact
- MAC, Inc. 410-742-0505
- For Caroline, Kent and Talbot Counties contact
- Upper Shore Aging 410-778-6000
- State Long Term Care Ombudsman 410-767-1108
- Statewide toll free 1-800-243-3425, extension 71108

Senior Information and Assistance Local Offices

Senior Information and Assistance is a statewide program that provides a single point of entry into the aging network and offers convenient access to information on services and benefits for older persons, their families and caregivers. This includes, but is not limited to information on transportation, income and financial aid, senior citizens centers and clubs, daily meals, pharmacy assistance, housing, volunteer opportunities, and more!

There are 120 local Senior Information and Assistance offices throughout the state. The friendly, trained staff at each office can also provide assistance in determining need for services and make referrals to appropriate agencies and offer case management/coordination for persons requiring ongoing services.

For inquiries or assistance at any time, please contact the office nearest you or call the Maryland Department of Aging at 1-800-243-3425, weekdays between 8:00 a.m. and 5:00 p.m.

Click here for a listing of Senior Information and Assistance offices

Senior Health Insurance Assistance Program

The Senior Health Insurance Assistance Program (SHIP) meets one of the most universal needs of Medicare beneficiaries , including those <u>under 65</u> years of age — **understanding their health insurance benefits, bills and rights**. The Maryland SHIP program provides trained staff and volunteer counselors in all 24 counties. Counselors provide in-person and telephone assistance in the following general areas:

- Medicare Prescription Drug Coverage Program (Medicare Part D)
- Medicare supplements (Medigap Plans)
- Assistance for disabled Medicare beneficiaries (under age 65)
- Medicare Advantage Plans (HMOs, preferred provider organizations)
- Long Term Care Insurance
- Medical Assistance programs
- Assistance for low-income beneficiaries
- Assistance with denials, appeals and grievances
- Billing problems
- Health care fraud and abuse
- Volunteer counselor opportunities
- Free community presentations and much, much more!

The Maryland Department of Aging receives funding for this program from the Centers for Medicare & Medicaid Services, the State of Maryland and local governments. **SHIP counseling services are confidential and free of charge**.

Maryland Senior Medicare Patrol

Most SHIP offices are open Monday through Friday during normal business hours.

Contact a local SHIP Office:

- Allegany 301-777-5970 ext. 110
- Anne Arundel 410-222-4464
- Baltimore City 410-396-2273
- Baltimore County 410-887-2059
- Calvert 301-855-1170 & 410-535-4606
- Caroline 410-479-2535
- Carroll 410-386-3806 & 1-888-302-8978
- Cecil 410-996-8169
- Charles 301-934-0118 & 301-870-3388 ext 5118
- Dorchester 410-376-3662 ext. 106
- Frederick 301-600-1604
- Garrett 301-334-9431 & 1-888-877-8403
- Harford 410-638-3025
- Howard 410-313-7392
- Kent 410-778-2564
- Montgomery 301-590-2819
- Prince George's 301-265-8471 & 301-265-8450
- Queen Anne's 410-758-0848 ext.2724
- Somerset 410-742-0505 ext. 106
- St. Mary's 301-475-4200 ext. 1064
- Talbot 410-822-2869
- Washington 301-790-0275 ext. 208
- Wicomico 410-742-0505 ext. 106
- Worcester 410-742-0505 ext. 106

Senior Legal Assistance

Senior Legal Assistance provides legal advice, counseling and representation to older Marylanders. The Area Agencies on Aging contract with local attorneys for service. Priority is given to issues involving the following:

- Income maintenance
- Disability benefits
- Health care
- Protective services
- Abuse
- Institutionalization

- Guardianship
- Housing

Caregiver Resources: http://www.aging.maryland.gov/caregiver.html

A page mostly devoted to caregiving and some form of semi-independent living, although not particularly at home or by a family member.

Massachusetts

For Residents:

http://www.mass.gov/?pageID=mg2constituent&L=2&L0=Home&L1=Resident&sid=massgov2

Elders:

http://www.mass.gov/?pageID=mg2topic&L=3&L0=Home&L1=Resident&L2=Elders&sid=massgov2

Elders

- **Caregiver Support**

The Massachusetts Family Caregiver Support Program offers caregivers assistance and support to ease the strain and reduce the challenges of caregiving.

- **Discrimination, Fraud and Abuse**

Information on how to prevent, protect and eliminate the mistreatment of elders.

- **Health Care**

Review the different health care options available for elders to see which option works best for your situation.

- **Home Care**

The Massachusetts Home Care Program provides support services to elders with daily living needs to remain at home in their communities.

- **Housing**

Learn about the different types of housing options available to you.

- **Long-Term Care**

Information on nursing facilities, residential care homes, assisted living facilities and other supervised living facilities for older adults.

- **Meals and Nutrition**

Peruse the various types of meal programs that can supplement your nutrition.

- **Retirement**

Information about compensation and benefits and planning for your post-work life.

- **Service Organizations and Advocates**

A number of resources are available to you in the event that you need some type of assistance.

- **Taxes**

Information for Senior Citizens and Retirees.

- **Transportation**

  Programs that provide transportation for individuals with special transportation needs such as special arrangements for older adults, people with disabilities and people transitioning into the workforce.

- **Volunteer and Work**

  Interested in volunteering or finding some type of work? Here are some resources that can point you in the right direction.

Caregiver Support:
http://www.mass.gov/?pageID=elderstopic&L=2&L0=Home&L1=Caregiver+Support&sid=Eelders

Caregiver Support
The Massachusetts Family Caregiver Support Program offers caregivers assistance and support to ease the strain and reduce the challenges of caregiving. Caring for a loved one can often be difficult and frustrating. We recognize the potential emotional, physical and financial strain of caregiving, as well as its pleasures. This site was designed to help you care for your loved one and yourself.

Are you a spouse, daughter, son, grandchild or friend who is caring for an adult age 60 or older? Do you care for someone with Alzheimer's disease? Or are you 55 years or older and raising a grandchild, young relative or caring for a disabled person? We are here to help — there is local help for you!

- **Program Overview**

  The Massachusetts Family Caregiver Support Program empowers elders and caregivers by providing information, education, support, and services that enhance quality of life.

- **Caregiving Resources**

- **Caring for Elders**

  Learn how to connect with community resources and support groups. Our tip sheets provide several "how-to's," as well as checklists for things like home safety and forms you can use to gather information for doctors visits, or to provide instructions for substitute caregivers. And we provide an extensive list of links to helpful external web resources.

- **Grandparents Raising Grandchildren**

- **Care for the Caregiver**

  Regardless if you are just starting out in a caregiving role or continuing to care for an older person whose needs are increasing—you first need to care for yourself. Find tips for preserving your physical and emotional health, community supports that make it possible for you to take a break from your daily responsibilities, and links to resources for fitness advice, health tools and newsletters

- **What Employers Can Do**

Learn about local and national resources that will help you understand and support the special issues faced by your employees who are caregivers.

- **Professional Resources**

- **Web Resources**

Caregiver Resources:
http://www.mass.gov/?pageID=eldersterminal&L=2&L0=Home&L1=Caregiver+Support&sid=Eelders&b=terminalcontent&f=csp_caregiving_resources&csid=Eelders

Family Caregiver Support Program:
http://www.mass.gov/Eelders/docs/caregiver_support_group_tipsheet.pdf Basically advice concerning choosing a caregiver support group

Websites: http://www.mass.gov/Eelders/docs/caregivers_useful_websites_family.pdf Like it says, websites that (might be) useful...

Disabilities:
http://www.mass.gov/?pageID=mg2topic&L=3&L0=Home&L1=Resident&L2=Disabilities&sid=massgov2

Disabilities

- **Civil Rights Laws and Regulations**

Massachusetts has a rich and exemplary history in promoting maximum levels of independence and inclusion in all aspects of society for people with disabilities.

- **Disability Services**

Blind, Deaf, Head Injury, Learning Disability, Mental Health, Intellectual Disability, and more.

- **Discrimination**

If you believe you have been treated differently because of a disability you may want to file a complaint. We have provided a list of resources available to assist you.

- **Equipment & Technology**

For those who need assistive technology or are trying to resolve a problem with their equipment.

- **General Information & Services**

Learn about laws, statistics, and how to combat abuse or neglect, among other things.

- **Housing**

Here you will find information about housing modifications, housing rights, different housing options available to you, and how to weatherize your home.

- **Independent Living**

Resources to help individuals with disabilities reach independence and full community participation.

- **Perinatal, Early Childhood, and Special Health Needs**

Information and programs available to those with young children with special needs.

- **Service Animals**

Find information about hearing ear dogs and guide dogs that can assist those in need.

- **Special Education**

The Special Education Planning and Policy Development is part of the Department of Education. It focuses on interagency and special education policy and planning and personnel development. The site provides links to special education information, documents, and resources.

- **Taxes**

Here you will find a listing of tax credits and exemptions available to those with disabilities.

- **Vehicles & Transportation**

A good resource for reviewing parking laws, finding appropriate public paratransit, and enrolling in the travel transit program.

- **Vocational Rehabilitation**

Rehabilitation services are designed to help people with disabilities enter and stay in the work force.

Disabled Home Care Assistance Program:
http://www.mass.gov/?pageID=eohhs2subtopic&L=6&L0=Home&L1=Consumer&L2=Disability+Services&L3=In-home+and+Community+Living+Supports&L4=Home+Care&L5=Home+Care+Assistance+Program+(HCAP)+for+Those+Under+60&sid=Eeohhs2

Home Care Assistance Program (HCAP) for Those Under 60
links:

- **Factsheets About Homecare**
- **What We Do**
- **Who is Eligible**
- **How to Apply**
- **What Else You Should Know**
- **Frequently Asked Questions About HCAP**
- **Home Care Assistance Program Handbook**

The Family Caregiver's Survival Guide ©2112 Revised 2015

- **The Resource Newsletter**

Michigan

Health and Services: http://mi.gov/som/0,1607,7-192-29942_32836---,00.html

Department of Human Services: http://mi.gov/dhs/0,4562,7-124-5453_5526---,00.html

This section is slightly abbreviated to what appear to be the pertinent departments and/or areas...

At the time of this writing, Michigan seems to be working towards some sort of coordinated independent living consensus, as detailed at: http://www.misilc.org/

State Disability Assistance

State Disability Assistance (SDA) Overview
Cash assistance for disabled adults who do not have dependent children.

State Disability Assistance (SDA) Overview
The State Disability Assistance (SDA) program provides cash assistance to disabled adults to help them pay for living expenses such as rent, heat, utilities, clothing, food and personal care items. A person is considered **disabled** for SDA purposes if he/she:<>

- Receives certain other disability-related benefits (such as Medicaid based on disability or blindness).
- Resides in a special facility (such as a licensed Adult Foster Care Home).
- Is certified by DHS medical consultants as unable to work due to a mental or physical disability for at least 90 days.

SDA may also be provided to the caretaker of a disabled person or to a person age 65 or older. An SDA group can be either a single person or spouses who live together.

• SDA Eligibility Requirements
Your disability, income and assets must be evaluated for the SDA program.

SDA Eligibility Requirements
"Disabled" for SDA Purposes
A person is considered "disabled" for SDA purposes if he/she:
- receives certain other disability-related benefits (such as Medicaid based on disability or blindness, or SSI, etc.), or
- resides in a special facility (such as a licensed Adult Foster Care Home, or a Substance Abuse Treatment Center), or
- is certified by DHS medical consultants as unable to work due to a mental or physical disability for at least 90 days.

SDA Residency Requirements
A person must be a Michigan resident and intend to remain in Michigan and **not** be receiving cash assistance from another state.

Citizenship Requirements

A person must be a U.S. citizen or have an acceptable alien status to qualify for SDA.

Asset Limits

Assets are cash or any other personal or real property you own. The asset limit for SDA is $3,000. Only cash assets are counted, such as:

- Cash on hand
- Bank and credit union accounts
- Investments
- Retirement plans
- Trusts

Assets such as your home, vehicles and personal belongings are not counted.

Countable Income

Most types of earned and unearned income are counted. Countable income is considered when determining the amount of SDA you are eligible to receive. Some examples of countable income are:

- Wages
- Self-employment earnings
- Rental Income
- Social Security Benefits
- Veterans benefits

Potential Benefits

SDA clients must apply for any other benefits they may be able to receive, such as:

- Retirement, Survivors, and Disability Insurance (RSDI)
- Supplemental Security Income (SSI)
- Worker's Compensation Benefits
- Veteran's Administration Benefits
- Railroad Retirement Benefits
- Other types of benefits (e.g., Black Lung benefits, Railroad unemployment benefits, Pension payments, Disability or retirement benefits, Earned but unpaid wages, Strike pay, Vacation pay or Supplemental unemployment benefit)

SDA clients must also be willing to sign an agreement to repay SDA benefits, when required, if lump sums or retroactive payments are expected.

There are other eligibility requirements you must meet to receive SDA that are not outlined here.

Only an Eligibility Specialist at DHS can accurately determine your family's eligibility for SDA. Ask for details when turning in a completed application at your local DHS County Office**.**

- Disability Determination Services

The Social Security Disability program provides benefits to persons with severe disabilities whose impairments prevent them from performing gainful work.

Disability Determination Services

The Disability Evaluationunder the Social Security Administration is the process which may allow benefits to be provided to persons with severe disabilities whose impairments prevent them from performing gainful work. In each of the six states within the Chicago Region, claims for the federal disability program are administered through the state. These State Disability Determination Services are 100 percent federally funded and make their decisions according to federal rules and regulations. In Michigan, the Department of Human Services is the parent agency for the DDS agencies.

The DDS agencies are responsible for developing medical evidence and rendering the initial determination on whether the claimant is or is not disabled or blind. DDS also determines continuing disability/blindness when a medical review is required

DHS Eligibility Determination
DHS clients who receive State Disability Assistance and disability-related Medicaid (e.g., MA-P) must apply for Supplemental Security Income (SSI) through the Social Security Administration. Other DHS cash programs may also require a client claiming disability to apply for SSI as an alternative source of income based on their inability to participate with work requirements. If an SSI application is denied, the client must pursue his appeal rights in order to remain eligible for SDA.

Your DHS specialist will work with you to obtain obtain medical evidence from your current doctor first. If that evidence is unavailable or insufficient to make a determination, the DDS may request and authorize a consultative examination in order to obtain the additional information needed either from your doctor or from a recommended doctor.

After completing the initial development of information, the DDS makes the disability determination. The determination is made by a two-person team consisting of a medical or psychological consultant (physician or psychologist) and a disability examiner. If this team finds that additional evidence is still needed, your DHS specialist will contact you and ask for more medical information.

After the DDS makes the disability determination, the documentation is returned to the local DHS office for appropriate action depending on whether the claim is allowed or denied.

• Disability Determination Services Customer Satisfaction Survey
This survey will help the Michigan Disability Determination Services improve service and make the process easier for you.

• Disability Determination Services (DDS) Office Locations

Disability Determination Services (DDS) Office Locations
The Social Security Disability program provides benefits to persons with severe disabilities whose impairments prevent them from performing gainful work. In each of the six states within the Chicago Region (Illinois, Indiana, Michigan, Minnesota, Ohio and Wisconsin), claims for the federal disability program are administered through the state. These State Disability Determination Services (DDS) agencies are 100 percent federally funded and make their decisions according to federal rules and regulations.

Michigan office locations are found below:

Four DDS Office Locations in Michigan
Lural Baltimore, Area Administrator
Disability Determination Service
P.O. Box 30011
Lansing, MI 48909
1-800-366-3404

John DeSpelder, Area Administrator
Disability Determination Service
P.O. Box 1200
Traverse City, MI 49685
1-800-632-1097

Randy Griswold, Area Administrator
Disability Determination Service
P.O. Box 4020
Kalamazoo, MI 49003
1-800-829-7763

Otis Kern, Area Administrator
Disability Determination Service
P.O. Box 345
Detroit, MI 48231
1-800-383-7155

Michigan Disability Determination Service Executive Office
Charles A. Jones, Interim Director
Michigan Disability Determination Service
P.O. Box 30011
Lansing, MI 48909
1-800-366-3404

Supplemental Security Income

• Supplemental Security Income (SSI) Overview
Supplemental Security Income (SSI) provides financial assistance to people who are aged, blind or disabled. Funding is primarily federal and is administered through the Social Security Administration.

Energy Assistance Programs

Low Income Home Energy Assistance Program (LIHEAP)
Designed to help eligible low-income households meet the high cost of home heating.

Other Sources of Income

Resources
Other sources of income are available outside of DHS.

Minnesota

Department of Human Services:
http://www.dhs.state.mn.us/main/idcplg?IdcService=GET_DYNAMIC_CONVERSION&RevisionSelection
Method=LatestReleased&dDocName=Home_Page

MinnesotaHelp.info website features community resources: http://www.minnesotahelp.info/Public/

1) Aging: http://www.minnesotahelp.info/Public/default.aspx?se=senior

2) Disabilities: http://www.minnesotahelp.info/Public/default.aspx?se=dlink

Caregiver

- ⊟ Adult Day Services
  - o Adult Day Health Programs
  - o Adult Day Program Centers
  - o Adult Day Programs (All)
  - o Family Adult Day Program Homes
- ⊟ Education, Counseling and Training
  - o Caregiver Consultant
  - o Caregiver Counseling
- ⊟ Respite Care
  - o Adult In Home Respite Care
  - o Adult Out of Home Respite Care
  - o Respite Care (All Adult Respite Care)
  - o Respite Care Volunteers
- ⊟ Support Groups
  - o Caregiver Support Groups
  - o Health Related Support Groups
  - o Mutual Support Group Clearinghouses
  - o Relatives as Parents Support Groups (Kinship)

Assistive Technology

- ⊞ Adapted Recreation
  - o Adapted Exercise Equipment
  - o Adapted Toys
  - o Sports/Leisure Aids
- ⊞ Assessment & Training
  - o Evaluation for Assistive Technology
  - o Training on using Assistive Technology
- ⊞ Communication Aids
  - o Speech Aids
- ⊞ Computer Donations

- o Adapted Computer Equipment
- o Computer Donation Programs
- ⊞ Control & Signaling Aids
  - o Control and Signaling Aids
  - o Emergency Alert
- ⊞ Getting Equipment
  - o Equipment Loans
  - o Equipment Rental
  - o Help Paying for Equipment
  - o New Equipment Sales
  - o Used Equipment Sales
- ⊞ Hearing Devices
  - o Alerting Devices
  - o Closed Captioned Decoders
  - o Hearing Aids
  - o Listening Devices
  - o Specialized Telecommunications Equipment
- ⊞ Information
  - o AT information
- ⊞ Medical Equipment
  - o Medical Equipment/Supplies
  - o TENS Units (helps with pain)
- ⊞ Mobility Aids
  - o Automobile/Van Adaptations
  - o Blind Mobility Aids
  - o Electric Scooters
  - o Standing Aids
  - o Transfer Devices
  - o Walking Aids
  - o Wheelchairs
- ⊞ Modifying, Altering & Repairing
  - o Altering AT to Meet Your Needs
  - o AT Custom Design
  - o AT Repairs
- ⊞ Other Assistive Technology
  - o Adapted Clothing
  - o Assistive Devices for Daily Living Activities
  - o Cognitive/Learning Aids
- ⊞ Prosthetics, Orthotics, & Seating
  - o Orthopedic Devices
  - o Prosthetic Devices
  - o Seating/Positioning Aids
- ⊞ Vehicles
  - o Auto/Van Modifications
- ⊞ Visual and Reading Aids

Independent Living

- ⊟ Help to Stay in Your Own Home
    - o Home/Community Care Financing (waivers)
    - o Supportive Living Services for Adults
- ⊟ Independent Living Skills
    - o Daily Living Skill Instruction
    - o Evaluation of Daily Living Skills
    - o Independent Living Centers
    - o Travel Training
- ⊟ Maintaining Your Home, Self, & Family
    - o Errand Running & Shopping
    - o Falls Prevention
    - o Grocery Delivery
    - o Handy-person
    - o Home Safety Checks
    - o Housekeeping
    - o Major Household Repair
    - o Making Meals
    - o Painting your House
    - o Parenting with a Disability
    - o Yard Work
- ⊟ Moving from a Facility
    - o Long Term Care Consultation
- ⊟ Personal Care Assistants (PCAs) & Home Care Services
    - o Home Health Aid
    - o Home Nursing
    - o PCA Choice - self-directed
    - o Personal Care Assistant (PCA)
- ⊟ Preparing for the Future
    - o Life Care Planning
- ⊟ Social Support
    - o Disability Related Support Groups
    - o Peer Support

Mississippi

Aging and Adult Services: http://www.mdhs.state.ms.us/aas.html

Division on Aging and Adult Services: http://www.mdhs.state.ms.us/aas_mfcsp.htm

Family Caregiver Support Program

The Mississippi Family Caregiver Support Program is the first of its kind for the Division of Aging and Adult Services. The services are provided to the caregiver. Caregiver is defined as:

- any individual, regardless of age, providing care for a person 60 years or older, or
- a grandparent or other relative caregiver, 60 years or older, caring for a child 18 years or younger.

The Mississippi Family Caregiver works in partnership with the ten (10) Area Agencies on Aging and local community-service providers to provide five (5) basic services for family caregivers, including:

- Information to caregivers about available services
- Assistance to caregivers in gaining access to services
- Individual counseling, organization of support groups, caregiver training to assist the caregivers in making decisions and solving problems relating to their caregiving roles
- Respite care to enable caregivers to be temporarily relieved from caregiving responsibilities
- Supplemental services, on a limited basis, to complement the care provided by caregivers

Other Resources

Administration on Aging

Find a Free or Discounted Drug Program

Contact Information

Mississippi Department of Human Services
Division of Aging & Adult Services
(601) 359-4929

Area Agency on Aging	Director	Contact Information	Counties Served
Central MS Area Agency on Aging P.O. Box 4935 Jackson, MS 39296	Bettye Burgess	(601) 981-1511 1-800-315-3103	Copiah, Hinds, Madison, Rankin, Simpson, Warren, Yazoo
East Central Area Agency	Rosie Coleman	(601) 683-2401	Clarke, Jasper, Kemper,

Area Agency on Aging	Director	Contact Information	Counties Served
on Aging P.O. Box 499 Newton, MS 39345		1-800-264-2007	Lauderdale, Leake, Neshoba, Newton, Scott, Smith
Golden Triangle Area Agency on Aging P.O. Box 828 Starkville, MS 39760-0828	Bobby Gann	(662) 324-4650 (662) 332-2636 (toll free within a 55-mile radius) 1-888-324-9000	Choctaw, Clay, Lowndes, Noxubee, Oktibbeha, Webster, Winston
North Central Area Agency on Aging 711-B South Applegate Winona, MS 38967	Darlena Allen	(662) 283-2675 (662) 283-2771 (toll free within a 55-mile radius) 1-888-427-0714	Attala, Carroll, Grenada, Holmes, Leflore, Montgomery, Yalobusha
North Delta Area Agency on Aging P.O. Box 1488 Batesville, MS 38601-1488	Ann Marie Ross	(662) 561-4100 1-800-844-2433	Coahoma, Desoto, Panola, Quitman, Tallahatchie, Tate, Tunica
Northeast MS Area Agency on Aging P.O. Box 600 Bonneville, MS 38829	Linda Presley	(662) 728-7038 1-800-745-6961	Alcorn, Benton, Marshall, Prentiss, Tippah, Tishomingo
South Delta Area Agency on Aging P.O. Box 1776 Greenville, MS 38702-1776	Sylvia Jackson	(662) 378-3831 1-800-898-3055	Bolivar, Humphreys, Issaquena, Sharkey, Sunflower, Washington
Southern MS Area Agency on Aging 9229 Highway 49 Gulfport, MS 39503	Robert Moore	(228) 868-2326 1-800-444-8014 (nationwide) www.smpdd.com	Covington, Forrest, George, Greene, Hancock, Harrison, Jackson, Jefferson Davis, Jones, Lamar, Marion, Pearl River, Perry, Stone, Wayne
Southwest MS Area Agency on Aging 100 South Wall Street Natchez, MS 39120	Yolanda Campbell	(601) 446-6044 1-800-338-2049	Adams, Amite, Claiborne, Franklin, Jefferson, Lawrence, Lincoln, Pike, Walthall, Wilkinson
Three Rivers Area Agency on Aging P.O. Box 690 Pontotoc, MS 38663	Joseph Cleveland	(662) 489-2415 (662) 489-6911 (toll free within a 55-mile radius) 1-877-489-6911 (statewide) www.trpdd.com	Calhoun, Chickasaw, Itawamba, Lafayette, Lee, Monroe, Pontotoc, Union

Division of Aging and Adult Services: http://www.mdhs.state.ms.us/aas_info.html

Services Overview

With the population of Mississippi living longer and longer each year, specialized services for persons over 60 become increasingly important. The Mississippi Department of Human Services, Division of Aging and Adult Services is dedicated to keeping pace with the needs of the state's older citizens and to improving their quality of life.One of every six adults in Mississippi is over 60. In this population segment, about 79 percent own the homes in which they live. Their independence does not separate them far from their families, for more than two-thirds of this older generation live within 25 miles of relatives. As their numbers continue to grow, so does the need for providing specialized services for older adults.

How Services are Provided - for the most part, the Mississippi Department of Human Services, Division of Aging and Adult Services coordinates the delivery of services available to adults 60 years of age and older. Our programs work to assure quality of life and continued independence for the state's older citizens.

Transportation - continued independence of older adults in the state is facilitated by transportation services offered in their communities. Nearly 300 vehicles (from vans to mini-buses) take older adults where they want to go, whether to dental and medical appointments, shopping areas, senior centers, recreational areas, food stamp offices, social security offices or educational facilities. Transportation is provided by local civic or community groups and Area Agencies on Aging in coordination with programs funded by the Mississippi Department of Transportation.

Information, Assistance, Outreach and Local Focal Points - knowing where to turn for help is the first step toward getting it. That first step is made easier through information, assistance, outreach and local focal points designated by the Division of Aging and Adult Services or Area Agencies on Aging. These points for information and assistance usually are the Area Agencies on Aging, senior centers, adult day care centers, or community action agencies. They link older adults to needed services and follow up as necessary to ensure that needs are met. Visit www.AoA.gov.

- **Nutrition -** The Older Adult Nutrition Program (OANP) is more than a meal - a well-balanced meal which provides a minimum of one-third (1/3) of the nutrient-based Recommended Dietary Allowances (RDAs) for older adults and follows the food-based *Dietary Guidelines for Older Americans*. The OANP is, also, fellowship for the 29% of seniors who participate in the congregate program at senior center sites and help and hope for the 71% of frail elderly whose meals are delivered to their homes.
- **Legal Assistance -** For those times when older adults need legal advice, consultation or representation, legal assistance may be obtained from lawyers or paralegals who have agreed to provide services to the state's elderly. Many of the services are available without charge from *legal services programs*. In other cases, private attorneys have agreed to accept reduced fees for referred elderly clients. **Older persons with a legal problem should contact their Area Agency on Aging for more information about contacting a legal services office.**
- **Mississippi Medicare Assistance Patrol Project (MsMAPP) -** is a federally-funded project to provide information and outreach, educating seniors. SMP's goal is to increase public awareness of the potential for health care error and abuse in the Medicare system; to prevent healthcare fraud; to prevent improper payments in Medicare programs; to preserve public health programs

(Medicare/Medicaid) *for future generations*; and to recruit and train retired professionals and interested adults as dedicated volunteers who will educate Medicare beneficiaries, and their families, recognize and report discrepancies in their health care delivery that may be caused by simple error or by fraud, waste or abuse; and the importance of recognizing and reporting healthcare error, fraud and abuse *(Protect, Detect, Report).* SMP is volunteer-driven. Because expediency often requires face-to-face contact, SMPs nationwide recruit and train some 5,000 volunteers every year to help in the effort.

- **Senior Community Service Employment Program (SCSEP) -** Adults 55 and above are working throughout the state through assistance from the Senior Community Service Employment Program. The program identifies employment opportunities for older persons whose incomes place them at or below the federal poverty level; who are unemployed or underemployed; or who have difficulty finding a job.Adults in the program generally work an average of 20 hours a week, receiving at least minimum wage.

Services For The Frail Elderly

Case Management - The frail elderly need special assistance to remain independent as long as possible. They receive it through case management - the planning, arrangement and coordination of appropriate community- based services. A network of public services is established, along with an informal support system of family members, friends, neighbors, churches, civic clubs and concerned citizens. Case managers identify the needs of frail elderly adults through a comprehensive assessment completed in the homes of clients. The assessment is followed by the development of a care plan, with the input of family members. The case manager arranges for appropriate services and does ongoing monitoring and adjustment to ensure proper care.

In-Home Services - Many older adults get the help they need to stay in their homes through the In-Home Services Program. The Homemaker program gives older citizens the option of having homemakers perform the housekeeping tasks they can no longer do or need assistance in doing. Homemakers perform routine household tasks such as cooking, cleaning, mending, grocery shopping, laundry, consumer education, bathing, dressing, safety education and oral hygiene assistance. The amount of time spent in homes depends on the needs of the older adult and the availability of the homemaker service. This service is provided at no cost to the older person, although contributions are solicited to help expand the availability of the service. Home-delivered meals provide basic nutrition for the frail homebound elderly. In some areas home health and respite care are also provided in the home.

Adult Day Care - Adult day care centers specialize in supervised care for functionally impaired elderly adults. Their programs focus on health maintenance, prevention/intervention and rehabilitation needs of older adults capable of only limited self-care. The centers care for adults four or more hours a day while their family members work or enjoy a respite from their role as caretaker. Center services are individualized, based on a systematic evaluation of each person's needs and strengths. Care is guided by an individual plan which outlines long and short term goals. The plan is reviewed periodically with family members for refinement and adjustment.

Ombudsman Program - The Ombudsman Program provides... *A Voice for Residents*. The ombudsman serves as a resident advocate and supports residents' highest possible quality of life and care and is responsible for investigating, and attempting to resolve concerns and complaints and by, or on behalf of, residents of long-term care facilities. Additional ombudsman services include answering questions and providing information and referral about long-term care residents; coordinating efforts with other agencies and organizations concerned with long-term care, while respecting the privacy and confidentiality of residents.Ten (10) local ombudsman programs are located throughout the state in the 10 Planning and Development Districts. Within each local ombudsman program, a full-time certified ombudsman is responsible for program components. Volunteers are also an integral part of the ombudsman program.

General Information

Homestead Exemption - Persons in the state who are 65 or older do not have to pay taxes on their homes and land if the **assessed value** is $7,500 or less. An older person with property **valued on the market** at $75,000 or less does not have to pay taxes. For the older person with homes and land **market valued** at more than $75,000, taxes are required only on the amount above $75,000. To get this tax advantage, residents over 65 must file for homestead exemption with their county tax assessor's office.

Recreation - The state's mild climate, with an average temperature of 63 degrees and yearly rainfall of about 50 inches, facilitates outdoor recreation year round. Mississippi has 17 state parks offering boating, camping, fishing, nature trails and refreshment facilities. Historic sites, arts and crafts shows and festivals featuring everything from Blues to strawberries offer additional opportunities for Mississippians to relax and have fun. Fresh and salt water fishing provides another recreation or outlet, as does hunting small game, deer and wild turkey. Persons 65 and above may obtain a free hunting and fishing license from their circuit clerk's office. Recreation in the state also includes various sporting events of the Southeastern Conference, the Southwestern Athletic Conference and professional baseball and hockey.Older adults also have special opportunities to participate in events such as Senior Olympics, a statewide athletic event designed for this age group.

Volunteer Program - The person delivering meals to homebound elderly adults, assisting at community focal points, providing insurance counseling and assistance, or serving as an ombudsman to residents of long-term care facilities could very well be a volunteer. In fact, many older adults are volunteering to perform services such as these and many, many more. They are doing so through the Division of Aging and Adult Services Volunteer Program, finding satisfaction in donating time to others. Contact your Area Agency on Aging for more information about how you can volunteer.

Contact Information

Mississippi Department of Human Services
Division of Aging & Adult Services
(601) 359-4929

Missouri

Senior Health and Safety: http://www.mo.gov/living-in-missouri/senior-health-safety/

Accessibility

Disabled parking permits

Assistance Programs

Benefitscheckup.org

Medicare basics

Medicare supplements

Elderly Care

Different types of nursing homes

How to select a nursing home

How nursing homes are inspected

Long-term Care Facility inspection results

Home health agencies

Find an Adult Day Care

Find a retirement home

Health Facilities and Services

Choosing a hospital

Dialysis facilities

Find a Missouri Aging Agency

Hospice

Prescriptions

AARP Rx Snapshot

Medicare Part D

MoRx pharmacy assistance program

Programs and services

Elderly advocacy and assistance

Insurance for seniors

Medicare supplement insurance

Missouri aging information network

Safety

AARP driving safety course

Elder abuse

Missourians Stopping Adult Financial Exploitation

Protecting Missouri's Seniors, Attorney General

Medicaid Fraud

Senior Lifestyle

Best counties for seniors

Missouri State Senior Games/Olympics

Nutrition

Volunteering

Pain and symptom management

Senior citizen discounts

Health and Senior Services: http://health.mo.gov/seniors/index.php

Help for Independent Living: http://health.mo.gov/seniors/independentliving.php

Getting Help at Home

As we age, many activities of daily living can become more difficult. But many people prefer to stay in their homes rather than move to a residential setting with a full-time staff to help them. Older people may choose to live independently in their homes with the help of **support services**.

For low-income older people, **Medicaid** pays for some of the services. Individuals **must pay** for others.

Information for Providers of Home-Based Services

The Department of Health and Senior Services **oversees individuals and companies** that provide home-based services to older adults and people with disabilities.

Jobs for Seniors

Training and job placement services are available to low-income Missourians age 55 or older.

Nutrition

Older adults can receive **nutritious meals at senior centers** or buy the food they need with **food stamps**.

They can also improve their diets with **U.S. Department of Agriculture commodity foods**.

Housing, Assisted Living, Adult Day Care

Missouri's housing guide describes housing options, affordable housing programs and services to help people stay in their homes.

Other programs like **adult day care**, **adult day health care**, and **assisted living**, also help individuals remain in their homes or in homelike settings as long as possible.

Transportation

OATS helps people all over Missouri get to work, doctor appointments, or do essential shopping. Reduced bus fares also help seniors get around in **Columbia**, **Kansas City**, **Springfield** and **St. Louis**.

Keeping Active

Exercise helps people stay fit and active and **prevent falls.strength training** and **Tai Chi** are especially good for older adults.

Related Links

- **Adult Day Health Care**
- **Adult Protective Services**
- **Advocacy for Persons with Disabilities**

  - **Missouri Protection and Advocacy Services**
  - **Paraquad**
  - **The Whole Person**
    Aging and Disability Resource Center
    Alzheimer's Safe Return Program
    Caregiver Support (Shared Care)
    Centers for Independent Living
    Home-Delivered Meals
    Medicaid Services
    Prescription Drug Plans
  - **Missouri Rx Plan**
  - **Medicare Part D**
    Preventing Falls
    Social Security Administration
    U.S. Dept. of Health and Human Services

Home and Community Based Services: http://health.mo.gov/seniors/hcbs/

Home and community based care providers play an integral role in allowing the Department of Health and Senior Services (DHSS) to provide home-based services to eligible individuals who wish to remain in a community setting.

All potential contractors must submit a proposal outlining their business practices and demonstrating an ability to serve the needs of the frail populations served by DHSS. Home and community based care providers must also make assurances regarding compliance with applicable federals and state laws, regulations, and orders relative to the provision of services.

The information provided on this site is intended as a resource for current home and community based care providers and potential contractors. You may click on any of the links listed to obtain additional information.

Home Health: http://www.missouriclaim.org/?q=medicare/compare-hh

If you are recovering from an illness, wound, surgery, stroke, or other disabling event, your doctor may prescribe home healthcare.

Home healthcare provides skilled nursing care, physical and occupational therapy, speech-language therapy, and medical social services in the comfort of home.

Home healthcare is prescribed by your doctor and is provided by a variety of healthcare professionals. Medicare covers home healthcare that is temporary and part-time.

Home health professionals may teach you, or your caregivers, how to care for wounds and manage medication. The goal is to help you reach and keep your best physical, mental and social well-being.

To help you make an informed decision, Medicare provides quality of care information for all Medicare-certified home health agencies. You can compare how well agencies in your area help patients get better in:

- taking oral medicines
- correctly dressing themselves
- level of confusion
- getting to and from the toilet
- pain when moving around
- mobility
- admission rate to the hospital
- getting in and out of bed

- the need for urgent, unplanned care

For more information call toll-free (800) MEDICARE (800-633-4227) or click here to get information about the quality of care in home health agencies in your area. You can use that site to find and compare home health agencies in your area.

Caregiving: Agencies on Aging Can Help: https://www.mosers.org/en/Retirees/Newsletters/Fall-2009/Agencies-on-Aging-Can-Help.aspx

In later years, when cooking meals, cleaning the house, driving to doctors' appointments, caring for a loved one, or being lonely becomes too much, it is nice to find someone who understands. Whether you are an older adult or someone concerned about the well-being of an older person, the staff at Missouri's ten Area Agencies on Aging understand what you are experiencing and can help you find answers.

Information

The Missouri Aging Information Network provides helpful tools, data and tips on hiring in-home caregivers, comparing nursing homes and home health agencies, and finding any of a wide variety of services in your county.

Care Coordination

Retirees often say that making all the arrangements for an aging parent or loved one becomes their new full-time job in retirement. If you are facing a complex situation that requires more than a phone call or web search, your Agency on Aging may be able to lend a hand by providing care coordination. A care coordinator will arrange an in-person visit and draw up a plan of action which specifies what services are needed, how to obtain them, and if financial assistance is available to pay for services. A typical service plan may include any of the following:

- Home-delivered meals
- Respite care and support for family caregivers
- Personal care
- Transportation
- Legal services
- Homemaker assistance
- Applying for public benefits
- Making referrals to other agencies

These services may also be available on an as-needed basis by contacting the Agency on Aging or the local senior center directly and may not require enrollment with a care coordinator.

Senior Centers with Noon Meals

Gathering together for a good meal at a local senior center provides the physical and social nourishment that many seniors crave. The noon meal program at most senior centers includes a lunch buffet with soup, a hot entrée, side items, dessert and drink for a suggested donation of $3.00 per person for people age 60 and older. Typical serving time is from 11:00 a.m. to 12:30 p.m. In addition to the meal, senior centers also provide:

- A variety of recreational and social activities
- Health education and screening programs
- Exercise classes
- Information and assistance services
- Volunteer opportunities for people of all ages

Find the senior center in your area by calling the Missouri Alliance of Area Agencies on Aging at 800-497-0822 or going online at *http://moaging.com.*

Home-delivered meals

Some senior centers deliver a week's worth of frozen meals and other food products like bread, desserts and fresh fruit. Others deliver hot meals daily. In some locations, a friend or family member may pick up a hot meal to take to someone who is homebound. You can make arrangements for home-delivered meals by contacting your local senior center directly or through the referral of a care coordinator.

Long-Term Care Ombudsman Program

An ombudsman is a specially trained volunteer who visits long-term care facilities such as nursing homes each week to talk with residents, and listen to their concerns, complaints or requests for help. The ombudsman will work with all the parties to try to reach a solution that is fair to everyone involved. The services of the ombudsman are free and confidential.

For more information or to request a visit from an ombudsman, write to the State Office of Long-term Care Ombudsman, P.O. Box 570, Jefferson City, MO 65102, or call 800-309-3282.

Support for Family Caregivers

If you are a caregiver for a parent, spouse or older person in your community, you know it is a big job that requires a tremendous amount of emotional, physical and mental energy and commitment. No matter how dedicated the caregiver is, sometimes he or she may need a break or a little extra support. The Agencies on Aging can help by providing caregivers with:

- Information and guidance
- Training in the proper way to provide care or administer medications
- Emotional support
- Periodic relief from care giving responsibilities

Area Agencies on Aging in Missouri

Southwest Office on Aging
Springfield • 800-497-0822
www.swmoa.com

Southeast Missouri Area Agency on Aging
Cape Girardeau • 800-392-8771
www.semoaaa.org

The Care Connection
Warrensburg • 800-886-4699
www.goaging.org

Northwest Missouri Area Agency on Aging
Albany • 888-844-5626
www.nwmoaaa.org

Northeast Missouri Area Agency on Aging
Kirksville • 800-664-6338
www.nemoaaa.com

Central Missouri Area Agency on Aging
Columbia • 800-369-5211
www.cmaaa.net

Mid-America Regional Council
Kansas City • 800-593-7948
www.marc.org

Mid-East Missouri Area Agency on Aging
Manchester • 800-243-6060
www.mid-eastaaa.org

St. Louis Area Agency on Aging
St. Louis • 314-612-5918
www.slaaa.org

Region X

Area Agency on Aging
Joplin • 417-781-7562
email: *aaax@aaaregionx.org*
www.aaaregionx.org

Montana

Department of Public Health and Human Services, Senior and Long Term Care:
http://www.dphhs.mt.gov/sltc/index.shtml

Senior & Long Term Care Division

Senior and Long Term Care

Mission
To advocate and promote dignity and independence for older Montanans and Montanans with disabilities by:

- Providing information, education, and assistance;
- Planning, developing and providing for quality long-term care services; and
- Operating within a cost–effective service delivery system.

Services
The division administers aging services, adult protective services, and the state's two veterans' homes. It also helps to fund care for elderly and disabled Montanans who are eligible for Medicaid and Supplemental Security Income (SSI).

The Office on Aging develops a State Plan on Aging and approves service delivery plans and programs developed by 10 Area Agencies on Aging located across Montana. Among the services provided by the area agencies are senior centers, Meals on Wheels, health services, transportation, home chore services, and information referral and assistance services. The Office on Aging houses the Long-Term Care Ombudsman, Elderly Legal Assistance, State Health Insurance and Assistance Program (SHIP).

The Long-Term Care Ombudsman is an advocate for all residents of long-term care facilities, especially nursing homes and personal care homes. The ombudsman can provide information or direct assistance related to the health, safety, and rights of residents.

The Legal Services Developer Program provides training for seniors, family members, and others on elder-specific laws. The program develops pro-bono and local legal service referrals, training materials, and telephone assistance to seniors.

The State Health Insurance Program (SHIP) provides Medicare and related health insurance information, counseling, assistance and advocacy to Montana Medicare beneficiaries, their family members, caregivers, and local professionals. statewide source of program information for beneficiaries of Medicare, Medicaid, Medicare supplemental policies, long-term care insurance, and other health insurance benefits.

The Information, Assistance and Referral Program is a service designed to link Montana seniors, their family members, and caregivers with needed services. Eighty-two technicians work through the local Area Agencies on Aging to provide information about service, make proper referrals, and do public education and outreach within their communities.

The Adult Protective Services Program employs 36 social workers across the state whose duties include investigating allegations of abuse, neglect, and exploitation for the elderly and people with disabilities. They also arrange for and coordinate a variety of support services aimed at protecting vulnerable people from abuse and neglect.

The Medicaid Community Services Program pays for personal care, skilled nursing care, home health aides, home dialysis attendants, and hospice care for elderly and disabled people eligible for Medicaid.

The Home and Community Based Services Program contracts with case managers in local communities to arrange for an array of in-home services to enable people in need of care to avoid a stay in a hospital or long-term care facility.

The Medicaid Nursing Facility Services Program pays for short-term and long-term nursing care for individuals eligible for Medicaid. Sixty percent of nursing care beds in Montana are funded through Medicaid.

The State Supplemental Payments Program supplements the Social Security Supplemental Security Income (SSI) of eligible individuals who live in designated residential care facilities. These facilities include community homes for individual with developmental or mental disabilities, group homes for individuals with severe disabilities, personal care homes, licensed foster homed, and transitional living homes.

Home and Community Based Services:
http://www.dphhs.mt.gov/sltc/services/communityservices/index.shtml

Home and Community

Based Services

Many individuals in need of long term care services choose to remain in their own homes or select other community options to meet their needs. The Community Services Bureau administers a number of

Medicaid-funded options that enable people who are aged or disabled and who have limited income and resources to remain in their homes, rather than receive services in a hospital or nursing facility. Those programs include the Home and Community-Based Services (HCBS) Waiver program, Personal Assistance Services, Home Health and Hospice.

A quick PDF overview of Community Services programs.

Community Alternatives - A wide range of community-based long term care services have been developed over recent years. They are designed to keep people as independent as possible in the community for as long as possible

The HCBS Waiver Program offers a variety of service and support choices to a limited number of individuals who are eligible for the program. To be eligible for the HCBS Waiver program, an individual must be elderly or disabled, Medicaid eligible, and require nursing facility or hospital level of care. The majority of the recipients served under this program require nursing facility level of care. A small percentage of individuals served at home are ventilator dependent and, without the HCBS Waiver program, would be in a hospital setting. In addition, the program serves a small number of individuals with a traumatic brain injury who would have been served in out-of-state rehab facilities, inpatient rehabilitation, or remained inappropriately placed in nursing homes, group homes, or other institutions were it not for the specialized services available under the HCBS Waiver program.

Personal Assistance Service, formerly known as Personal Care Service, is an entitled service which helps eligible people remain in their homes who need help with activities such as bathing, grooming, dressing and meal preparation. The goal of the Personal Assistance Services program is to prevent or delay nursing facility placement by providing medically necessary, long-term maintenance or supportive care in the home.

Home Health Services are part-time nursing and restorative therapy services provided in the home to eligible people who require these services. The goal of the Home Health Services Program is to avoid unnecessary hospital or nursing facility stays by providing skilled nursing or therapy services in the home.

Hospice provides a group of services to people who are terminally ill. Hospice services are mostly palliative in nature, striving to keep the person as comfortable as possible and helping their family cope with the death of a loved one. The goal of the Hospice Program is to provide health and support services to people who are terminally ill and their families.

Community Services Bureau staff people are located throughout the State, and help administer these programs. This includes monitoring services, training staff, helping people access services and implementing policy. Please click on the side menu to learn more about these Medicaid-funded programs and where staff are located.

Nebraska

Department of Health and Human Services: http://www.hhs.state.ne.us/HCS/Programs/DPFS.htm

Home and Community Services

Disabled Persons and Family Support Program

What is Disabled Persons and Family Support (DPFS)?

DPFS provides up to $300 a month of funding for services to individuals with disabilities to help them continue to live independently or help families stay together.

Who may need this program?

Those who need to maintain their independence, such as:

- Employed adults with disabilities
- Adults with disabilities who live independently
- Families who have a family member with disabilities living with them at home

What services may be available through DPFS?

The needs of the clients determine which services can be funded through DPFS. Some of the funded services include:

- Attendant/personal care
- Home health care
- Housekeeping
- Transportation
- Special equipment
- Home modifications

Who may be eligible for DPFS?

Persons may be financially eligible if their gross monthly income does not exceed the guidelines in the box below. A certain amount of your income will be disregarded or not counted in determining income. This is considered a disability-related deduction.

Family Size	Gross Monthly Income $
1	1364
2	1784
3	2203
4	2623
5	3043
6	3463

7	3541
8	3620
9 or more	3699

The maximum monthly benefit for attendant/personal care, home health care, housekeeping, or transportation is $300. For special equipment or home modification, the maximum yearly benefit is $3600.

DPFS cannot pay for services or items available from other sources. Persons who apply must explore all other possible funding sources.

How do I apply for DPFS?

To request an application for yourself or on behalf of another adult, contact:

Nebraska Department of Health and Human Services
Medicaid and Long-Term Care
Disabled Persons and Family Support
PO Box 95025
Lincoln, Nebraska 68509-5025
(402) 471-9310
Outside Lincoln call toll free 1-800-358-8802

OR: Download an application.

More questions and answers about DPFS

Information on becoming a provider of services

Contact someone who can answer your questions about DPFS:
800-358-8802

For children, contact a MHCP worker nearest you:

Grand Island	(800) 892-7922
Gering	(800) 477-6393
Lincoln	(877) 213-4754
Norfolk	(800) 704-0180
North Platte	(800) 778-1611
Omaha	(402) 595-2120

Staff of the Department of Health and Human Services will evaluate each application and approve or disapprove payments based upon need and available funds. You may be contacted if more information is needed to make a decision.

DPFS cannot pay for services available from other sources. Persons who apply must explore all other available funding sources.

FAQs

How does DPFS verify medical need?

DPFS uses the Disability Report which accompanies your application to verify medical need. This report should be completed by your doctor.

What rate can I pay my bath aide / housekeeper?

A monthly limit is established for each service, but you and your provider negotiate the rate of pay.

How are payments made?

There are two methods of payment. DPFS can pay providers directly or reimburse you. Payments are made monthly.

Can I keep the care provider I already have?

DPFS allows you to choose your own providers.

My mother (or adult child) lives with us. Do you count our income and resources?

Only the income and resources of the applicant and his/her spouse, if married, are considered.

Can DPFS pay my rent?

DPFS does not pay rent, utilities, or medical bills.

Where can I read the DHHS regulations about the DPFS Program?

Title 472   Disabled Persons and Family Support Program

Home and Community Services: http://www.hhs.state.ne.us/hcs/services/

Services help people who are aged or have disabilities to meet their needs. Services help Nebraskans achieve their goals in how to live and where to live.

First, a person must qualify for a program that offers a particular service. Each program has its requirements. Persons who qualify for a program are also called "clients." Not all services are available through all programs.

A client partners with a Services Coordinator or a Social Services worker to get the services s/he needs. They will assess the client's needs and determine if the client is eligible for a service/program.

Services we offer:

- Adult Day Services
- Adult Family Home
- Adult Protective Services (APS)
- Assisted Living Services, Medicaid Waiver
- Assistive Technology/Home Modification
- Child Care for Children/Youth with Disabilities
- Children's Specialized Health Care
- Chore Services (cleaning, shopping, preparing meals, etc.)
- Early Development Network Services
- Home Delivered Meals
- Home Health
- Hospice
- Identifying your child's medical condition
- Independence Skills Building
- Nutrition
- Personal Assistance Services
- Personal Emergency Response System
- Respite Care
- Services for Adults with Cystic Fibrosis, Hemophilia, and Sickle Cell Disease
- Transportation

Home and Community Service Programs: http://www.hhs.state.ne.us/hcs/programs/

What's a program?

A program is a group of services intended to meet a client's or family's need. The program helps people who are aged or have disabilities to meet their needs and achieve their goals in how to live and where to live.

First, a person must qualify for the program. Each program has its own requirements. Persons who are eligible for a program are called clients. Once eligible, clients will partner with a Services Coordinator or a Social Services Worker to get the services they need, and help achieve their goals.

Programs offered by Home and Community Services:

- Assistance to the Aged, Blind, or Disabled (AABD)
- Aged & Disabled Medicaid Waiver (AD Waiver)
- Autism Waiver
- Disabled Children's Program (DCP)
- Disabled Persons and Family Support Program
- Katie Beckett
- Lifespan Respite Subsidy Program
- Medically Handicapped Children's Program
- Social Services for Aged and Disabled (SSAD)
- Traumatic Brain Injury Waiver (TBI Waiver)

Home and Community Services
Assistance for Adults Over Age 65

Subscribe to this page

Home and community-based services enable persons who are aged to live in their own home or apartment.

First, a person must qualify for a program that offers services. After qualifying for a program, the "client" partners with a Services Coordinator. Together, they will assess the client's needs and determine if the client needs a particular service.

Services

I need help with housekeeping, laundry, meals, paying bills, essential errands and shopping, personal care, and minor home repairs or I may need supervision. Services

I need help bathing, dressing, walking, toileting, eating, shopping, and other activities so that I can live as independently as possible. Chore or Personal Assistance Services

My primary caregiver occasionally needs a short break from caring for me full-time, so that s/he can refresh, recharge, and continue as a good caregiver. Respite Services

I need transportation to medical appointments or to make essential trips to community services, grocery shopping, etc. Transportation Services

I'm unable to prepare my own meals, and there's no one else who can prepare my meals. Home Delivered Meals

I need changes made to my home, such as remodeling the bathroom or a ramp to get in and out of the house, that will help me live as independently as possible. I need assistive devices so that I can be as independent as possible in doing my daily activities. Home Modifications/Assistive Technology

I need to learn how I can become more independent in my daily activities and how to manage my physical disabilities. My caregiver may also need this training. Independence Skills Building

I know I need to improve what I eat and how I eat. I need information about the importance of food/nutrition as it relates to my disability. I need an expert to help me chose nutritious foods and develop healthy eating habits. Nutrition Services

I may need emergency help at any time while in my home. No one may be around to help me. I'm worried that I may not be able to use the phone to call for help. Personal Emergency Response System

I want to live in a home-like setting. However, I need to live in a facility where people assist with my personal care, day to day activities, and health maintenance. Assisted Living Service

I don't need 24-hour institutional care. However, because of my physical or mental impairment, I need a program of structured and monitored social, physical, and intellectual services or activities, in a group setting, for at least three hours a day. Adult Day Services

I can't live by myself and need some supervision, and I would prefer to live in a family setting. Adult Family Home

I have a terminal disease and need end-of-life care. Hospice

I am in need of skilled nursing or aide services so I can be healthy and safe at my home. Home Health

What programs may offer services that an adult with disabilities could need?

- Aged & Disabled Medicaid Waiver (AD Waiver)
- Social Services for Aged and Disabled (SSAD)
- Adult Protective Services (APS)
- Lifespan Respite Subsidy Program

I know someone who wants to become my service provider. How do they apply?

They would need to contact a "resource developer" in their area to apply.

Home and Community Services
Information for Providers

Are you interested in becoming a DHHS-approved services provider? It's a great community service you'll be performing for Nebraskans who are aged or experience disabilities. You'll be helping individuals to live independently in a home or community setting. You'll be helping spouses continue to care for their loved ones. You'll enable families to keep their children with disabilities in the home environment rather than an institution.

DHHS-approved service providers create choices for Nebraskans with disabilities in how to live and where to live. While no one gets rich as a DHHS-approved service provider, it pays a modest rate. Service providers are not State of Nebraska or DHHS employees. Rather, they work for the individual, and are paid by DHHS on behalf of the individual.

The service 'Area Agencies on Aging' is offered at the following sites:

- Aging Office of Western Nebraska (AOWN) - Central Office http://www.aown.org (external link)

- AREA AGENCY ON AGING

  CASE MANAGEMENT to assist elderly clients to remain in their own homes

ASSESSMENTS for those considering a nursing home to determine if home assistance or another alternative might be appropriate

COORDINATION OF CONGREGATE MEALS and home delivered meals in individual communities

TELEPHONE ASSURANCE Monday-Friday to verify the well being and safety of home bound individuals

HEALTH AND WELLNESS EDUCATION

LIFELINE EMERGENCY RESPONSE SYSTEM, an in-home service targeted at helping clients remain safe in their homes

INFORMATION AND REFERRAL

IN-HOME CAREGIVERS LIST who have had criminal background checks, to hire for private duty, and offers referral to respite providers for families and/or individuals in need

MEDICARE INSURANCE COUNSELING

IN-HOME CHORE AND HOUSEKEEPING

LOANING OF DURABLE MEDICAL EQUIPMENT

CAREGIVER support group

CONTRACTED HANDYMAN services offer homemaker/housekeeper duties, lawn mowing, and snow removal for individuals 60 years of age or older; suggested contributions are based on total cost of services, then applied to a sliding fee scale
Contacts:
Box Butte County (see listing for Alliance Senior Center)
Cheyenne County, contact Mike Hashman 308-254-4053
City of Kimball, contact Sheri Roberds, (308) 235-2688
Morrill County, contact Nancy Eichhaler, (308) 262-1846
Scotts Bluff County, contact Carol Prince, (308) 436-6687

o   Aging Office of Western Nebraska (AOWN) - Chadron http://www.aown.org (external link)
AREA AGENCY ON AGING

CASE MANAGEMENT to assist elderly clients to remain in their own homes

ASSESSMENTS for those considering a nursing home to determine if home assistance or another alternative might be appropriate

COORDINATION OF CONGREGATE MEALS and home delivered meals in individual communities

TELEPHONE ASSURANCE Monday-Friday to verify the well being and safety of home bound individuals

HEALTH AND WELLNESS EDUCATION

LIFELINE EMERGENCY RESPONSE SYSTEM, an in-home service targeted at helping clients remain safe in their homes

INFORMATION AND REFERRAL

IN-HOME CAREGIVERS LIST who have had criminal background checks, to hire for private duty, and offers referral to respite providers for families and/or individuals in need

MEDICARE INSURANCE COUNSELING

IN-HOME CHORE AND HOUSEKEEPING

LOANING OF DURABLE MEDICAL EQUIPMENT

CAREGIVER ASSISTANCE
o   Aging Office of Western Nebraska (AOWN) - Sidney http://www.aown.org (external link)
AREA AGENCY ON AGING

CASE MANAGEMENT to assist elderly clients to remain in their own homes

ASSESSMENTS for those considering a nursing home to determine if home assistance or another alternative might be appropriate

COORDINATION OF CONGREGATE MEALS and home delivered meals in individual communities

TELEPHONE ASSURANCE Monday-Friday to verify the well being and safety of home bound individuals

HEALTH AND WELLNESS EDUCATION

LIFELINE EMERGENCY RESPONSE SYSTEM, an in-home service targeted at helping clients remain safe in their homes

INFORMATION AND REFERRAL

IN-HOME CAREGIVERS LIST who have had criminal background checks, to hire for private duty, and offers referral to respite providers for families and/or individuals in need

MEDICARE INSURANCE COUNSELING

IN-HOME CHORE AND HOUSEKEEPING

LOANING OF DURABLE MEDICAL EQUIPMENT

CAREGIVER ASSISTANCE
- Aging Partners - Administration http://aging.lincoln.ne.gov (external link)
  PLANS, coordinates, and advocates for development and improvement of program, services and benefits for older persons

TECHNICAL support to publicly-funded local aging programs in Butler, Fillmore, Lancaster, Polk, Saline, Saunders, Seward and York counties.

LIVING WELL MAGAZINE is a quarterly magazine published to educate and inform persons on topics, programs, issues and activities that are a concern to the mature population, their families and community organizations. This magazine is for the 32,000 citizens, 60 years of age and older, who reside in the counties of Butler, Fillmore, Lancaster, Polk, Saline, Saunders, Seward and York

FINANCIAL MANAGEMENT including preparing budgets, monitoring revenues and expenses, and submitting financial reports to all funding sources
- Blue Rivers Area Agency on Aging http://www.braaa.org (external link)
  INFORMATION AND REFERRAL

RESPITE CARE

CARE MANAGEMENT for those age 60+

SENIOR CARE OPTIONS for those age 65+

AGED AND DISABLED MEDICAID WAIVER for those age 65+

OMBUDSMAN for long term care for those age 60+
- ENOA - Blair Office http://www.enoa.org (external link)
  CASE MANAGEMENT and information and assistance for programs in Washington County

RURAL transportation, minibus in Washington County; transports from Blair to Omaha or Fremont and from Fort Calhoun to Omaha
- ENOA - Cass County Office http://www.enoa.org (external link)
  TRANSPORTATION for older adults in rural areas of Cass, Sarpy, and Dodge Counties

INFORMATION AND ASSISTANCE for older adults in Cass County
- ENOA - Eastern Nebraska Office on Aging http://www.enoa.org (external link)
  SENIOR CENTERS noon meals for seniors - 444-6513 (see below for Omaha locations)

HOME DELIVERED meals for homebound elderly and disabled individuals certified by a case manager from ENOA or DHHS; clients receive 5-7 meals a week; sliding fee scale -

444-6444 or 444-6766

PUBLIC INFORMATION - New Horizons Newspaper - 444-6654

TRANSPORTATION, rural areas
402-721-7770 - Dodge County
402-426-9614 - Washington County
888-210-1093 - Cass, Douglas, and Sarpy Counties

HEALTH maintenance clinic - 444-6444

VOLUNTEERS ASSISTING SENIORS (VAS) - free assistance for people 55 years and older in insurance, legal and consumer issues, including Medicare counseling - 444-6617

HOMEMAKER services - 444-6444 ext 223

RETIRED SENIOR VOLUNTEER PROGRAM (RSVP) - 444-6444 Ext 224

FOSTER GRANDPARENTS provide service to children with special needs; volunteers who are age 60 and over and meet income guidelines agree to serve an average of 20 hours per week and receive a tax-free stipend of $2.70/hour and an array of benefits - 444-6444 Ext 246 or 245

SENIOR COMPANION Program provides individuals with special needs assistance in their homes or a facility; Companions receive a tax-free stipend of $2.70/hour and other benefits; must meet income guidelines - 444-6444 Ext 247 or 246

CASE MANAGEMENT - 444-6596

PERSONAL CARE services - 444-6444

DURABLE MEDICAL EQUIPMENT - 444-6444

SENIOR CARE OPTIONS - 546-1870

GRANPARENTS RESOURCE CENTER provides services for grandparents caring for their grandchildren - 444-6444 ext. 297

FAN program year round for people 60+years - 444-6596

VOLUNTEER Opportunities - 444-6444 ext. 221

SENIORHELP VOLUNTEER Program - 444-6444 ext. 238

LONG-TERM care ombudsman - 444-6444 ext 239

SENIOR EMPLOYMENT program is a referral, job search source for employment for individuals 50 years and older; offers subsidized employment for individuals 55 years and older who are unemployed and qualify at 125% of poverty guidelines - 444-6684

COMPUTER CLASSES for those 50 and older; $20 for 10 hours of instruction - 444-6684

AGED MEDICAID Waiver - 546-1870

CASE MANAGER coordinates services, working on behalf of older individuals; arranges for in-home services

INTERGENERATION Orchestra of Omaha combines volunteer musicians under 25 years of age and 50 years and over; auditions held each May - 444-6444 ext 221

DOUGLAS AND SARPY COUNTY SENIOR CENTER locations:
Bellevue Senior Center, 109 West 22nd Avenue, 68005 - 293-3041
Camelot Friendship Center, 9270 Cady Avenue, 68134 - 444-3091
Christ Child North, 2111 Emmet, 68110 - 453-6363
Corrigan Senior Center, 3819 X Street, 68107 - 731-7210
Florence Senior Center, 2920 Bondesson Street, 68112 - 444-6333
Heartland Family Service Senior Center, 2101 South 42nd Street, 68105 - 553-5300
Highland Tower Senior Center, 2500 B Street, 68105 - 444-6513
Immanuel Courtyard, 6757 Newport Avenue, Suite 100, 68152 - 829-2912
Intercultural Community Center, 2021 U Street, 68107 - 444-6529
LaVista Senior Center, 8116 Parkview Boulevard, 68128 - 331-3455
Millard/Montclair Center, 2304 South 135th Avenue, 68144 - 546-1270
Native American Elders Nutrition Program, 2240 Landon Court, 68102 - 346-0902
Papillion Senior Center, 1001 Limerick Road, 68046 - 597-2059
Park Tower Senior Center, 1601 Park Avenue, 68105 - 444-6513
Ralston Senior Center, 7301 Q Street, Suite 100, 68127 - 339-4926
Seven Oaks Lunch Club, 3439 State Street, 68112 - 451-4477
St Mary Magdalene Senior Center, 1817 Dodge Street, 68102 - 346-3234

DODGE COUNTY SENIOR CENTER locations:
Dodge, 226 Elm Street - (402) 693-2239
Fremont, 1730 West 16th Street - (402) 727-2815
Hooper, 208 North Main Street - (402) 654-2537
North Bend, 240 East 10th Street - (402) 652-8661
Snyder, 2nd and Elm Street - (402) 568-2245

CASS COUNTY SENIOR CENTER locations:
Eagle, 509 4th Street - (402) 781-2468
Elmwood, 144 North 4th Street - (402) 994-2145
Louisville, 423 Elm Street - (402) 234-2120
Nehawka, Community Center - (402) 227-9923
Plattsmouth, 308 South 18th - (402) 296-5800 x1
Weeping Water, 303 West Eldora - (402) 267-5303

WASHINGTON COUNTY SENIOR CENTER locations:

Arlington, 305 North 3rd Street - (402) 478-4774

Blair, 1278 Wilbur Street - (402) 533-9622 x1007

○ Midland Area Agency on Aging http://www.midlandareaagencyonaging.org (external link)

COMPREHENSIVE assessment done in the client's residence to identify client's needs and plan care

CHOICES case management services helps to coordinate and manage care on behalf of the client; evaluate needs, resources, and family support to help decide what plan of care is best for the individual, and assist in organizing and overseeing the home care plan

SENIOR CENTERS provide a variety of services including congregate and home delivered meals, social activities and educational programs.

VOLUNTEERS provide telephone reassurance and Senior Companion programs

HANDYMAN and homemaker services also available

○ Northeast Nebraska Area Agency on Aging (NENAAA) http://www.nenaaa.com (external link)

SENIOR CARE OPTIONS provides a nursing facility pre-admission screening to ensure Medicaid applicants in need of nursing facility care receive information on alternative choices appropriate to their level of care and assistance in finding and setting up the services needed

CARE MANAGEMENT provides a health, social,and functional assessment and helps plan for needed services; coordination of in-home services; on-going monitoring and follow-up; long term care facility information

IN-HOME SERVICES, including grocery shopping, cleaning, laundry, transportation, respite, lawn care, snow removal, and personal care

EMERGENCY RESPONSE SYSTEM may be available for persons who can benefit from the security of the system.

NUTRITION COUNSELING provides individual counseling to those at nutritional risk because of their physical health, diagnosis, medication, family finances, or family status change

CONGREGATE MEALS are provided to a qualified individual. The meal must meet 1/3 of the daily recommended dietary needs of adults 60 and over including the requirements of the Older Americans Act and state and local laws.

HOME-DELIVERED MEALS are provided to frail, homebound by reason of illness, disability or isolation. The meals must meet 1/3 of the daily recommended dietary needs of adults 60 years and over and the requirements of the Older Americans Act and state and local laws.

OMBUDSMAN advocates for the rights of residents of long term care facilities through empowerment, problem-solving, and conflict resolution

LEGAL ASSISTANCE on an individual basis, and educational programs at senior centers

AGED AND DISABLED MEDICAID WAIVER allows Medicaid dollars to be used for specific services for those with long term care needs; must be 65 or older, Medicaid eligible, with needs which would require nursing facility care and can by safely served at home at a cost not more than nursing facility care; services may include housekeeping, grocery shopping, respite, transportation, lifeline, and assisted living

HEALTH CLINIC services provided by a licensed health care professional designed to identify, prevent or treat physical or mental health problems

SUPPORTIVE services is a broad provision of health, social, educational services including recreational, general information, public information and publication.

OUTREACH identifies potential clients and encourages their use of existing services

INFORMATION AND ASSISTANCE provides information on available services, links individuals to the services and provides adequate follow-up procedures

TRANSPORTATION and ASSISTED TRANSPORTATION may be available to transport from one location to another

SHIIP Senior Health Insurance Information Program provides insurance information and counseling to older Nebraskans and person with disabilities regarding Medicaid, Medicare, and health insurance, including the Medicare Prescription Drug Plans; toll free hotline, public education, and educational literature also available - 800-234-7117

FAMILY CAREGIVER SUPPORT for those caring for an aging adult or grandparents caring for a minor child; provides information, assistance, training, support group, respite care, and supplemental services

o South Central Nebraska Area Agency on Aging http://www.agingkearney.org (external link)
INFORMATION and Assistance to assist individuals in securing needed information and/or services that cannot be offered through the agency

CARE MANAGEMENT to help seniors find in-home services and care providers to allow them to live independently for as long as possible, preventing premature nursing home placement

SENIOR CARE OPTION (SCO) will evaluate the long term care needs of persons over age 65 seeking Medicaid coverage for nursing facility care to determine if such care is needed or if other options are viable

HEALTH and nutrition programs include 20 congregate meal sites and home delivered meals through six sites; health and nutritional counseling may be provided to individual seniors, depending on available funding

LEGAL SERVICES for persons age 60 and over and their spouses; specializes in Elderlaw and provides assistance with simple wills, powers of attorney for health care, living wills, durable powers of attorney, Medicare/Medicaid, etc.

MEDICAID WAIVER in-home services, including assisted living, for those age 65 and older with care needs; must meet income and resource guidelines as well as other eligibility criteria

INSURACE ASSISTANCE - SHIIP (Senior Health Insurance Information Program) assists seniors regarding health insurance issues such as Medicare, Medicaid, Medicare supplemental insurance, long term care insurance, group health insurance, etc.

FAMILY CAREGIVER PROGRAM provides caregiver training and education, information on available services, caregiver support, and funding for emergency response systems

RESPITE CARE grants to provide temporary relief for the permanent caregiver; grant amounts vary and are provided through the Family Caregiver Program
- Southwest 8 Senior Services http://www.southwest8.org (external link)
SENIOR CENTERS offer recreation, education, and arts and crafts programs (see separate listings)

ADVOCACY through senior advocates

CONGREGATE MEAL SITES, homebound and frozen meals, nutrition education, and special diet counseling

OUTREACH

OLDER IOWA'S legislature

ELDER CARE FUNDING for in-home service, home-health, and adult day care

COMMUNITY-BASED adult services

ECONOMIC DEVELOPMENT activities

NEWSLETTER, The Senior Courier

CASEMANAGEMENT program

SHIIP - Senior Health Insurance Information Program - Medicare

INFORMATION and Assistance

FAMILY CAREGIVER support

ELDER ABUSE Initiative

SUPPORT GROUP Grandparents raising grandchildren

SENIOR VOLUNTEER PROGRAM Foster grandparent, Senior Companion

- West Central Nebraska Area Agency on Aging (WCNAAA) http://www.wcnaaa.org (external link)
SENIOR CARE OPTIONS provides a nursing facility preadmission screening to ensure Medicaid applicants in need of nursing facility care receive information on alternative choices to their level of care and assistance in finding and setting up the services needed.

CARE MANAGEMENT includes health, social and functional assessment and helps plan for needed services

HOUSEKEEPING and supportive services to include grocery shopping, cleaning, laundry, transportation and personal care

FAMILY CAREGIVER SUPPORT for those caring for an aging adult or grandparents caring for a minor child: provides information, assistance, support group, respite care and supplemental services

CONGREGATE MEALS are provided to persons 60 and older. The meal must meet 1/3 of the daily recommended dietary needs of adults including the requirements of the Older Americans Act and state and local laws.

HOME DELIVERED MEALS are provided to homebound by reason of illness, disability or isolation. The meals meet 1/3 of the daily dietary recommended needs of adults 60 years and over and the requirements of the Older Americans Act and state and local laws.

PUBLIC BENEFIT SERVICES, legal assistance, education, Medicare filing, and volunteer training through SHIIP

-

Nevada

Health and Social Services: http://nv.gov/residents/health/

Prescription Assistance/ Disabled: http://dhhs.nv.gov/DisabilityRx.htm

NEVADA DISABILITY RX

Effective January 1, 2007, the state of Nevada began providing assistance with the cost of prescription medicines to qualified individuals with disabilities. Eligibility requirements are:

- Age 18 through 61 with verifiable disability
- Nevada resident continuously for at least the last 12 months
- Annual income no more than $26,054 for singles and $34,731 for couples

Disability Rx Enrollment for Nevada's Disability Rx prescription program is open. Unfortunately, a limited amount of funding is available and a waiting list has been established. As funds become available, the lowest household income designated on the waiting list will receive priority for enrollment.

This is an on-line application. You can fill out the form on-line, print it, and then mail it to the address provided.

For an application or additional Disability Rx information, dial 687-4210, ext. 244 if calling from the Reno-Carson City-Gardnerville areas, or if outside this area call toll-free 1-866-303-6323.

Based on funding availability, the benefits are ...

For those who are Not Medicare Eligible:

- No monthly premium
- No deductible
- Co-payments of $10 for generics or $25 for preferred brands
- Annual coverage limit of $5,100

For those who are Medicare Eligible:

- Help with monthly premiums for Medicare Part D Prescription Drug Plan (if not qualified for maximum help from Medicare with that expense)
- Help with prescription costs after reaching the Medicare Part D coverage limit

If you think you qualify, click here for the PDF application.

This is an on-line application. You can fill out the form on-line, print it, and then mail it to the address provided

- OR -

You can print the application, fill it out, then mail it to the address provided.
For more information call:
1 - 866- 303-6323

Prescription Assistance/ Seniors: http://dhhs.nv.gov/SeniorRx.htm

Welcome to **Senior Rx**, Nevada's plan to provide Nevada seniors relief from the high cost of prescription medicine. **Senior Rx** provides assistance with Medicare Part D expenses for members who **ARE** eligible for Part D and a cost-sharing benefit for members who are **NOT** eligible for Part D.

Senior Rx is funded with a portion of Nevada's share of tobacco settlement funds and was passed into law during the 1999 legislative session. **Senior Rx** provides up to $5,100 in benefits per year depending on the member's situation. Many of the program's benefits are administered through a contracted pharmacy benefit manager called Catalyst Rx. Other benefits are coordinated directly with the Medicare Part D plans that serve as the first prescription drug resource for enrolled members.

For details about **Senior Rx** benefits, click on Senior Rx Plan Design.

Effective July 1, 2011,
the maximum annual household income for singles is $26,054,
and the maximum annual household income for married couples is $34,731.

Senior Rx Enrollment for Nevada's Senior Rx prescription program currently has a waitlist. The persons with lowest household income designated on the waiting list will always receive priority for enrollment.

If you think you qualify, click here for the PDF application.
This is an on-line application. You can fill out the form on-line, print it, and then mail it to the address provided.

For an application or additional **Senior Rx** information, dial **687-4210, ext. 244** if calling from the Reno-Carson City-Gardnerville areas, or if outside this area call toll-free

Aging and Disabled Services Division: http://aging.state.nv.us/index.htm

Aging and Disabled Resource Center: http://www.nvaging.net/adrc/home.htm

Aging and Disability Resource Center (ADRC) Program Overview

Provides citizen-centered "one-stop" entry points into the long-term support system
Serves individuals in need of long-term support, caregivers, and those planning for future long-term

support needs

ADRC Functions

Awareness and Information

- Public education

- Information on long-term support options

Assistance

- Long-term support options counseling

- Benefits counseling

- Employment options counseling

- Referral to other programs and benefits that can help people remain in the community, including programs to assist in obtaining and sustaining paid employment

- Crisis intervention

- Assistance in planning for future long-term support needs

Access

- Eligibility screening

- Assistance in gaining access to long-term support services that may be paid with private funds

- Comprehensive assessment of long-term support needs and care planning

- Programmatic eligibility determination for long-term support services, including the Medicaid long-term care level of care determination

- Medicaid financial eligibility determination that is wither integrated or so closely coordinated with the ADRC that applicants experience a seamless interaction

- One-stop access to all public programs for community and institutional long-term support services administered by the state under Medicaid, Older Americans Act programs devoted to long-term support services, and any other publicly funded services the state determines should be accessed through the ADRCs

For more information, please contact:

Aging and Disability Services Division - Carson City
(775) 687-4210
adsd@adsd.nv.gov

Or visit NevadaADRC.com

Assistance for Caregivers: http://www.nevadacareconnection.org/

Welcome!

The purpose of this website is to provide up-to-date resources and information that will support and assist caregivers as they care for family members and friends that are frail or disabled.

If you know of someone who would benefit from this information but does not have access to the Internet, please feel free to print out the material.

Overview of Information

• Resources available by city, county and/or zip code that contain pertinent information and current contact information.

• Search Box at the top locates community resources or general information.

• Special events, current classes and workshops, new programs, and support group information to assist caregivers and care-receivers.

• Calendar of Events - North and Calendar of Events - South to view at a glance not only what is happening in the current month, but also future months.

• Links to state, and national websites that provide assistance to caregivers.

• Tips & Tools sections where experts offer caregiving tips, information and programs. A special section for caregivers caring for seniors with Alzheimer's Disease or Dementia.

• A glossary that contains definitions of words and terms that would be helpful to caregivers.

• A help page that explains how to use this site.

• A map of what is on this site.

• A feedback page for you to share ideas and comments to improve the quality in this site.

New Hampshire

Residents-Living: http://www.nh.gov/residents/living.html

Disabled

- Governor's Commission on Disability
- Developmental Disabilities Council
- Developmental Services for Adults
- Web Accessibility Initiative

Seniors
- Prescription Drug Assistance for Seniors
- ServiceLink
- Assisted Living and Residential Services
- Glencliff Home for the Elderly

Health and Safety
- Physician Finder
- Healthy NH 2010
- Medicine Cabinet
- Medicare Program
- Medicaid Program
- NH HealthCost

Bureau of Elderly and Adult Services: http://www.dhhs.nh.gov/dcbcs/beas/index.htm

The Bureau of Elderly and Adult Services (BEAS) provides a variety of social and long-term supports to adults age 60 and older and to adults between the ages of 18 and 60 who have a chronic illness or disability.

Mission Statement

A variety of social and long-term services and supports can be accessed through the ServiceLink Resource Centers and the NH DHHS District Offices. Services and supports are intended to assist people to live as independently as possible in safety and with dignity. Examples include:

o   Home care

- o Meals on wheels
- o Transportation assistance
- o Long Term Care-Nursing home and community based care
- o Information and assistance regarding Medicare and Medicaid
- o Information about volunteer opportunities
- o Investigation of reports of abuse, neglect or exploitation of incapacitated adults

BEAS Locations

BEAS staff are located at DHHS District Offices and ServiceLink Resource Centers throughout NH and coordinate services to seniors and adults with disabilities and chronic illnesses who meet certain eligibility criteria. BEAS also has a main office, located in Concord, responsible for administrative support and general program and financial planning.

ServiceLink Resource Centers

A major partnership between BEAS and local communities is the ServiceLink Resource Centers, a statewide network of community-based resources for seniors, adults living with disabilities and their families. The ServiceLink Resource Centers are available to anyone who needs assistance, advice, help finding services or support with an issue relating to a senior member or disabled adult living in our community. ServiceLink partners promote the independence and well-being of the people they serve at thirteen primary locations and many satellites throughout NH.

Community-Based Provider Network

A critical component of the BEAS statewide delivery system is its community based provider network; many of these providers are nonprofit agencies. BEAS coordinates long-term care support services through contracts at the local level, thus reflecting the commitment of DHHS to strengthen the autonomy of local communities and to direct resources to where they are needed most.

Program Information
Community Based Care
Services
Adult Protection
Audits
Catastrophic Illness Program
Community Passport
Elder Abuse Advisory Council

Family Caregivers
Home & Community Care
Housing
Nursing Home Care
Outreach
Prescription Drug Assistance
Publications
State Committee on Aging
State Registry
Transportation
Contact Elderly & Adult
Services

Family Caregiver Support Services: http://www.dhhs.nh.gov/dcbcs/beas/familycaregivers.htm

Support services are available to family members, partners and other informal caregivers who are providing day to day care to a frail older adult, an adult with a diagnosis of Alzheimer's disease or other related disorders, an adult with disabilities who needs assistance with daily living activities, and grandparents and relative caregivers raising children.

Who are Family Caregivers?

A family caregiver is anyone who provides regular care for a relative, a partner or a friend. The amount of care that the family member or other individual provides may have increased over time, or they may have found themselves in that role suddenly, without notice. For many it is a labor of love but it can also be physically and emotionally demanding. It is important to keep a balance between caring for another individual while caring for oneself.

The NH Family Caregiver Support Program

Through the National Family Caregiver Support Program, the Bureau of Elderly and Adult Services and the NH ServiceLink Resource Centers provides the following services for family caregivers. These services can Include:

- Information about community programs and local resources.
- Assistance in assessing individual caregiving needs, help in identifying options, and accessing local providers.
- Individual counseling and access to support groups.
- Education and training to help develop caregiving skills.

o Respite care services to provide a temporary break for eligible full time family caregivers, and limited services that complement the care the family caregiver is providing that can include: chore services, assistive equipment, home modifications, and transportation services.

o For more information contact ServiceLink toll free at: 1-866-634-9412.

Alzheimer's Disease and Related Disorders

Services and resources to help persons with Alzheimer's Disease and Related Disorders (ADRD) and their family caregivers. These programs include:

o Respite care services to provide a temporary break for family caregivers who live with and care for an individual diagnosed with Alzheimer's disease or other related disorder.

o Information and referrals to resources for families.

For Alzheimer's or dementia specific information contact the Alzheimer's Association via their toll free 24/7 helpline: 1-800-272-3900. For more information contact ServiceLink toll free at: 1-866-634-9412.

Grandparents and Relatives Raising Children

Through the NH Family Caregiver Support Program eligible grandparents and relatives can receive respite services such as in-home child care, after school programs and camps.

o Families and Children

o Family Assistance

o Women, Infants and Children Nutrition Program

A Resource Guide for NH Relative Caregivers

In New Hampshire, there are more than 4,000 children living with grandparents without either parent present. There are over 2,300 children living in households headed by other relatives. Children and their caregivers are often eligible for state and federal benefits; however, finding those benefits can often be confusing and frustrating. This booklet can guide you in the right direction, help you ask the right questions, and help you find the answers you need.

Transitions in Caregiving Demonstration Project

The Transitions in Caregiving demonstration project funded by the Administration on Aging is changing the way services are provided to family caregivers of older adults in New Hampshire. The new consumer-directed model allows eligible family caregivers more flexibility, choice and control over the services they receive, as well as providing more comprehensive supports. The ServiceLink Resource

Centers provide the single point of entry for services for family caregivers. This model of support has been recognized by the Council of State Governments with their <u>2010 Innovation Award for the Eastern Region</u>.

Publications

<u>NH Family Care Guide: Alzheimer's Disease and Related Disorders</u> - a comprehensive guide for family caregivers and others who are dealing with effects of Alzheimer's disease or other types of irreversible dementia. The companion guide <u>Sources of Help</u> provides additional information for family members and others in making long term care plans. These are available for free to family caregivers by download, or print copies can be obtained by request by calling the Bureau of Elderly and Adult Services at (800) 351-1888, ext. 4680

Division of Family Assistance: http://www.dhhs.nh.gov/dfa/index.htm

The Division of Family Assistance administers programs and services for eligible NH residents by providing financial, medical, food & nutritional assistance, help with child care costs and emergency help to obtain and keep safe housing. Family Assistance staff determines initial and continuing eligibility, the amount of benefits and deliver benefits using federal and NH guidelines and policies.

Food & Nutrition Programs

o   Food Stamp Program

Medical Coverage

o   Medicaid
o   Medicare Beneficiaries Savings Program
o   NH Healthy Kids Programs

State Supplemental Programs (SSP - Cash)

o   Old Age Assistance (OAA)
o   Aid to the Permanently and Totally Disabled (APTD)
o   Aid to the Needy Blind (ANB)

Temporary Assistance for Needy Families (TANF)

o   NH Employment Program

- o   Family Assistance Program
- o   Child Care Assistance
- o   Emergency Assistance
- o   Employment and Training Programs and Support Services

Cash Assistance Programs: http://www.dhhs.nh.gov/dfa/cash/index.htm

Cash Assistance is provided through Division of Family Assistance (DFA) in two general program areas, the Temporary Assistance for Needy Families (TANF) and State Supplemental Programs (SSP) for the Needy Blind (ANB), Permanently and Totally Disabled (APTD) and Old Age Assistance (OAA).

State Supplemental Programs (SSP-Cash)

State Supplemental cash assistance supports elderly adults, individuals that are physically disabled, mentally disabled or legally blind. Eligibility and benefit amounts for the State Supplement Programs depend on the individual and spouse's income, resources and on living arrangement. Services are provided for eligible individuals through the following programs:

- o   Aid to the Permanently and Totally Disabled (APTD)
- o   Aid to the Needy Blind (ANB)
- o   Old Age Assistance (OAA)

Temporary Assistance for Needy Families (TANF)

TANF provides assistance to needy families with dependent children with a network of employment support through the NH Employment Program. Services are provided for families with dependent children through the following TANF and related programs:

- o   Family Assistance Program (FAP) or
- o   New Hampshire Employment Program (NHEP)
- o   Child Care Assistance
- o   Emergency Assistance
- o   Employment and Training Programs and Support Services

Seniors: http://www.dhhs.nh.gov/foryou/seniors.htm

Wellness
- Drug & Alcohol
- Fruits & Vegetables
- Hand Washing
- Immunizations
- Minority Health

Nutrition & Physical Activity
- Obesity Prevention
  - Oral Health
  - Tobacco

Safety
- Adult Protection
- Domestic Violence
- Food Protection
- Injury Prevention

Long-Term Care Ombudsman
- Suicide Prevention

Diseases and Conditions
- Asthma
- Avian Flu
- Diabetes

Eastern Equine Encephalitis & West Nile Virus (EEE & WNV)
- Hepatitis A
- Hepatitis C
- Human Immunodeficiency Virus (HIV)/Acquired Immune Deficiency Syndrome (AIDS)
- Influenza (Flu)
- Lyme Disease
- Measles
- Meningitis
- Mumps
- Pertussis (Whooping Cough)
  - Rabies
  - Salmonella
  - Staph

Sexually Transmitted Diseases (STDs)
- Tuberculosis

Support Services
- Administrative Appeals
- Aid to the Needy Blind

Aid to the Permanently and Totally Disabled
- Behavioral Health
- Catastrophic Illness

Commodity Supplemental Food
- Developmental Services
- Emergency Assistance
- Family Caregivers

Farmers' Market Nutrition
- Food Stamps

Home & Community Care
- Housing Services

Medical Assistance-Medicaid

Medicare Beneficiaries Savings
- Medicare Part D
- Nursing Home Care
- Old Age Assistance
- Prescription Drugs

People with Disabilities: http://www.dhhs.nh.gov/foryou/disabilities.htm

Support Services
- Acquired Brain Disorders
- Administrative Appeals
  - Adult Services
  - Aid to the Needy Blind
- Aid to the Permanently and Totally Disabled
  - Area Agencies
  - Behavioral Health
- Children & Adolescent Services
- Community Mental Health Centers
- Family Centered Early Supports & Services
  - Family Support
- Medicaid for Employed Adults with Disabilities

- o <u>Ombudsman</u>
- o <u>Special Medical Services</u>

New Jersey

Community and Wellness: http://www.newjersey.gov/nj/community/

Senior Services: http://www.newjersey.gov/nj/community/senior/

Senior Services

Directories
- Getting Answers – Contact Directory
- Listing of NJ Senior Services
- County Directory of Offices on Aging
- Aging & Disability Resource Connection
- Information For Caregivers

Health & Wellness
- Staying Healthy
- Medicare
- State Health Insurance Assistance Program (SHIP)
- Pharmaceutical Assistance to the Aged and Disabled (PAAD) program
- Senior Gold Prescription Discount Program
- Get Flu Ready NJ
- Osteoporosis
- Hearing Aid Assistance to the Aged and Disabled (HAAAD)

Housing Options and Assisted Listing
- Global Options (GO) for Long-Term Care
- Community Choice
- Guide to Community-Based Long Term Care in NJ
- Report Abuse/Neglect at Nursing Homes or Long Term Care Facilities
- HMFA Affordable Rentals for Seniors
- NJ Lifeline – Utilities Assistance Program

Safety & Legal
- Protect Yourself From Elder Fraud [pdf - 645.47 KB]
- Office of The Public Guardian

- Adult Protective Services (APS)

  Benefits & Assistance
- Statewide Benefits for Older Persons

- Federal Programs For Older Persons

- Division of Senior Benefits and Utilization Management

- Tax Information For Seniors

- Free Tax Preparation Services

- Special Automobile Insurance Policy (SAIP), *also known as Dollar a Day, is a new initiative to help make limited auto insurance coverage available to drivers who are eligible for Federal Medicaid with*

Division of Aging and Community Services: http://web.doh.state.nj.us/adrcnj/

Services and Resources: http://web.doh.state.nj.us/adrcnj/resources.aspx

Information by Topic
Do you want websites or printable information related to an older adult, a person with a disability, or a caregiver? **General topics** are defined and listed by category A to Z.

Caring For Others
Caregiving is the active, unpaid, and continuous help provided to a person with a disability, or to a person who is frail or elderly. Through this door you will find general information on topics of particular interest to caregivers and some tools that will help you evaluate your needs.

Screening Tools/ Application Forms
Enter this door to find program applications that can be printed or completed online. You will also find online screening tools that will help you learn if you are eligible for some programs.

Quick Links
Click here for quick access to websites for many New Jersey agencies, facilities and toll-free numbers.

Division of Disability Services:
http://www.state.nj.us/humanservices/dds/home/cntrindlivindex.html

Centers for Independent Living

Centers for Independent Living, many of them funded through the Division of Vocational Rehabilitation Services, in the Department of Labor & Workforce Development, are community-based, consumer-driven organizations that provide information and referral, peer counseling, skills training, advocacy and a variety of services based on individual needs.

STATEWIDE INDEPENDENT LIVING COUNCIL (SILC)

PROGRESSIVE CENTER FOR INDEPENDENT LIVING (PCIL)
1262 Whitehorse-Hamilton Sq. Road., Bldg. A, Suite 102
Hamilton NJ 08690
Telephone: (609) 581-4500 (877) 917-4500
TDD: (609) 581-4550
www.njsilc.org

ALLIANCE FOR DISABLED IN ACTION (ADA)

(Middlesex, Somerset, Union Counties)
629 Amboy Avenue, Edison, NJ 08837
Telephone: (732) 738-4388
TDD: (732) 738-9644
www.adacil.org

CAMDEN CITY INDEPENDENT LIVING CENTER

(City of Camden)
2600 Mt. Ephraim Avenue, Suite 413
Camden, NJ 08104
Telephone: (856) 966-0800
TDD: (856) 966-0830
www.camdencityilc.org

CENTER FOR INDEPENDENT LIVING OF SOUTH JERSEY, INC. (CIL-SJ)

(Camden and Gloucester Counties)
1150 Delsea Drive, Suite 1
Westville, NJ 08093
Telephone: (856) 853-6490
Toll free: (800) 413-3791
TDD: (856) 853-7602

DIAL, INC.

(Essex and Passaic Counties)
2 Prospect Village Plaza, First Floor
Clifton , NJ 07013
Telephone: (973) 470-8090
TDD: (973) 470-2521
www.dial-cil.org

DAWN, INC.

(Morris, Sussex and Warren Counties)
30 Broad Street, Suite 5
Denville, NJ 07834
Telephone: (973) 625-1940 (888) 383-DAWN
TDD: (973) 625-1932
www.dawncil.org

HEIGHTENED INDEPENDENCE & PROGRESS (HIP)

(Bergen County)
131 Main Street, Suite 120
Hackensack, NJ 07601
Telephone: (201) 996-9100
TDD: (201) 996-9424
www.hipcil.org

HEIGHTENED INDEPENDENCE & PROGRESS-HUDSON

(Hudson County)
26 Journal Square, Suite 602
Jersey City, NJ 07306
Telephone: (201) 533-4407
TDD: (201) 533-4409
www.hipcil.org

OCEANS CENTER FOR INDEPENDENT LIVING

(Monmouth and Ocean County)
279 Broadway, Second Floor, Suite 201
Long Branch, NJ 07740
Telephone: (732) 571-4884
TDD: (732) 571-4878
www.moceans.org

PROGRESSIVE CENTER FOR INDEPENDENT LIVING (PCIL)

(Hunterdon and Mercer Counties)
1262 Whitehorse-Hamilton Sq. Rd., Bldg. A, Suite 102
Hamilton NJ 08690
Telephone: (609) 581-4500 (877) 917-4500
TDD: (609) 581-4550
Hunterdon County Branch: Telephone:(908) 782-1055
(877) 376-9174
TDD: (908) 782-1081

www.pcil.org

RESOURCES FOR INDEPENDENT LIVING (RIL)

(Burlington County)
351 High Street, Suite 103
Burlington, NJ 08016
Telephone: (609) 747-7745
TDD: (609) 747-1875
www.rilnj.org

TOTAL LIVING CENTER, INC. (TLC)

(Atlantic County)
The Courtyard, Suite B-8
707 Whitehorse Pike
Absecon, NJ 08201
Telephone: (609) 645-9547
TDD: (609) 645-9593
www.tlcenter.org

TRI-COUNTY INDEPENDENT LIVING CENTER, INC.

(Cape May, Cumberland, Salem Counties)
120 North High Street, Suite 12
Millville, NJ 08332
Telephone: (856) 327-5177
TDD: (856) 327-5328
www.tricountycil.org

Office of Home and Community Services: http://www.state.nj.us/humanservices/dds/ohcs/

When Medicaid was enacted by Congress in 1965, people with severe disabilities almost always lived in institutions. Since then, new medical treatments and the growing number of services that are available in the community have meant that it is now often possible for people with even the most severe disabilities to continue to live at home, as long as they have the support services they need.

Personal Care Assistant (PCA) Services

Personal Care Assistant (PCA) Services. This is an optional benefit offered to New Jersey Medicaid beneficiaries who are experiencing some functional impairment and need a Personal Care Assistant to help them with some aspects of daily living such as dressing or bathing.

Recipients must have a doctor's order to receive this service, but they do not have to be permanently disabled. An estimated 27,000 people receive this service at any given time.

Section 1915[c] of the federal Social Security Act now allows states to "waive" requirements of the original Medicaid legislation and create so-called waiver programs that provide care in the home and in the community, as an alternative to institutional care.

DDS administers 3 Medicaid Waiver programs...

In New Jersey, the Division of Disability Services administers three home- and community-based services, or waiver programs. These are:

AIDS Community Care Alternatives Program (ACCAP). At any one time this program can serve a maximum of 750 people statewide, including those of any age with AIDS and children up to age 13 who are HIV positive. It provides full Medicaid benefits plus case management, private-duty nursing, medical day care, and personal care assistant services. Children receive additional benefits, including placement in a specialized group foster care home or reimbursement to their foster parents, through DYFS.

Community Resources for People with Disabilities Waiver (CRPD). The waiver is designed to provide services in addition to full Medicaid benefits to people who otherwise would be unable to live in the community and would probably have to move into a nursing home or other institution. Additional services included in the waiver are case management, environmental/vehicle modifications, community transitional services and personal emergency response systems (PERS).

TBI (Traumatic Brain Injury) Waiver. This waiver program can serve up to 350 people between the ages of 21 and 64 who have survived a traumatic brain injury after the age of 21. People in the program receive full Medicaid benefits plus additional services, including: case management, a structured day program, respite care, and night supervision.

Medicaid Personal Care Assistant (PCA) Services:
http://www.state.nj.us/humanservices/dds/ohcs/pca/index.html

Program Description
The Personal Care Assistant (PCA) Program is an optional statewide service offered to New Jersey Medicaid recipients who are experiencing some functional impairment and need a personal care assistant to help them with some aspects of daily living, such as dressing or bathing.

The purpose of the program is to accommodate long-term chronic or maintenance health care, as opposed to short-term skilled care as is provided under Medicaid's home health program. PCA services are non-emergency health related tasks done by qualified staff in a medically eligible beneficiary's home.

An estimated 22,000 people receive this service at any given time. The program is administered by the Division of Disability Services, Office of Home and Community Services.

Qualifications

In order to qualify for PCA services recipients must be:

Participating on Medicaid Plan A or G of the New Jersey FamilyCare program;

> Have a doctor's order to receive this service, but they do not have to be permanently disabled;
> Live in a community-based residence (private home, apartment, rooming house, or boarding home) or group home, skill development home, supervised apartment or other congregate living program where personal care **is not** provided as a part of the service package included in the living arrangement; and
> Have a documented need for hands-on personal care.

Services

Services include assistance with activities of daily living (ADLs) and household duties essential to the patient's health and comfort. PCA services are performed under the supervision of a registered professional nurse employed by a Medicaid provider.

Services may be provided by community-based home care agencies under contract with Medicaid or by independent clinics under contract to the Division of Mental Health Services (DMHS).

PCA services must be prior authorized by the Division of Disability Services.

Accessing PCA Services

Recipients may contact community-based home care agencies under contract with Medicaid directly in order to select an agency to provide services.

Community-based home care agencies listed by New Jersey county may be obtained by contacting DDS, Office of Home and Community Services (OHCS) at (609) 292-4800. Information may be sent to requesters by fax, email or regular mail.

Eligibility Determination

Upon selection of a community-based home care agency by the recipient the following process will occur in order to determine eligibility and award of services:

Provider agency will obtain necessary personal and medical information to verify Medicaid eligibility;

> A nurse will visit the recipient's home to perform an assessment of need for personal care assistance;
> Provider agency will submit a prior authorization request to the Division of Disability for review upon the results of the assessment; and

Division staff will review the request and notify the provider agency of the decision on eligibility and number of hours awarded per week.

The final decision on award of service hours is made by the Division of Disability Services professional staff based on the nursing assessment and the recipient's need for personal care assistance.

Division of Aging and Senior Services: http://nj.gov/health/senior/index.shtml

The New Jersey Division of Aging and Community Services (DACS) administers programs designed to make it easier for seniors to get the help they need to support their well-being and maintain themselves in the community for as long as possible with independence, dignity and choice.

Our Website has been designed with you, the consumer, in mind.

- Under **Getting Answers** you will find out whom to contact at the State or in your community to learn about and access senior and caregiver services.

- Under Staying Healthy you will get information about Medicare options, nutrition, health education and other programs that help you maintain and improve your health.

- Getting Help at Home details programs that help people in need of long-term care services get help in their home or a community setting rather than in a nursing home.

- Staying Safe explains how vulnerable adults living at home or in institutions are protected from abuse, neglect and exploitation.

- If you do not find the information you are looking for here, please call us toll-free at **1-800-792-8820**, (or at 609-943-3437 for out-of-state callers). For information on services available within your county, call NJEASE toll-free at **1-877-222-3737**.

Getting Help at Home: http://nj.gov/health/senior/help.shtml
- Program Administration
- Toll-Free Telephone Numbers
- Long-Term Care Planning
- Adult Day Care
- Home and Community-Based Programs

Program Administration

Office of AAA Administration

Most senior services in New Jersey are administered locally by county-based Area Agencies on Aging (AAAs). Click here to find the AAA in your county.

Office of Community Choice Options

Most seniors and people with disabilities in need of long-term care services prefer to get help in their home or in a community setting rather than in a nursing home. This office helps individuals learn about and access those services.

Office of Global Options for Long-Term Care & Quality Management

This office administers a number of home and community-based programs that help seniors, people with disabilities and their caregivers.

Return to Top

Toll-Free Telephone Numbers

NJEASE

New Jersey Easy Access, Single Entry (NJEASE) is our state's senior service delivery system. Your best first step to finding out about in-home services is a call to NJEASE toll-free at 1-877-222-3737.

Return to Top

Long-Term Care Planning

A Guide to Community-Based Long Term Care in New Jersey

It is important to plan now for long-term care needs you may encounter as you age. This on-line guide can help you make the right choices now for a secure future.

Return to Top

Adult Day Care

Adult Day Health Services

Adult Day Health Services provide a safe environment for frail elderly during the day when their caregivers are at work. Some health-related services are provided.

Alzheimer's Adult Day Services

This program partially subsidizes the purchase of adult day care services for persons with Alzheimer's disease or a related dementia.

Social Adult Day Care

This adult day care option is for individuals who do not need medical attention during the day, but may need supervision to ensure their safety and well-being.

Return to Top

Home and Community-Based Programs

Global Options (GO) for Long Term Care
On January 1, 2009, three Medicaid-supported home and community-based service programs were combined to create GO. This consolidation improves access to a wider range of services for a greater number of seniors and adults with physical disabilities who meet the income, asset and nursing facility level of care requirements established by Medicaid. GO participants will have the options to hire and direct their own service providers.

Congregate Housing Services Program
This program provides supportive services to individuals who are elderly and disabled residing in selected subsidized housing facilities.

JACC (Jersey Assistance for Community Caregiving)
JACC is a state-funded program similar to GO, but for individuals with slightly higher incomes.

Money Follows the Person (MFP)
This is a federal demonstration project that helps eligible individuals who have been residing in nursing facilities and developmental centers for six months or more to move into a community setting.

Program of All-inclusive Care for the Elderly (PACE)
PACE is an innovative Medicare program that provides frail individuals age 55 and older comprehensive medical and social services coordinated and provided by an interdisciplinary team of professionals in a community-based center and in their homes. PACE helps participants delay or avoid long-term nursing home care.

Statewide Respite Care Program
This program provides relief for unpaid caregivers by ensuring their loved ones are cared for while the caregiver takes personal time.

New Mexico

Aging and Long Term Services Department:
http://www.nmaging.state.nm.us/ALTSD_second_page.html

Aging and Long Term Resource Center: http://www.nmaging.state.nm.us/Resource_Center.html

Aging Network Division: http://www.nmaging.state.nm.us/Aging_Network_Division.html

Elderly and Disabled Services:
http://www.nmaging.state.nm.us/EDSD/Elderly_Disability_Services_Division.html

Elderly and Disability Services
For Information regarding Long-Term Services in your area, please contact
the Aging & Disability Resource Center (ADRC) at 1-800-432-2080,
if you are in Santa Fe please call 505-476-4846.

The Elderly and Disability Services Division has moved to the Human Services Department (HSD). HSD is responsible for the administration of the Coordination of Long-Term Services Program, the CoLTS C waiver (formerly known as the Disabled and Elderly Waiver) program, the Personal Care Option program, the Program of All-inclusive Care for the Elderly (PACE), the Traumatic Brain Injury program, the GAP Program, and Mi Via, New Mexico's Self-directed Waiver program. These programs provide support to enable older adults and individuals with disabilities to remain in their own homes and communities or to return to their homes from a nursing facility or institution. The programs advocate for each consumer to live in the least restrictive environment, and provides education and training for consumers, case managers, and direct service providers.

LINKS TO RELATED PAGES

Library for the Blind and Physically Handicapped
Governor's Commission on Disability
Emergency Preparedness planning kit for individuals living with a disability
Cornell University's 2008 Disability Status Report for New Mexico*
Back In Use is dedicated to helping New Mexicans with disabilities get the equipment

CoLTS program (Coordination of Long-Term Services)
CoLTS C Waiver (formerly D&E Waiver)
Brain Injury Services Program
Personal Care Option (PCO)
Mi Via
Program of All-Inclusive Care for the Elderly
GAP Program
Money Follows the Person
All EDSD programs

they need either for free or at very little cost Links marked with an asterisk (*) are Adobe Acrobat pdf files. If necessary, click here to download Adobe Acrobat Reader at no charge.

Independent Living Centers in New Mexico Spinal Cord Injury Awareness

New Mexico Human Services Department: http://www.hsd.state.nm.us/isd/tanf.html

General Assistance: http://www.hsd.state.nm.us/isd/ga.html

The objective of general assistance is to provide cash assistance to dependent needy children and disabled adults who are not eligible for assistance under a federally matched cash assistance program, such as New Mexico works (NMW) or the federal program of supplemental security income (SSI).

Basic General Assistance Rules

- You must provide your SSN within 60 days of approval.
- You must be:
  - a citizen of the United States;
  - a naturalized citizen;
  - an alien that entered the United States as a legal permanent resident or PRUCOL before August 22, 1996; or
  - an alien who entered the United States on or after August 22, 1996, and who meets the definition of a qualified alien, and is subject to the five-year bar from participation in the federally funded TANF cash assistance program.
- You must be living in the state of New Mexico, and have demonstrated an intent to remain in the state.
- You CANNOT be:
  - included as a benefit group member and receiving cash assistance from another department cash assistance program;
  - an SSI recipient;
  - a recipient of benefits from a federally-funded TANF program (including a tribal program) or BIA-GA program;
  - a recipient of a government-funded adoption subsidy program; or
  - a recipient of benefits from a TANF or GA program in another state.
- You may not be the payee for more than one GA cash assistance payment.

- The Supplemental Nutrition Assistance program, Medicaid, LIHEAP and other similar programs are not considered concurrent assistance and shall not make an individual ineligible for GA cash assistance programs.

For more details please contact your <u>nearest office</u>.

Governor's Commission on Disability: http://www.gcd.state.nm.us/

Disability Links: http://www.gcd.state.nm.us/links.htm

New York

-A lot of drop down menus, but not bad for navigation...

Family: http://www.nysegov.com/citGuide.cfm?superCat=82

Aging: http://www.nysegov.com/citGuide.cfm?superCat=82&cat=388&content=main

Assisted Living
- Find Long-Term Care Insurance - PlanAheadNY.com
- Home Health and Hospice Profile
- New York State Partnership for Long-Term Care
- New York State Veterans Homes
- Osteoporosis
- Senior Citizens Insurance Resource Center
- Senior Programs Locator for New York City Residents
- Contact Your Local Office for the Aging
- Critical Questions to Ask About Senior Housing
- Eat Well to Age Well
- Explore Aging Facts, Figures & Reports
- Find Long Term Care Services
- Finding a Nursing Home in New York State
- Food Stamps (En Español)
- Foster Grandparent Programs
- Get Medicare Beneficiary Insurance Information
- Health Insurance Information, Counseling and Assistance Programs (HIICAP)
- Home Energy Assistance Program (HEAP) (En Español)
- Long Term Care Insurance Information
- Medicare Information & Assistance at HIICAP
- myBenefits.ny.gov (En Español)
- Retired and Senior Volunteer Programs
- Senior Citizen Resource Guide
- Senior Companion Program
- Senior Housing Definitions
- Stay Active & Fit for Healthy Aging
- Support for Families & Caregivers
- Utility Programs and Protections for Senior Citizens

Caregiving Support: http://www.aging.ny.gov/Caregiving/Index.cfm

Program For Families and Caregivers

Programs For Families & Caregivers

There are a variety of programs that support and assist caregivers. Such programs exist at the county offices for the aging, Alzheimer's Association, Red Cross, Cooperative Extensions, and other community and faith-based organizations. On-line resources are plentiful and easily accessible for people who cannot leave their loved one to attend a local training or support group.

New York Elder Caregiver Support Program

The New York Elder Caregiver Support Program assists informal caregivers - spouses, adult children, other family members, friends and neighbors in their efforts to care for older persons who need help with everyday tasks. Because of the assistance they receive, these older persons with chronic illnesses or disabilities are able to remain in their own homes in the community. Some local programs also assist grandparents and other older relative caregivers of children and promote the retention of the children in a nurturing family environment instead of placement in foster care. Informal caregivers are an invaluable resource to their loves ones and to the United State's health care system because of the care they provide.

While caregivers choose to support their loved ones, it is often challenging and can create physical, emotional and financial strains on the caregiver. Caregivers can turn to the New York Elder Caregiver Support Program for help and support with their unique caregiving circumstances. <u>Local offices for the aging</u> are ready to serve caregivers in their communities. Local caregiver support programs provide:

- **Information** about available services
- **Assistance** in gaining access to services
- **Individual Counseling, Support Groups, and Training** to assist caregivers in the areas of health, nutrition and financial literacy and to make decisions and solve problems relating to their caregiver roles.
- **Respite** to temporarily relieve caregivers from their responsibilities by providing a short-term break through home care, overnight care in an adult home or nursing home, adult day care and other community-based care.
- **Supplemental Services** to complement the care provided by the caregiver, such as a Personal Emergency Response System, assistive technology, home modifications, Home Delivered Meals, transportation.

New York@Home Programs and Services Supporting New York's Caregivers:
http://www.aging.ny.gov/NYSOFA/Programs/CaregiverSVCS/NYHomeCaregivers.cfm

1. Caregiver Resource Centers
2. Family Caregiver Council Information
3. Alzheimer's Disease Coordinating Council
4. Regional Caregiver Centers of Excellence
5. Social Adult Day Services Program
6. Respite Programs
7. NY Connects – Choices for Long Term Care

8. <u>NYS Senior Citizens Helpline</u>
9. <u>Alzheimer's Disease Supportive Services Program</u>
10. <u>Supplemental Nutrition Assistance Program(SNAP) and Older Americans Act Title IIIC-2 home-delivered meals</u>
11. <u>Older Americans Act Title IIIC-1 congregate nutrition program</u>
12. <u>Older Americans Act Title IIIE</u> - New York Elder Caregiver Support Program – Title III-E of the Older Americans Act

---

NewYork@Home Programs and Services Supporting New York's Caregivers

For additional information and resources - http://www.aging.ny.gov/Caregiving/Index.cfm

Informal caregivers – families, friends, neighbors, and loved ones of the growing aging population – play a critical role in helping older persons who need support with tasks of everyday living to remain at home in the community, maintain their independence, and the quality of their lives. In fact, informal caregivers are recognized as the bedrock of community care, providing 75 to 80 per cent of the daily assistance needed by those who need long-term care.

In New York State, there are an estimated 2.2 million family caregivers providing care, at an estimated value of $24 billion. This unpaid care saves billions of dollars in state and federal funds. Furthermore, caregiving is a fundamental aspect of family and community life; it is one way of expressing commitment to those one cares about, and gives meaning to human relationships. Informal caregivers are an invaluable resource for their loved ones and to the United State's health care system because of the care they provide. However, caregiving often comes at a price; it is challenging work, creating physical, emotional, and/or financial strains on the caregiver.

Housing Options: http://www.aging.ny.gov/Housing/HousingResources/Housing.cfm

Housing options for older people in New York State

The overwhelming preference of older people is to age in place in their own homes and apartments, and most older people are able to do that.

Aging in place can be a safe and successful experience if the physical aspects of a home accommodate a resident's physical and mental frailties, if the home is affordable, and if residents have easy access to necessary services and activities.

For some older people, changes in their physical, emotional, or mental health, or in their family, social, or financial situations may compromise their ability to continue living where they are. Such changes may persuade an older person to consider relocating to a more supportive living environment.

Whether choosing to age in place . . . or to relocate to another living environment, being an informed consumer-by gathering appropriate information-is critical to making the best housing choice, one that meets a person's needs and preferences.

Staying in your Own Home provides brief descriptions of a variety of programs and strategies that older people can employ to make "aging in place" a safe, successful option.

Descriptions-Retirement Housing Options provides brief descriptions of the major types of retirement housing that are available for older people in New York State.

Relocating-Critical Questions to Ask provides information on a number of topics that should be considered when making a decision to relocate from your own home into other types of retirement housing.

For a list of retirement housing options, information about housing-related programs, and information about in-home and community-based services available for older people in your county, please contact your local Office for the Aging.

Staying in Your Own Home: http://www.aging.ny.gov/Housing/Resources/Index.cfm

A major preference of older people is to continue living in their own homes for as long as possible. Sometimes, frailty or affordability issues compromise an older person's ability to age in place safely and successfully.

Service providers and advocates can assist older people and their caregiver families find access to programs and strategies that will enable older homeowners to remain living in their own homes. These options include the conversion of a home's equity into a source of additional monthly income, home repair programs, physical design modifications of an existing home to make it more useable by frail older people, and a variety of in-home and community-based supportive assistance programs. To view brief descriptions of these options, click on the following topics:

1. Reverse Mortgage
2. Property Tax Deferral
3. Property Tax Abatement
4. Sale/Leaseback
5. STAR (New York School Tax Relief Program)
6. Tax Form IT-214 (Circuit Breaker Program)
7. Home Energy Assistance Program (HEAP)
8. Utility Energy Assistance
9. Access to Home (modification) Program
10. RESTORE Home Repair Program
11. Weatherization Program
12. Section 504 Home Repair Program
13. Affordable Home Ownership (home rehabilitation) Program
14. Subsidized Housing
15. Section 8 Rental Assistance Program
16. Rent Control and Rent Stabilization
17. Senior Citizen Rent Increase Exemption (SCRIE)
18. Housing Counseling
19. In-Home and Community-Based Services

And under Staying in your Own Home:

http://www.aging.ny.gov/NYSOFA/Programs/CommunityBased/NYHomeCommunityBased.cfm

1. NY Connects: Choices for Long-term Care
2. Expanded In-Home Services for the Elderly Program (EISEP)
3. Community Services for the Elderly Program and Older Americans Act Title IIIB
4. Supplemental Nutrition Assistance Program (SNAP) and Older Americans Act Title IIIC-2
5. Congregate Services Initiative (CSI)
6. Transportation Operating Program
7. Naturally Occurring and Neighborhood Naturally Occurring Retirement Communities (NORCs & NNORCs)
8. Elder Abuse Outreach and Prevention
9. Long Term Care Ombudsman Program (LTCOP)
10. Social Adult Day Services Program (SADS)
11. Respite and Caregiver Support Programs
12. Nursing Home Diversion-Community Living Program and Aging and Disability Resource Center (ADRC) Expansion
13. Older Americans Act Title IIIC-1 congregate nutrition program
14. Farmers Market Nutrition Program

Disability Issues (Family):

http://www.nysegov.com/citGuide.cfm?superCat=82&cat=444&content=main

- Disability and Health in New York State
- Disability and the Law Video Series
- Financial Planning for Persons with Disabities
- Find Long-Term Care Insurance - PlanAheadNY.com
- Home Ownership for New Yorkers with Disabilities
- Taining and technical Assistance
- Forms of the Commission on Quality of Care
- Addresses and phone numbers for OMRDD Developmental Disabilities Services Offices (DDSO).
- Advance Directives for Mental and Physical Health Care
- Advocacy Services for Persons with Disabilities
- Blindness Services
- Commission for the Blind and Visually Handicapped Area Offices
- Complaints About Care and Treatment for People with Disabilities
- Developmental Disabilities Services Listing and Map
- Directory of Services for Persons with Developmental Disabilities
- Disability Benefits Qualification and Determination (En Español)
- Forms for OMRDD providers.
- Future Planning for a Child with a Developmental Disability
- Guardianship for a child with a Developmental Disability
- Investigation of Deaths in the Mental Hygiene System
- Long Term Care Insurance Information
- Office of Mental Retardation and Developmental Disabilities (OMRDD).
- Online (PDF) Forms for Workers' Comp\Disability Benefits Transactions
- Qualification for Disability Assistance (En Español)

◆Reporting Fiscal Fraud, Waste or Abuse in Mental Hygiene Programs
◆Rewarding Opportunities in Direct Support.
◆Rights\Obligations Under Workers' Compensation and Disability Benefits Laws
◆Services for people with mental retardation and developmental disabilities.
◆Surrogate consent for mentally disabled persons
◆The Commission on Quality of Care's Speakers Bureau.
◆The Handbook for Utility Customers with Disabilities
◆VESID - Assisting NYS Businesses Seeking Employees
◆Vocational and Educational Services for Individuals with Disabilities (VESID)
◆Vocational Rehabilitation District Office Information
◆What residential opportunities are available for people with disabilities.

Client Assistance Program (Cap): http://cqc.ny.gov/advocacy/protection-advocacy-programs/cap

The Client Assistance Program (CAP) is a federal program administered by the Commission to assist with problems encountered by individuals with disabilities seeking vocational rehabilitation, employment, and independent living services from the NYS Vocational and Educational Services for Individuals with Disabilities (VESID) or the Commission for the Blind and Visually Handicapped (CBVH). . There is also a list of local legal assistance and outreach contact offices.

CAP Brochure (English) (Spanish)

Informed Consumers Make Our Best Clients

The Client Assistance Program (CAP) provides New Yorkers who have any type of disability with information and assistance in securing training and services leading to employment and independent living. A CAP advocate near you can provide you with information on funding and services to assist you in achieving your employment and independent living goals.

The Commission administers the Client Assistance Program (CAP), as authorized and funded by the Rehabilitation Act, as amended. The Rehabilitation Act provides federal funding for states to provide a broad range of services leading to employment and independent living. The Scope of Services section of the Rehabilitation Act provides a summary of these training and service options available to meet the individualized needs of New Yorkers with disabilities.

A CAP program that provides legal and advocacy services to persons receiving services must be available to applicants and consumers of vocational rehabilitation services in order to receive Rehabilitation Act funds.

The Commission's CAP program is available free of charge to adults seeking information and referral, applying for Office of Vocational and Educational Services for Individuals with Disabilities (VESID) and Commission for the Blind and Visually Handicapped (CBVH) services, or in the process of receiving VESID or CBVH services. CAP is also available to assist students in transition from school to adult life with training and services leading to employment, and in resolving complaints with Independent Living Centers.

CAP Services

- Public Education on Vocational Services
- Information & Referral Individualized Advocacy Services
- Representation at Mediation, Administrative Reviews, Fair Hearing & Court

CAP Areas of Expertise

- VESID and CBVH Policies and Practices
- Student Loan Default Resolution
- Social Security Work Incentives Assessment & Referral
- Assistance with Transition from School to Adult Life
- Assistance in Transition from Sheltered Employment to Supported Employment
- Informational Trainings Targeting Undeserved Populations
- Assessment and Referral of Related Services Leading to Employment

CAP Network

Almost all the Commission's CAP funding is used to support regionally subcontracted offices. The system is designed to provide for individualized advocacy, "outreach" and legal support. Most CAP outreach offices are located in Independent Living Centers where there is access to related services that promote successful employment. The bulk of CAP day-to-day business is assisting persons with disabilities in getting vocational rehabilitation services and employment services from VESID or CBVH.

Individualized Advocacy Services & Representation

Usually the CAP advocate will learn about the consumer's goals, interests and abilities. CAP will then discusses with the consumer their rights under the Rehabilitation Act and the Individualized Plan for Employment (IPE). CAP advocates make every effort to inform consumers of services available through VESID/CBVH including but not limited to Evaluations, Supported Employment, College Training, Vocational Training, On The Job Training, Transition Services, Self Employment Services etc.

If a consumer is experiencing a conflict, the CAP advocate will contact the VESID or CBVH counselor to negotiate a resolution. When a negotiated settlement is not possible, CAP can represent consumers of service at formal mediation, administrative reviews, fair hearings and in court. Common issues addressed by CAP are:

- Agreement on an Employment Objective: when VESID or CBVH do not agree with the consumer that a particular objective is achievable;
- Appropriateness of Training: disagreements on where what type of training should be pursued;
- Evaluations: contested inaccurate or incomplete evaluations, or a consumer is seeking a customized assessment;
- Denial of Services: consumer is found not eligible for services, denied specific services, offered less-than-adequate services to meet needs,
- Employment/Placement: consumer wants assistance in finding employment, an integrated placement as opposed to a sheltered workshop setting, wants to be trained for a career rather than an entry level position; and
- Technology Issues: i.e., client needs adaptive equipment or services, to be employed or benefit from vocational rehabilitation services.

VESID & CBVH

In New York the State Education Department provides vocational counseling and services for New Yorkers with disabilities through the Office of Vocational and Educational Services for Individuals with Disabilities (VESID). For New Yorkers who are blind, the NYS Department of Children and Family Services provides vocational counseling and services through the Commission for the Blind and Visually Handicapped (CBVH).

Office for People With Developmental Disabilities

Putting People First: Housing Initiative: http://www.opwdd.ny.gov/housing/index.jsp

Welcome to OPWDD's Housing Initiatives

Home is truly where the heart is – and OPWDD realizes this vision for people with developmental disabilities as a "home of choice" outcome and offers a series of activities, projects, and strategies promoted by OPWDD and its partners to increase access to a variety of living arrangements both within the family home and beyond.

OPWDD is in the process of transforming its Home of Your Own Program (HOYO) to include a greater reliance on public/private partnerships to act as a catalyst to expand the supply of affordable and accessible housing for people with developmental disabilities, their income-eligible parents or legal guardians, and OPWDD's workforce.

These public/private partnerships will serve as the catalyst to convene other grassroots and regional housing stakeholders. The partnership will study local, regional, State and federal housing programs and policies. This will increase local understanding of the programs and policies available to assist people with developmental disabilities to address their housing needs. The partnerships will provide training and technical assistance to nonprofit and other organizations and act as an advocate for the expansion of affordable and accessible housing opportunities. This public/private partnership is in direct line with OPWDD's mission, vision and guiding principles – it Puts People First.

In addition, OPWDD's Office of Housing Initiatives offers a variety of supports and services to men and women who are interested in living more independently, or in realizing the American Dream of homeownership.

Housing Options Through OPWDD
Home of Your Own Program
Realizing the Dream
Mortgage Products
Upcoming Events
Home Grant Program
News and Press Releases
NY Housing Matters Newsletters
Additional Housing Information
Contact Us

North Carolina

To Live:

http://www.northcarolina.gov/1,1,North_Carolina_A_better_place_to_live,North_Carolina_A_better_place_to_live.html

Disability Services
  - Health and Human Services Info for People with Disabilities
  - Assistance for Persons with Disabilities
  - Services for the Blind and Visually Impaired
  - Services for the Deaf and Hard of Hearing
  - Vocational Rehabilitation Services
  - Obtain Assistance Living Alone
  - Governor Morehead School for the Blind
  - Social Security Disability Benefits
Health and Human Services for Older Adults
  ⊞ Services
  - County Health Departments
  - Federal Government Information for Seniors
  - Financial Assistance
  - Health and Human Services for Seniors
  - Resources for Finding Available Services
  - Retiring In North Carolina
  - Senior Tar Heel Discount Card
  - Services for Older Adults
  - Social Security
  - Tax Assistance
  ⊞ Healthcare
  - Diabetes
  - Heart Disease and Stroke Prevention
  - Immunizations for Adults
  - Mental Health Counseling Contacts
  - Nursing Home Complaint Hotline
  ⊞ Housing and Meals
  - Adult Care Home Case Management
  - Contacts for Congregate Meals
  - Contacts for Home Delivered Meals
  - Long Term Care Options
  - Low Income Energy Assistance Program
  ⊞ Work

Division of Aging and Adult Services: http://www.ncdhhs.gov/aging/service.htm

Services

The Division of Aging and Adult Services supports older and disabled adults and their families through a community-based system of opportunities, services, benefits, and protections.

Services for Older and Disabled Adults		
adult care home case management	health promotion *disease prevention evidence based medication management*	mental health counseling
adult day care		personal and family counseling
adult day health care	health screening	project care
adult placement services	health support services	respite - group / institution
adult protective services	home delivered meals	senior centers
at-risk case management	home health	senior companion
care management	housing and home improvement	state-county special assistance for adults
congregate nutrition	individual and family adjustment services	state-county special assistance for adults in-home program
family caregiver support		transportation *general medical*
foster care services for adults	in-home aide	
guardianship services	legal	

Directories
Aging Services

By County
(PDF)

By Service
(PDF)

County Fact Sheet

County Departments of Social Services

Caregiver Support: http://www.ncdhhs.gov/aging/services/fcsvc.htm

AAA Family Caregiver Resource Specialists

Region	Area Agency on Aging / Counties Served	Family Caregiver Specialist
A	Southwestern Commission Cherokee, Clay, Graham, Haywood, Jackson, Macon, Swain	Cindy Miles 828-586-1962, ext. 218 cindy@regiona.org
B	Land-of-Sky Regional Council Buncombe, Henderson, Madison, Transylvania	Carol McLimans 828-251-6622, ext 119 carol@landofsky.org
C	Isothermal Planning & Development Commission Cleveland, McDowell, Polk, Rutherford	Michelle Templin 828-287-2281, ext. 1258 mtemplin@regionc.org
D	High Country Area Agency on Aging Alleghany, Ashe, Avery, Mitchell, Watauga, Wilkes, Yancy	Brenda Reece 828-265-5434, ext. 128 breece@regiond.org
E	Western Piedmont Council of Governments Alexander, Burke, Caldwell, Catawba	Mary Mitchell 828-485-4256, ext. 256 Mary.mitchell@wpcog.org
F	Centralina Council of Governments Anson, Cabarrus, Gaston, Iredell, Lincoln, Mecklenburg, Rowan, Stanly, Union	Dawn Gartman 704-372-2416 dgartman@centralina.org
G	Piedmont Triad Regional Council Alamance, Caswell, Davidson, Davie, Forsyth, Guilford, Montgomery, Randolph, Rockingham, Stokes, Surry, Yadkin	Blair Barton-Percival (336) 294-4950 bbpercival@ptrc.org Holli Ward 336-761-2111 hward@nwpcog.org
J	Triangle J Council of Governments Chatham, Durham, Johnston, Lee, Moore, Orange, Wake	Ellison Jones 919-558-9391 ejones@tjcog.org
K	Kerr Tar Regional COG	Melissa Jones 252-436-2051

	Granville, Franklin, Vance, Warren, Person	mjones@kerrtarcog.org
L	Upper Coastal Plain Council of Governments Edgecombe, Halifax, Nash, Northhampton, Wilson	Kim Emory 252-234-5952 Kim.emory@ucpcog.org
M	Mid-Carolina Council of Governments Cumberland, Harnett, Sampson	Barbara White 919-323-4191, ext. 28 bwhite@mccog.org
N	Lumber River Council of Governments Bladen, Hoke, Richmond, Robeson, Scotland	Anne Oglesby 919-618-5533, ext. 3006 aco@mail.lrcog.dst.nc.us
O	Cape Fear Council of Governments Brunswick, Columbus, New Hanover, Pender	Holly Henderson 910-395-4553, ext. 204 Hhenderson@capefearcog.org
P	Eastern Carolina Council Carteret, Craven, Duplin, Greene, Jones, Lenoir, Onslow, Pamlico, Wayne	Mineko Holloway 252-638-3185, ext. 3011 mholloway@eccog.org
Q	Mid-East Commission Beaufort, Bertie, Hertford, Martin, Pitt	Sallie Williamson 252-974-1800 swilliamson@mideastcom.org
R	Albemarle Commission Camden, Chowan, Currituck, Dare, Gates, Hyde, Pasquotank, Perquimans	Catherine Smith 252-426-5753 csmith@albemarlecommission.org

Family Caregiver Support Program: http://www.ncdhhs.gov/aging/fchome.htm

North Carolina's Family Caregiver Support Program

Families are the major provider of long-term care in America. In 2008, about 20% of adult North Carolinians reported providing care or assistance to a family member or friend with a long-term illness or disability.

In an effort to help family and informal caregivers care for their loved ones at home for as long as possible, The National Family Caregiver Support Program (NFCSP), established in 2000, provides grants to States and Territories to fund a range of supports that assist these caregivers.

As the State Unit on Aging, the NC Division of Aging Adult Services administers the State's Family Caregiver Support Program. Services are provided locally through 17 Area Agencies on Aging.

The NFCSP offers a range of services to support family caregivers. Specific services vary by county but generally include:

- Information to caregivers about available services,
- Assistance to caregivers in gaining access to the services,
- Individual counseling, organization of support groups, and training to assist caregivers in the areas of health, nutrition, and financial literacy, and in making decisions and solving problems about their caregiving roles
- Respite care to enable caregivers to be temporarily relieved from their caregiving responsibilities; and
- Supplemental services, on a limited basis

These services can work in conjunction with other State and Community-Based Services to provide a coordinated set of supports. Studies have shown that these services can reduce caregiver depression, anxiety, and stress and enable them to provide care longer, thereby avoiding or delaying the need for costly institutional care.

FCSP Serves the Caregiver

Eligible family caregivers are:

- A caregiver of any age providing care for an older adult age 60 or older OR providing care for a person with Alzheimer's Disease or related brain disorder
- A caregiver (who is not the birth or adoptive parent), age 55 or older, raising a related child age 18 and under or an adult with a disability

For More Information

Contact the Area Agency on Aging that serves your County.

People With Disabilities: http://www.ncdhhs.gov/disabilities/index.htm

Services, Hotlines, Fact Sheets, Advocacy

Everything from A to Z

- Adjustment to Vision Loss
- Adult Care Home Case Management
- Adult Care Home Penalties
- Adult Day Services
- Adult Placement Services
- Adult Protective Services
- Alzheimer's Support Program
- Assistive Technology (For People with Disabilities)
- At-Risk Case Management (Services to

Services

Expand All Items Below | Collapse Items Below
 (Since your browser is not JavaScript-enabled, the Expand and Collapse links do not work. All items below are expanded by default.)

Advocating for People with Disabilities

- Children Services: Prenatal, Infants, and Preschool

Prevent Abuse, Neglect, or Exploitation)
- Boards and Commissions
- Business Enterprise Program (Employment for the Visually Impaired in Vending and Food Service)
- Child Service Coordination
- Client Assistance Program (Accessing and Understanding Disability Services)
- Community Alternative Programs (Help to Stay in the Home)
- Consumer-Directed Supports (Choices for Home Based Services)
- Counseling Services at Departments of Social Services
- Deaf Services
- Deaf/Blind Services from the Division of Services for the Deaf
- Deaf-Blind Services from the Division of Services for the Blind
- Developmental Centers:
    - Caswell Developmental Center
    - J. Iverson Riddle Developmental Center
    - Murdoch Developmental Center
- Developmental Disabilities Contacts (Local Management Entity Directory)
- Early Hearing Detection and Intervention (Newborn Hearing Screening and Followup)
- Early Intervention for Deaf and Hard of Hearing
- Eastern NC School for the Deaf
- Emergency Preparedness and Public Safety for the Deaf and the Hard of Hearing
- Employment Services for People with Disabilities
- Employment Services for the Visually Impaired and Deaf/Blind
- Family Caregiver Support
- Food and Nutrition Services (Formerly Food Stamps)

- Children Services: 5 to 22 years
- Communication and Technology, All Ages
- Developmental Disabilities and Special Needs, All Ages
- Employment Info for Job Seekers (ages 16 and up)
- Family Supports, All Ages
- Institutional Care, All Ages
- Living Independently
- Income Support
- Medical Services
- Residential Care
- **Hotlines**

- CARE-LINE Information and Referral Service (Help finding the programs and people to help you): **1-800-662-7030**
- Children with Special Health Care Needs Helpline: **1-800-737-3028**
- Home Health and Health Care Complaint Line (For nursing homes, hospitals, group homes, and other health care facilities): **1-800-624-3004**

Facts and Fact Sheets about People with Disabilities

- Governor Morehead Preschool (For the visually impaired)
- Governor Morehead School for the Blind
- Governor Morehead School Outreach Program
- Guardianship and Alternatives to Guardianship
- Hard of Hearing Services
- Heating and Cooling Assistance (Crisis Intervention)
- Housing and Home Improvement
- Independent Living for People with Disabilities
- Independent Living Services for the Visually Impaired and Deaf/Blind
- In-Home Aides
- Interpreters for the Deaf
- Long-Term Care Ombudsman (Advocacy for residents in long-term care facilities)
- Medicaid for Long-Term Care
- Medical Eye Care Program (Preserving or Improving your Vision)
- Nursing Home and Health Care Complaint Line (For hospitals, group homes, and other health care facilities): **1-800-624-3004**
- NC School for the Deaf
- Psychiatric Hospitals
    - Broughton Hospital
    - Central Regional Hospital
    - Cherry Hospital
    - John Umstead Hospital
- Regional Resource Program for the Deaf and Hard of Hearing
- Special Supplemental Nutrition Program for Women, Infants, and Children (WIC)
- State-County Special Assistance (For adult care home residents)
- State Facilities (alcohol and drug abuse treatment, developmental centers, neuromedical treatment, psychiatric

- Disaster Preparedness (1.6 MB PDF)
- Long-Term Care, About
- Medical Care Decisions and Advance Directives
- See also: Disability Statistics and Publications

Community Advocacy: How to get Involved

- Boards and Commissions
- Grant Opportunities

Divisions that Serve People with Disabilities

- Medical Assistance
- Mental Health, Developmental Disabilities and Substance Abuse Services
- Services for the Blind
- Services for the Deaf and Hard of Hearing
- Vocational Rehabilitation

hospitals)
- Telecommunications Access for the Deaf and Hard of Hearing
- Traumatic Brain Injury
- Vision and Hearing Loss Services
- Whitaker School (Long-term treatment program for emotionally handicapped adolescents)
- Wright School (Mental health treatment for children with serious emotional and behavioral disorders)
- Neuro-Medical Treatment Centers
  - Black Mountain Neuro-Medical Treatment Center
  - O'Berry Neuro-Medical Treatment
  - Longleaf Neuro-Medical Treatment
- Vocational Rehabilitation: General Services for People with Disabilities
- Vocational Rehabilitation: Employment Services for the Visually Impaired and Deaf/Blind

North Dakota

Department of Human Services: http://www.nd.gov/dhs/

Adult and Aging Services: http://www.nd.gov/dhs/services/adultsaging/

The Department of Human Services administers programs and services that help older adults and people with physical disabilities to live safely and productively in the least restrictive, appropriate setting.

- Publications
- Related Links

Services

Assisted Living Services

Family Caregiver Support Program

> Federally funded under the Older Americans Act, this program offers help to caregivers.

Home and Community-Based Care

> North Dakota provides home and community-based services through several programs, which each serve different needs.

- Service Payments for the Elderly and Disabled Program
- Expanded Service Payments for the Elderly and Disabled Program (Ex-SPED)
- Medicaid Waiver for Home and Community Based Services
- Older Americans Act Services

Information and Assistance - Aging and Disability Resource-LINK

> The Department of Human Services operates an Aging and Disability Resource-LINK funded under the Older Americans Act.

Long Term Care Ombudsman Program

> Individuals residing in nursing homes, assisted living facilities, basic care homes, or hospital swing bed, transitional and sub-acute settings may have concerns about their care. This program is intended to help resolve concerns.

Qualified Service Providers

- Find a Qualified Service Provider (database)

Information about how an agency or individual can enroll as a Qualified Service Provider (QSP) to provide personal or attendant care services, homemaker services and other approved services to eligible individuals.

Vulnerable Adult Protective Services

The North Dakota Legislature passed the Vulnerable Adult Protective Service Law in 1989. The law authorized the Department of Human Services to develop, administer, and implement a program of protective services for vulnerable adults.

Aging Services Division Contact Information:

Aging Services Division

Jan Engan, Director

N.D. Department of Human Services

1237 W Divide Ave, Suite 6

Bismarck ND 58501

Phone: 701.328.4601 / ND Relay TTY: 1.800.366.6888

Fax: 701.328.8744

E-Mail: dhsaging@nd.gov

Family Caregiver Support Program: http://www.nd.gov/dhs/services/adultsaging/caregiver.html

- **Fact Sheet**: ND Family Caregiver Support Program (68kb pdf)

Federally funded under the Older Americans Act, this program offers help to caregivers who are:

- Caring for an adult age 60 or older, or
- Age 60 years or older and caring for grandchildren or other young relatives who are age 18 or younger

Services Available

- Information about local services and supports
- Assistance from a trained Caregiver Coordinator to help caregivers assess needs and access support services
- Individual and family counseling, support groups, and training
- Respite care for caregivers

Services are provided FREE to qualifying participants. There is no means test. Individuals must be given the opportunity to contribute to the cost of the services; however, no one can be denied service due to inability or unwillingness to contribute.

Seeking Local Services

For information about the family caregiver support program and services in your area, contact a caregiver coordinator at your Regional Human Service Center.

Aging Services Division Contact Information:

Aging Services Division

1237 West Divide Avenue, Suite 6

Bismarck, ND 58501

Phone: (701) 328-4601

TTY: (701) 328-3480

Fax: (701) 328-4061

dhsaging@nd.gov

ND Aging and Disability Resource-LINK (800) 451-8693 [National]

Services to Individuals With Disabilities: http://www.nd.gov/dhs/services/disabilities/index.html

Services to Individuals with Disabilities

Disability Services Division in the Department of Human Services was formed in July 1996, through the merger of the Division of Developmental Disabilities and the Division of Vocational Rehabilitation.

Division of Vocational Rehabilitation

Division of Vocational Rehabilitation provides training and employment services to individuals with disabilities so they can become and remain employed.

Developmental Disabilities

Developmental Disabilities services provide support and training to individuals and families in order to maximize community and family inclusion, independence, and self-sufficiency; to prevent institutionalization; and to enable institutionalized individuals to return to the community.

Other programs within the realm of Disability Services

Disability Determination Services

Disability Determination Services provides eligibility decisions on behalf of applicants to the Social Security Administration.

Early Intervention Program

The Early Intervention Program is designed to identify in the earliest stages children at risk of developmental delays and to provide early assistance because the right help can make all the difference.

Vision Services

Vision Services help individuals with visual impairments so they can maintain independence in their home environments.

Independent Living Services

The purpose of Independent Living Services is to eliminate barriers and to provide assistance to individuals with disabilities so they can live and work more independently in their homes and communities.

Business Services

Business Services provides consultation, technical assistance and information to businesses so they can have an available source of qualified employees and receive solutions to disability-related issues.

Client Assistance Program (CAP)

The Client Assistance Program (CAP) provides advocacy, consultation, education, and referral to individuals who are seeking or receiving vocational rehabilitation services and independent living services so they can resolve issues and receive the services they are eligible to receive.

Other programs

Interagency Program for Assistive Technology (IPAT)

> Interagency Program for Assistive Technology (IPAT) is an independent entity. It provides education, consultation, and referral to people with disabilities so they can access assistive technology (AT) services and devices such as communication devices, adaptive computer equipment, seating systems, magnifying equipment, and much more.

Please select one of the above programs for more information.

Disability Services Division

1237 W Divide Ave, Suite 1A
Bismarck, ND 58501-1208
Phone: (701) 328-8930
Toll Free: (800) 755-8529
TTY: (701) 328-8968
Fax: (701) 328-8969
dhsds@nd.gov

ND Vocational Rehabilitation

(dba Rehabilitation Consulting & Services)

1237 W Divide Ave, Suite 1B
Bismarck, ND 58501-1208
Phone: (701) 328-8950
Toll Free: (800) 755-2745
TTY: (701) 328-8968
Fax: (701) 328-8969
dhsds@nd.gov

Ohio

Living in Ohio: http://ohio.gov/living/

Senior Resources

Adult Care and Planning [-]

- o Adult Protective Services
- o Alzheimer's Respite Care and Assistance
- o Long Term Care Guide
- o Long-term Care Ombudsman Programs
- o PASSPORT In-home Care
- Area Agency on Aging Directory
- Department of Aging

Golden Buckeye Card (Senior Discounts) [+]
- o Health and Nutrition [-]

- o Nutrition Services
- o Ohio's Best Rx
- o Ohio Senior Health Insurance Information Program - OSHIIP
- o Senior Farmer's Market Nutrition Program

Housing [-]

- o Energy Assistance Programs
- o Homestead Exemption
- o U.S. Department of Housing and Urban Development Information for Senior Citizens
- o Housing and Home Repair

Medicare [-]

- o Medicare Premium Assistance Program
- o Medicare / Medicare Part D Information
- Senior Centers
- Volunteer Opportunities

Long Term Care Consumer Guide: http://www.ltcohio.org/consumer/index.asp

Home Care and Other Options: http://aging.ohio.gov/resources/assessments/

Home and Community Based Services:
http://www.ltcohio.org/consumer/index.asp?html=homecare#HomeCareHead

National Family Caregiver Support Program:
http://aging.ohio.gov/resources/nationalfamilycaregiversupport/

Ohio Department of Aging National Family Caregiver Support Program

Are You A Caregiver?

Approximately 1.3 million Ohioans provide some level of care for a loved one who is older or who has a disability. You may be a caregiver if:

- You feel like you've swapped roles with a parent, spouse or other family member.
- You help someone with chores like cleaning, grocery shopping, cooking or transporation.
- You help someone with daily activities, such as bathing, dressing and eating.
- You help someone manage his finances, file insurance claims or pay bills.
- You skip meals or forgo exercise and the things you enjoy because someone needs you.

Brochure: 10 Questions That May Change Your Life (and the lives of the people in it)

Whom Does Caregiving Affect?

In Ohio, family caregivers provide care that, if provided by paid caregivers, would cost $14.2 billion each year. Caregivers are spouses, children, grandchildren, grandparents, brothers, sisters, aunts, uncles, friends, neighbors and more.

Approximately 60 percent of family caregivers are women, many of whom have their own families and jobs. More than three out of five workers have had to make some adjustment to their work life, from reporting late to giving up work entirely, to care for a loved one. Ten percent of family caregivers go from full-time to part-time jobs because of caregiving responsibilities.

Fact sheet: Whom Does Caregiving Affect?

Recognizing Elder Caregivers

Each year, the Ohio Department of Aging presents a handful of devoted caregivers with the Elder Caregiver Award. It is our way to honor them for the work they do to make Ohio a better place, while symbolically recognizing the combined value of all informal caregivers throughout the state.

Year of the Family Caregiver

The U.S. Administration on Aging has proclaimed 2011 the Year of the Family Caregiver to commemorate the 10th anniversary of the National Family Caregiver Support Program and spotlight the important role of family caregivers. Learn more at www.celebratingfamilycaregivers.org

Get Help

According to the National Family Caregivers Association, more than 90 percent of people who recognize themselves as caregivers become more proactive, engaged and confident, and provide better care as a result. Caregivers who access and use support services also report fewer negative emotions, such as depression, anxiety and anger. Through the National Family Caregiver Support Program, your Area Agency on Aging is ready to assist you with supports that may include:

- Care training, resources and information;
- Caregiver support groups;
- Respite care;
- Adult day services;
- Home delivered meals programs;
- and more.

Kinship Care

Caregiving has many faces in Ohio, and includes situations in which grandparents or other relatives or friends become primary caregivers for children when their parents are unable or unavailable to do so. These arrangements can be temporary, but often are permanent. In a system that typically favors the immediate family, these "extended" families often face unique challenges. The Department of Aging proudly supports KinshipOhio, a collaborative effort to ensure all kin caregivers are directed toward and able to access available supports.

Lifespan Respite Care

The Department of Aging is working with the Ohio Family Children First Council and the newly formed Ohio Respite Coalition to enhance respite services across Ohio. Lifespan respite care programs are coordinated systems of accessible, community-based respite care services for family caregivers of children or adults with special needs. For more information, on lifespan respite and caregiver support programs visit www.caregiver.org and www.archrespite.org.

In March 2011, state partners held the Ohio Respite Summit to support Ohio's lifespan respite grant application to be submitted to the Administration on Aging in spring 2011.

- Summit Summary Report
- Presentation by ARCH National Respite Network and Resource Center
- Presentation by Down Syndrome Association of Greater Cincinnati

Ohio Department of Aging Long-term Care Assessments

Planning ahead for long-term health care needs can reduce stress and ensure that personal choices are observed and that financial resources are put to best use. Planning ahead is never easy, but skilled staff at your Area Agency on Aging can help you explore your options and develop a care plan.

A professional long-term care assessment consultant (most often a nurse or social worker) will meet with you and your family for a free in-home evaluation of your current situation and future options. He or she will explain services available, discuss eligibility requirements and financial resources required, and help determine your needs and wishes.

Contact your Area Agency on Aging and ask for a free personal assessment today!

Area Agencies on Aging: http://aging.ohio.gov/resources/areaagenciesonaging/

About Area Agencies on Aging

Created by the Older Americans Act of 1965, Area Agencies on Aging respond to the needs of the elderly in the communities they serve. They are advocates, planners, funders and educators, as well as providers of information and referral services. Area agencies work with public and private partners to respond to the unique needs of older citizens and families in their areas.

Ohio has twelve area agencies, each serving a multi-county planning and service area. Agencies create local plans based on the population and resources in their communities.

While many state and federally funded programs operate the same way across the state, area agencies often have latitude in customizing their service delivery to provide the most appropriate system of care for their communities. The Department of Aging and other funding sources routinely monitor the area agencies, and the agencies in turn monitor their local partners who provide direct services.

Area agencies distribute federal, state and local funds to service providers. With few exceptions, area agencies do not provide direct in-home and community-based services. However, they do provide assessment and case management of consumers as well as provide information and referral to service agencies. Many also make available educational trainings and workshops for the citizens and professionals in their areas. The area agencies also house or coordinate with regional long-term care ombudsman programs, which assist consumers of long-term care services with choices and concerns.

The Ohio Association of Area Agencies on Aging serves as the collective voice for area agencies in the state.
Find them on Facebook.

In addition, Ohio has several County and Municipal Offices on Aging.

Find Your Area Agency

Council on Aging of Southwestern Ohio
Serving Butler, Clermont, Clinton, Hamilton & Warren counties
175 Tri County Parkway
Cincinnati, OH 45246
1-800-252-0155
www.help4seniors.org
Find them on Facebook.

Area Agency on Aging, PSA 2
Serving Champaign, Clark, Darke, Greene, Logan, Miami, Montgomery, Preble & Shelby counties
40 W. Second Street, Suite 400
Dayton, OH 45402
1-800-258-7277

www.info4seniors.org

Find them on Facebook.

Area Agency on Aging 3
Serving Allen, Auglaize, Hancock, Hardin, Mercer, Putnam & Van Wert counties
200 E. High St./2nd Fl.
Lima, OH 45801
1-800-653-7723
www.aaa3.org

Find them on Facebook.

Area Office on Aging of Northwestern Ohio, Inc.
Serving Defiance, Erie, Fulton, Henry, Lucas, Ottawa, Paulding, Sandusky, Williams & Wood counties
2155 Arlington Avenue
Toledo, OH 43609-0624
1-800-472-7277
www.areaofficeonaging.com

Find them on Facebook.

Ohio District 5 Area Agency on Aging, Inc.
Serving Ashland, Crawford, Huron, Knox, Marion, Morrow, Richland, Seneca & Wyandot counties
780 Park Avenue West
Mansfield, OH 44906
1-800-860-5799
www.aaa5ohio.org

Find them on Facebook.

Central Ohio Area Agency on Aging
Serving Delaware, Fairfield, Fayette, Franklin, Licking, Madison, Pickaway & Union counties
174 East Long Street
Columbus, OH 43215
1-800-589-7277
www.coaaa.org

Find them on Facebook.

Area Agency on Aging District 7, Inc.
Serving Adams, Brown, Gallia, Highland, Jackson, Lawrence, Pike, Ross, Scioto & Vinton counties
University of Rio Grande/F32
160 Dorsey Drive
P.O. Box 500
Rio Grande, OH 45674-0500
1-800-582-7277
www.aaa7.org

Find them on Facebook.

Area Agency on Aging 8
Serving Athens, Hocking, Meigs, Monroe, Morgan, Noble, Perry & Washington counties
1400 Pike Street
Marietta, OH 45750
Send mail to:
P.O. Box 370
Reno, OH 45773
1-800-331-2644
www.areaagency8.org
Find them on Facebook.

Area Agency on Aging Region 9, Inc.
Serving Belmont, Carroll, Coshocton, Guernsey, Harrison, Holmes, Jefferson, Muskingum & Tuscarawas counties
60788 Southgate Road
Byesville, OH 43723
1-800-945-4250
www.aaa9.org

Western Reserve Area Agency on Aging
Serving Cuyahoga, Geauga, Lake, Lorain & Medina counties
925 Euclid Avenue/#600
Cleveland, OH 44115
1-800-626-7277
www.psa10a.org
Find them on Facebook.

Area Agency on Aging 10B, Inc.
Serving Portage, Stark, Summit & Wayne counties
1550 Corporate Woods Parkway, Suite 100
Uniontown, OH 44685
1-800-421-7277
www.services4aging.org
Find them on Facebook.

Area Agency on Aging 11, Inc.
Serving Ashtabula, Columbiana, Mahoning & Trumbull counties
5555 Youngstown-Warren Road
Suite 2685 Second Floor
Niles, Ohio 44446
1-800-686-7367
www.aaa11.org

Residential State Supplement: http://aging.ohio.gov/services/residentialstatesupplement/

The Residential State Supplement (RSS) program provides a monetary supplement to low-income adults with disabilities who do not require nursing home care. The supplement, along with the consumer's income, pays for an approved living arrangement.

With the passage of H.B. 153, Ohio's 2012-2013 biennial operating budget, RSS officially transferred from the Ohio Department of Aging to the Ohio Department of Mental Health (ODMH), effective July 1, 2011. During this transition every effort is being made to ensure continuity for residents' payments and placements. As information about the program becomes available it will be distributed via ODMH's RSS web page.

Please call 1-855-777-6364 for more information and assistance.

Oklahoma

Residents: Seniors and Retirement: http://www.ok.gov/section.php?sec_id=35

- Seniors & Retirement
  - Adult Protective Services
  - Arthritis Prevention and Education
  - DisabilityInfo.gov - Federal Resource for Amercians with Disabilities
  - File an Insurance Complaint
  - Firefighters Pension and Retirement System
  - Heart Disease and Stroke Prevention
  - In-Home Care for Elderly and Disabled Persons
  - Law Enforcement Retirement System
    - Licensed Long Term Care Facilities Directory
    - Long Term Care Complaint Registry
  - Long Term Care Insurance
  - Medicare, Medicaid Fraud Resources
  - Police Pension and Retirement System
  - Programs and Services for Older Oklahomans
  - Public Employees Retirement System
  - Report Insurance Fraud
  - Senior Health Insurance Counseling Program - Medicare
  - Senior Insurance Buying Guides
  - Social Security Benefits Calculator
  - Teachers' Retirement System
  - Transportation Services
  - Volunteer Opportunities for Older Persons
  - Weather Notifications for Deaf and Hard-of-Hearing

In Home Care For Elderly and Disabled Persons: Aging Services: Advantage Services:
http://www.okdhs.org/programsandservices/aging/adw/default.htm

Service Information

The ADvantage Program of the Home-and Community-Based Services provides Medicaid services to help people stay at home instead of going to a nursing home. The program assists frail elders and adults who have physical disabilities.

A person must first qualify for Medicaid, a low income service, prior to receiving ADvantage. ADvantage cannot be provided for children or those individuals with mental retardation.

Online Services

- Community Services Worker Registry

Frequently Asked Questions: http://www.okdhs.org/programsandservices/aging/docs/#find

- Find what services are available through the AD*vantage* Services
- Get additional information

Contact Information

AD*vantage* Services Intake Line:
1-800-435-4711

AD*vantage* Services Consumer Inquiry System (CIS) Line:
1-800-435-4711

Aging: Frequently Asked Questions
AD*vantage* Services Intake Line:
1-800-435-4711

AD*vantage* Services Consumer Inquiry System (CIS) Line:
1-800-435-4711

OASIS:
(405) 271-6302
1-800-426-2747

Senior Infoline:
1-800-211-2116

RX for Oklahoma:
(405) 701-8216
1-800-RX4-OKLA

Transportation:
(405) 521-4214
1-800-498-7995
How Do I...
Adult Day Services:

- *Apply for Services?*
  To apply for services, contact the <u>OKDHS Human Services Center</u> nearest you.

- *Get a license?*
  <u>Adult Day Services</u> **is a structured, comprehensive program that provides a variety of health, social, and related support services in a protective setting for some portion of a day. Individuals who participate in adult day services attend on a planned basis during specified hours. If you are interested in providing day services, please contact the Oklahoma Department of Health.**

- *Learn about the requirements of a center, including a participants' rights?*

The rights of a participant in Adult Day Services and the requirements of any center can be found at <u>Adult Day Center Regulations</u> (Link opens in new window), information provided by the Oklahoma State Health Department.

ADvantage Services

- *Find what services are available through the ADvantage Services?*
  When you apply for AD*vantage* by calling one of the contact lines or going to your local county OKDHS office, you will be set up for an "assessment." A nurse will come to your home to complete the assessment. At that time, the nurse will determine if you are medically eligible for ADvantage. During the same time period, an OKDHS social worker will decide if you are financially eligible for ADvantage. If you are financially and medically eligible, a case manager will help decide what services you need and will develop a treatment plan for you. The case manager will also help to arrange the services. Services may include:

  - Adult day health care
  - Case management
  - Consumer directed personal assistance services & supports
  - Home-delivered meals
  - Home modification
  - Hospice
  - Occupational therapy
  - Personal care
  - Physical therapy
  - Prescription drugs
  - Specialized equipment and supplies
  - Speech therapy
  - Supported restorative assistance

- *Get additional information by calling the following numbers:*
  - AD*vantage* Services Intake Line:
    1-800-435-4711
  - AD*vantage* Services Consumer Inquiry System (CIS) Line:
    1-800-435-4711

- <u>The ADvantage Administration Unit Question site for OKDHS Employees</u> -

  The AD*vantage* Administration Unit has developed an improved form of communication for OKDHS employees, allowing them the opportunity to ask questions of the AD*vantage* Administration Unit regarding policies, procedures, programs and Member issues.

  We will answer your inquiry as promptly as possible. Please provide as much Member specific information as possible, to aide in our research. Please note that there is a maximum 24 hour turn around time during business days, for all inquiries.

Area Agencies on Aging:

- *Find out what kind of services are available?*

Services available at the <u>Area Agencies on Aging</u> (AAA) are numerous. Services are provided by <u>Older Americans Act</u> funds. Services are provided to seniors 60 and over, as well as to disabled or low-income individuals. Learn about the various services available:

- **Congregate and Home Delivered Meals:**
  Over four million meals are served each year, at 234 local nutrition sites throughout Oklahoma, and to homebound individuals. Meals are planned by a Registered Dietitian and must meet one-third of the recommended daily requirement.

- **Health Promotion:**
  Often located at the local nutrition site, health promotion services include provision of educational presentations, exercise programs, and health screening activities to persons sixty and older.

- **Nutrition Education:**
  Information on the benefits of healthy eating and exercise are provided to congregate and homebound meal participants.

- **In-Home Assistance:**
  Local projects are funded by Area Agencies on Aging to provide chore services, personal care, housekeeping, and home repair.

- **Outreach:**
  Skilled outreach personnel in each county provide one-on-one assistance to help older persons make informed choices.

- **Legal Services:**
  Educational presentations on legal issues of interest to older adults are provided, as well as individual legal assistance. Legal assistance is provided through the Legal Aid Services of Oklahoma.

- **Transportation:**
  Trips to the nutrition site, the bank, the doctor's office or grocery store allow older persons who no longer drive to remain independent in their communities.

- **Caregiver Assistance:**
  Services, education and support groups are available to family members who are caring for older persons.

- **Grandparents Raising Grandchildren:**
  A number of services are available to grandparents raising grandchildren. Educational opportunities, conferences and support groups are available.

- **Respite:**
  Respite care is a temporary break from long and arduous caregiving duties. Respite vouchers help caregivers pay someone who has temporarily taken their place as a care provider.

- **Long-Term Care Ombudsman:**
  Ombudsman advocate for the rights of residents in long-term care facilities.

- *Locate an Area Agency on Aging?*
  There are 11 Area Agencies on Aging throughout the state. Service areas are composed of counties. To locate a service area:
  - <u>Area Agencies on Aging locations</u>
  - <u>Area Agencies on Aging Key Personnel</u>

Caregiver Initiative:

- *Apply for services?*
  Services are funded and provided through the 11 <u>Area Agencies on Aging</u>.

- *Find out what type of services are available?*

  - *Assistance with access to community services*
  - *Counseling*
  - *Support groups*
  - *Training for caregivers*
  - *Respite services for caregivers*
  - *Other supplemental services*

Grandparent Initiative:

- *Find out about grandparent support groups?*
  The number of support groups for grandparents raising grandchildren is increasing in Oklahoma. Many of them offer child care so that both grandparents and their grandchildren have a chance to participate in the group. Support groups can offer: emotional support, guidance, assistance, advice, resources and information.

  The <u>Oklahoma Areawide Services Information System</u> (OASIS) (Link opens in new window) has a list of grandparent support groups within the state and contact information.

- *Get information about services for grandparents raising grandchildren?*
  A number of services are available to grandparents raising grandchildren (and other relatives serving as parents). To learn about services, resources and to get a manual entitled "Starting Points for Grandparents Raising Grandchildren," contact <u>OASIS</u> (Link opens in new window). OASIS serves as the grandparent clearinghouse for information in Oklahoma. The OASIS contact numbers are: 1-800-426-2747 or (405) 271-6302.

The <u>Community Relations Unit</u> of the <u>Aging Services Division</u> also presents two conferences per year to give grandparents information about resources and services. To get information about the conferences, contact the Community Relations staff.

Housing:

- *Find out about housing options?*

  - Assisted Living:
    Assisted Living may provide assistance with personal care, medications and ambulation. The center may also provide nursing supervision and information or unscheduled nursing care. The assisted living center cannot provide 24-hour skilled nursing care as is provided in a nursing facility.

- **Continuum of Care:**
  Continuum of Care combines the services of a nursing facility with an assisted living center and/or an adult day care center.

- **Independent Senior Housing:**
  This housing option offers various combinations of meal plans, housekeeping, laundry services, recreation and transportation services. No personal care such as bathing assistance is provided. Retirement communities may or may not include assisted living and nursing facility care on the same campus.

- **Nursing Facilities:**
  Nursing Facilities provide 24-hour skilled care and related services for residents who require medical or nursing care.

- **Residential Care Facilities:**
  This type of facility offers or provides residential accommodations, food service and supportive assistance. A residential care home may provide assistance with meals, dressing, bathing and other personal needs, and it may assist in the administration of medication. However, it cannot provide medical care.

Get a list of various facilities and regulations from the <u>Oklahoma Department of Health Long-Term Care Service</u> (Link opens in new window)

Legal Services:

- *Find out how to get legal services?*
  Information about legal services can be obtained through the <u>Area Agencies on Aging</u> (AAA), or by contacting the <u>Legal Services</u> Developer at the Aging Services Division. Helpful documents, such as Do Not Resuscitate, guardianship information and end-of-life forms are available through <u>Publications</u>.

Long-Term Care Ombudsman:

- *Become a volunteer Ombudsman?*
  The ombudsman program is supported by local volunteers who are committed to improving the lives of older persons in institutions. The <u>Area Agencies on Aging</u> Ombudsman Supervisors train, supervise and support the volunteers. Persons interested in volunteering should contact the <u>Ombudsman Supervisor</u> in their area, or state office <u>personnel</u>.
- *Compare Nursing Homes?*
  <u>Medicare</u> (Link opens in new window) provides information to help individuals decide what nursing home will meet their needs. The "Nursing Home Compare" allows searches by state, county, name of facility or proximity.

- *File a complaint with an Ombudsman?*
  To file a complaint, simply contact the <u>Ombudsman Supervisor</u> in the <u>Area Agencies on Aging</u> in which the long-term care facility is located.

- *File a complaint with the Health Department?*
  Long-term care facilities must be licensed by the Oklahoma Department of Health to provide care. Complaints can be made directly to the Health Department (.pdf, 1 pp, 23.1KB).

- *What does the ombudsman do with a complaint?*
  A long-term care ombudsman is a person who receives complaints from residents of long-term care facilities, their friends or relative and attempts to resolve those complaints within the facility. The Ombudsman has the authority to explore problems and recommend corrective action to the facility.

Pharmacy Connection Council:

- *Get cheap or no-cost prescription drugs?*
  The Central Oklahoma Community Action Agency, the Retired and Senior Volunteer Program and Oklahoma Pharmacy Connection Council have joined together to help inform Oklahomans of prescription drugs that may be of no charge to them. The RX for Oklahoma (Link opens in new window) Program connects persons who qualify for assistance with cheap or no-cost drugs from the drug manufacturers.

Respite:

- *Apply for services?*
  The Oklahoma Areawide Services Information System (OASIS) (Link opens in new window) can: answer respite questions, give qualifying information and send out applications for service.

- *Find out how much voucher money, will be received?*
  The voucher amounts for respite services range from $200 to $400, depending upon the funding source and availability of funds. The vouchers are good for three months. Once the vouchers expire, the caregiver can reapply by contacting OASIS.

  Vouchers are given to caregivers to buy respite from whomever they wish, as long as the person chosen is at least 18 years of age and does not live in the home of the caregiver or care receiver. If the caregiver does not have anyone to provide respite care, OASIS may be able to assist in locating a provider.

- *Learn more about respite?*
  The respite program lets caregivers take a break away from the duties of taking care of another person. Caregivers can use respite hours in the manner that best meets personal needs and desires. Respite can be used to visit family or friends, to run errands, spend an evening at the movies, to take a vacation, or to just catch up on much needed rest.

There is no income limit for:

  - Persons caring for individuals 60 and over

- Grandparents 55 or older raising grandchildren

RSVP

- *Learn about the volunteer programs of the Senior Corps?*
  The Aging Services Division has a publication that explains the different volunteer programs for older Oklahomans. The publication also gives contact information for all of the Senior Corps (SC) (Link opens in new window) sites within the state.

The three Senior Corps volunteer opportunities for older persons include:

- RSVP - matches persons 55 or older Oklahomans with local problems in their communities
- Foster Grandparent Program - Persons 60 and over provide valuable assistance to children with special needs
- Senior Companion Program - Volunteers 60 and over provide comfort and in-home assistance with daily living tasks to frail, homebound elderly persons.

State Plan Personal Care:

- *Qualify for services?*
  To see if you or someone you know might qualify for personal care service or other programs, contact your local county OKDHS Human Services Center. Your income will be a factor, as well as your physical condition. State plan personal care is available to persons of all ages who qualify financially and medically.

Transportation:

- *How to get a van?*
  The Capital Assistance Program provides vehicles for private non-profit organizations and public agencies (under certain conditions) for the transportation of older persons and persons with disabilities.

  Private non-profit organizations and public agencies may apply for a van by contacting the Support Services Unit staff of the Aging Services Division.

- *Become eligible?*
  In order to qualify entities must meet one of the following criteria's:

  1. Be a private non-profit corporation or association;
  2. Be a public body approved by the State to coordinate services for elderly and persons with disabilities;
  3. Be a public body which certifies to the Governor that no non-profit corporations or associations are readily available in the area to meet special

needs of the elderly and persons with disabilities.

Aging Services: Area Agencies on Aging: Contact information:
http://www.okdhs.org/programsandservices/aging/aaa/docs/contact.htm

Please note: The areas cover the following parts of the state:
<u>Area 1</u> is located in the northeastern part of the state and includes Craig, Delaware, Mayes, Nowata, Ottawa, Rogers and Washington counties.
<u>Area 2</u> is the mid-eastern part of the state and includes Adair, Cherokee, McIntosh, Muskogee,Okmulgee, Sequoyah and Wagoner counties.
<u>Area 3</u> is located in the southeastern part of the state and includes Choctaw, Haskell, Latimer, LeFlore, McCurtain, Pittsburg, and Pushmataha counties.
<u>Area 4</u> is located in the south central part of the state and includes Atoka, Bryan, Carter, Coal, Garvin, Johnston, Love, Marshall, Murray and Pontotoc counties.
<u>Area 5</u> is located in the east central part of the state and includes Hughes, Lincoln, Okfuskee, Pawnee, Payne, Pottawatomie and Seminole counties.
<u>Area 6</u> is the greater Tulsa metro and includes Creek, Osage and Tulsa counties.
<u>Area 7</u> is located in the north central part of the state and includes Alfalfa, Blaine, Garfield, Grant, Kay, Kingfisher, Major and Noble counties.
<u>Area 8</u> is the Oklahoma City metro and includes Canadian, Cleveland, Logan, and Oklahoma counties.
<u>Area 9</u> is located in the southwestern part of the state and includes Caddo, Comanche, Cotton, Grady, Jefferson, McClain, Stephens and Tillman counties.
<u>Area 10</u> is located in the southwestern part of the state and includes Beckham, Custer, Greer, Harmon, Kiowa, Jackson, Roger Mills and Washita counties.
<u>Area 11</u> is located in the northwestern part of the state and includes Beaver, Cimarron, Dewey, Ellis, Harper, Texas, Woods and Woodward counties.

Area	Counties	Agency	Address	Additional Contacts
1	Craig, Delaware, Mayes, Nowata, Ottawa, Rogers and Washington	Grand Gateway Area Agency on Aging (Link opens in new window)	333 S. Oak St. P.O. Box Drawer B Big Cabin, OK 74332-0502	• Area Agency on Aging Key Personnel • Area Ombudsman Supervisors
2	Adair, Cherokee, McIntosh, Muskogee,Okmulgee, Sequoyah and Wagoner	Eastern Oklahoma Development District (EODD) Area Agency on Aging (Link opens in new window)	1012 N. 38th St. P.O. Box 1367 Muskogee, OK 74402-1367	• Area Agency on Aging Key Personnel • Area Ombudsman Supervisors

3	Choctaw, Haskell, Latimer, LeFlore, McCurtain, Pittsburg and Pushmataha	Kiamichi Economic Development District of Oklahoma (KEDDO) Area Agency on Aging (Link opens in new window)	1002 HWY 2 North WILBURTON, OK 74578-3607	• Area Agency on Aging Key Personnel • Area Ombudsman Supervisors
4	Atoka, Bryan, Carter, Coal, Garvin, Johnston, Love, Marshall, Murray and Pontotoc	Southern Oklahoma Development Association (SODA) Area Agency on Aging (Link opens in new window)	224 W. Evergreen Durant, OK 74701	• Area Agency on Aging Key Personnel • Area Ombudsman Supervisors
5	Hughes, Lincoln, Okfuskee, Pawnee, Payne, Pottawatomie and Seminole	Central Oklahoma Economic Development District (COEDD) Area Agency on Aging (Link opens in new window)	400 N. Bell P.O. Box 3398 Shawnee, OK 74802-3398	• Area Agency on Aging Key Personnel • Area Ombudsman Supervisors
6	Creek, Osage and Tulsa	Indian Nations Council of Governments (INCOG) (Link opens in new window)	2 West Second Street, Ste. 800 Tulsa, OK 74103	• Area Agency on Aging Key Personnel • Area Ombudsman Supervisors
7	Alfalfa, Blaine, Garfield, Grant, Kay, Kingfisher, Major and Noble	Northern Oklahoma Development Authority (NODA) Area Agency on Aging (Link opens in new window)	2901 N. Van Buren Enid, OK 73703-2505	• Area Agency on Aging Key Personnel • Area Ombudsman Supervisors
8	Canadian, Cleveland, Logan and Oklahoma	Areawide Aging Agency (Link opens in new window)	4101 Perimeter Center Drive #310 OKC, OK 73112	• Area Agency on Aging Key Personnel • Area Ombudsman Supervisors
9	Caddo, Comanche,	Association of	802 Main St.	• Area Agency on

	Cotton, Grady, Jefferson, McClain, Stephens and Tillman	South Central Oklahoma Governments (ASCOG) Area Agency on Aging (Link opens in new window)	P.O. Box 1647 Duncan, OK 73533-1647	Aging Key Personnel • Area Ombudsman Supervisors
10	Beckham, Custer, Greer, Harmon, Kiowa, Jackson, Roger Mills and Washita	South Western Oklahoma Developmental Authority (SWODA) Area Agency on Aging (Link opens in new window)	Sherman Industrial Air Park Building 420 Sooner Dr. P.O. Box 569 Burns Flat, OK 73624-0569	• Area Agency on Aging Key Personnel • Area Ombudsman Supervisors
11	Beaver, Cimarron, Dewey, Ellis, Harper, Texas, Woods and Woodward	Oklahoma Economic Development Authority (OEDA) Area Agency on Aging (Link opens in new window)	330 Douglas Ave. P.O. Box 668 Beaver, OK 73932-0668	• Area Agency on Aging Key Personnel • Area Ombudsman Supervisors

Aging Services

Programs Information: http://www.okdhs.org/programsandservices/aging/

The OKDHS Aging Services Division (ASD) helps develop systems that support independence and help protect the quality of life for older persons as well as promotes citizen involvement in planning and delivering services.

Services

- Adult Day Services
- ADvantage Services
- Area Agencies on Aging
- Evidence-Based Fitness Programs (Link opens in new window)
- Grandfamilies
- Legal Assistance
- Long-Term Care Ombudsman
- Oklahoma Senior Corps Program
- Pharmacy Connection Council
- Respite
- State Plan Personal Care
- Transportation

Online Services
Contact Information

Phone: (405) 521-2281
Fax: (405) 521-2086

Mailing Address
2401 N.W. 23rd St., Ste. 40
Oklahoma City, OK 73107

- Contact local Area Agencies on Aging

Programs and Services for Persons with Disabilities
Quick Links
Programs and Services

- Adults
- Business and Employers
- Children/Youth
- Communities
- Families
- Health and Medical
- Older Oklahomans

Persons with Disabilities: http://www.okdhs.org/programsandservices/docs/disabilities.htm

- Adult Protective Services (APS) - Information about the program that investigates reports of abuse, neglect or exploitation of vulnerable adults, including persons with developmental disabilities.
- ADvantage Waiver - Provides Medicaid services to help people (including older Oklahomans and adults who have physical disability) stay at home instead of going to a nursing home. The program does not cover children or persons with mental retardation.
- Child Support Services - Services designed to help children get the support they need, including locating the non-custodial parents' addresses and employers, establishing legal paternity, establishing child and medical support orders, enforcing support for married, separated or divorced parents and modifying support orders.
- Developmental Disabilities Services - Provides services to persons ages 3 and older who have a primary diagnosis of mental retardation (IQ of 70 or below). The persons served may also have other developmental or physical disabilities in addition to mental retardation.
- Early and Periodic Screening, Diagnosis and Treatment (EPSDT) - Services that have an established schedule of exams to ensure the continued health of Medicaid eligible individuals up to age 21.
- Refugee Assistance - Cash and medical assistance programs are available to eligible refugees for

up to eight months after they arrive in the United States.

- Resource Centers - Public residential facilities that provide a full array of medical, therapeutic and vocational services as well as around-the-clock care for residents.
- SoonerStart - Oklahoma's early intervention program for infants and toddlers with disabilities and developmental delays.
- Supplemental Nutrition Assistance - Also known as the "nutrition safety net of the nation," these benefits help raise nutritional levels of low-income households.
- Supplemental Security Income - Disabled Child Program (SSI-DCP) - Services that assist children from birth to age 18, who receive a Supplemental Security Income Disability Payment, in getting needed equipment and services. This includes adaptive equipment and specialty formula from birth to age 18 and diapers from age 4 to age 18.
- Tax Equity and Fiscal Responsibility Act (TEFRA) - Program that allows children with physical or mental disabilities, who would not ordinarily be eligible for Supplemental Security Income benefits because of their parent's income or resources, to become eligible for Medicaid.
- Temporary Assistance for Needy Families (TANF) - provides temporary cash assistance in meeting basic needs, training leading to employment, employment services and child care assistance for qualified families
- Transportation - Provides funding for specialized public transportation services to the elderly and persons with disabilities. Grants are awarded in the form of vehicles to private, non-profit applicants in urban and rural areas.
- Utility Assistance Get information about cash assistance to help low income households to pay winter heating and summer cooling bill, and to provide help for families who have received utility cut-off notices.

Oregon

Department of Human Services: http://www.oregon.gov/DHS/index.shtml

Seniors and People With Physical Disabilities: Help in Your Home:
http://www.oregon.gov/DHS/spwpd/ltc/inhome.shtml

- Overview
- Client-employed Providers and Homecare Workers
- Independent Choices
- Oregon Project Independence
- Spousal Pay
- In-home services survey results (12/2004)

Overview
Seniors and people with physical disabilities can receive services while living in their own homes. These services include personal assistance, nursing tasks and help with housekeeping. Home-delivered meals can also be arranged. Medicaid may be able to pay for some of these services for eligible individuals.

Services may include help with:

- Bathing, dressing and personal hygiene
- Mobility and transfers
- Getting to and from the bathroom
- Housekeeping and laundry
- Meal preparation or delivery (Meals on Wheels)
- Memory and confusion
- Shopping and transportation
- Medical equipment
- Assistance with medications

For further assistance and information contact an Area Agency on Aging (AAA) or Department of Human Services (DHS) local office in your area.

Client-Employed Provider Program (CEP)
The Client-Employed Provider Program (CEP) allows Medicaid clients to select and hire their own care providers, called home care workers. Home Care Workers may be friends, neighbors, or relatives. For more information about employing someone to help you in your home, see the CEP Employers Guide (pdf). The case manager at your Area Agency on Aging (AAA) or Department of Human Services (DHS) local office may also have a list of care providers in your area.

If you are interested in becoming a Homecare Worker, you will find more information in the Home Care Worker Guide (pdf).

We can help

DHS wants clients to be actively involved in directing their care. The CEP Program offers the client the opportunity to control the selection and employment of a service provider. DHS and AAA case managers can help you arrange the services you need.

The case manager can help the client:

1. Select a qualified provider,
2. Get the provider enrolled as a Homecare Worker in the CEP Program,
3. Obtain a list of enrolled Homecare Workers,
4. Know what services are authorized,
5. Provide a task list for the Homecare Worker,
6. Identify potential risks and safety hazards in the home, and
7. Identify medical equipment to increase independence at home.

Independent Choices

This program offers you, the consumer, more choice in the way you receive your in-home services. The program turns control over to you, so that you can choose to purchase services as you need them. You will be able to manage your own care in ways that better meet your needs. Download the brochure (pdf)

To determine if you qualify, or for further assistance and information, contact the Area Agency on Aging (AAA) or Department of Human Services (DHS) local office in your area.

Back to top

Oregon Project Independence

Oregon Project Independence (OPI) serves individuals who are 60 years of age or older or who have been diagnosed with Alzheimer's disease or a related disorder, meet the requirement of our long-term care services priority rule and are not receiving Medicaid long-term care services except Food Stamps, Qualified Medicare Beneficiary or Supplemental Low Income Medicare Beneficiary Program benefits.

These services are provided statewide through Area Agencies on Aging local offices. Clients with net incomes between 100 percent and 200 percent of Federal Poverty Level (FPL) are expected to pay a fee toward their service, based on a sliding fee schedule. Families with net incomes above 200 percent FPL pay the full hourly rate of the service provided. Allowable services include personal care, homemaker/home care services, chore services, assisted transportation, adult day care, respite, case management, registered nursing services and home delivered meals.

Spousal Pay

The Spousal Pay Program is an In-Home Support Services program that allows payment for services that are provided by the spouse of an eligible person.

Individuals must be eligible for <u>Medicaid</u> and qualify for in-home services. They must also have a medically diagnosed, progressive, debilitating condition, which limits their <u>activities of daily living</u>, or a spinal cord injury or similar disability, which permanently impairs their ability to perform activities. Individuals on this program must need full assistance from others in at least four of the following six areas:

- Bathing
- Dressing and grooming
- Eating
- Cognition
- Elimination (going to the bathroom)
- Mobility.

Spouses must provide services that exceed what would usually be expected of a husband or wife. The spouse must be capable of meeting the individuals service needs.

For further assistance and information contact the Area Agency on Aging (AAA) or Department of Human Services (DHS) <u>local office</u> in your area.

Area Agencies on Aging and Seniors & People with Disabilities Services - Local Offices:
http://www.oregon.gov/DHS/spwpd/offices.shtml

Baker County
Baker SPD
3165 10th Street, Ste 400
Baker City, OR 97814
Phone: 541-523-5846
FAX: 541-524-0441
Community Connection of Northeast OR, Inc.
2810 Cedar Street
Baker City, OR 97814
Phone: 541-523-6591
FAX: 541-523-6592

^ *Back to top*

Benton County
OR Cascades West Council of Governments
1400 Queen Avenue SE, Ste 206
Albany, OR 97322
Toll free: 800-638-0510
Phone: 541-967-8630
FAX: 541-967-6423

^ *Back to top*

Clackamas County
Clackamas Area Agency on Aging
2051 Kaen Road, 1st Floor
PO Box 2950
OR City, OR 97045-0295
Phone: 503-655-8640
FAX: 503-650-5722
Canby SPD
214 SW 2nd
Canby, OR 97013-4140
Phone: 503-263-6700
FAX: 503-263-6655
TTY: 503-263-6654
Estacada SPD
320 SW Zobrist St
Mailing address:
PO Box 370
Estacada, OR 97023
Phone: 503-630-4605
FAX: 503-630-5600
TTY: 503-630-4702
Milwaukie SPD
4382 SE International Way, Ste C
Milwaukie, OR 97222-4627

Phone: 971-673-6600
FAX: 971-673-6637
TTY: 971-673-6639
Oregon City SPD
221 Molalla Ave, Ste 104
Oregon City, OR 97045
Phone: 971-673-7600
FAX: 971-673-7637
TTY: 971-673-7638
Clatsop County
Northwest Senior and Disability Services
(NWSDS)
2002 SE Chokeberry Road
Warrenton, OR 97146
Phone: 503-861-4200
Fax: 503-861-0934
Toll free: 800-442-8614

^ Back to top

Columbia County
Area Agency on Aging
125 N. 17th St
St Helens, OR 97051
Phone: 503-397-3511
FAX: 503-397-3290
St. Helens SPD
500 N Highway 30, Suite 240
St. Helens, OR 97051-1200
Phone: 503-397-5863
Voice/TTY: 503-397-2797
FAX: 503-397-0389

^ Back to top

Coos County
Area Agency on Aging
93781 Newport Lane
Post Office Box 1118
Coos Bay, OR 97420-4030
Toll-free: 800-858-5777
Phone: 541-269-2013
FAX: 541-267-0194
TTY: 541-267-4477
Coquille SPD
341 Second Street
Coquille, OR 97423

Phone: 541-396-7282
FAX: 541-396-2962
North Bend SPD
3030 Broadway
North Bend, OR 97459
Phone: 541-756-2017
FAX: 541-756-1861
TTY: 541-756-8799

^ Back to top

Crook County
Prineville SPD
457 NE Ochoco Plaza Drive, Ste C
Prineville, OR 97754
Phone: 541-447-4511
FAX: 541-447-8010

^ Back to top

Curry County
Area Agency on Aging
93781 Newport Lane
PO Box 1118
Coos Bay, OR 97420-4030
Toll free: 800-858-5777
Phone: 541-269-2013
FAX: 541-267-0194
Brookings SPD
586 5th Street, Suite 200
Brookings, OR 97415
Toll free: 800-419-1371
Phone: 541-469-9299
FAX: 541-469-0632
Gold Beach SPD
94145 West Fifth Place
PO Box 1170
Gold Beach, OR 97444-1170
Toll free: 800-257-1385
Voice/TTY: 541-247-4515
FAX: 541-247-5938

^ Back to top

Deschutes County
Central OR Council on Aging
1135 SW Highland Ave.
Redmond, OR 97756

Phone: 541-548-8817
FAX: 541-548-2893
COG Office
1135 SW Highland Ave.
Redmond, OR 97756
Phone: 541-548-8817
FAX: 541-548-3826
Bend SPD
1300 NW Wall St., Suite 102
Bend, OR 97701
Toll free: 800-452-5684
Phone: 541-388-6240
FAX: 541-388-6490
La Pine SPD
16493 Bluewood Pl, Suite 1
PO Box 98
La Pine OR 97739
Phone: 541-536-8919
FAX: 541-536-8798
Redmond SPD
1135 SW Highland
Redmond, OR 97756-2650
Phone: 541-548-2206
FAX: 541-548-6026

^ Back to top

Douglas County
Douglas County Senior Services
621 W. Madrone Street, Room 316
Post Office Box 2189
Roseburg, OR 97470-3093
Toll free: 800-234-0985
Phone: 541-440-3580
FAX: 541-440-3599
TTY: 541-440-3548
E-mail: seniors@co.douglas.or.us
West Office - Reedsport
Douglas County Senior Services
680 Fir Avenue
Reedsport, OR 97467-1431
Phone: 541-271-4835
FAX: 541-271-5039
Roseburg Disability Services
251 NE Garden Valley Blvd., Suite A
Roseburg, OR 97470-0321
Toll free: 800-548-3381

Phone: 541-440-3427
FAX: 541-440-3482

^ Back to top

Gilliam County - See Wasco County

^ Back to top

Grant County
Grant County Services
Area Agency on Aging
142 NE Dayton
John Day, OR 97845
Phone: 541-575-2949
FAX: 541-575-2248
John Day/Grant SPD
725 W Main, Suite E
John Day, OR 97845
Toll free (Voice/TTY): 800-358-6267
Phone: 541-575-0255
FAX: 541-575-2910

^ Back to top

Harney County
Harney County Senior Citizens, Inc.
17 S Alder Street
Mailing address: P.O. Box 728
Burns, OR 97720-2048
Phone: 541-573-6024
FAX: 541-573-6025
SPD Office:
Burns/Harney
809 W Jackson, Suite 300
Burns, OR 97720
Toll free: 800-442-2867
Voice/TTY: 541-573-2691
FAX: 541-573-5823

^ Back to top

Hood River County - See Wasco County

^ Back to top

Jackson County

Rogue Valley Council of Governments
Central Point
155 N. First Street
PO Box 3275
Central Point, OR 97502-2209
Phone: 541-664-6674
FAX: 541-664-7927
Medford Senior Services Office
2860 State Street
Medford, OR 97504-8474
Phone: 541-776-6222
FAX: 541-776-6215
TTY: 541-732-1801
Medford Disability Services Office
28 W 6th, Suite D
PO Box 880
Medford, OR 97501-0063
Toll free: 800-336-8204
Phone: 541-776-6210
FAX: 541-776-6251

^ Back to top

Jefferson County
Madras SPD
678 NE Highway 97, Suite D
Madras, OR 97741
Phone: 541-475-6773
FAX: 541-475-3012
TTY: 541-475-2292

^ Back to top

Josephine County
Rogue Valley Council of Governments
155 N. First Street
PO Box 3275
Central Point, OR 97502-2209
Phone: 541-664-6674
FAX: 541-664-7927
Grants Pass Senior & Disability Services Office
2166 NW Vine Street, Suite J
Grants Pass, OR 97526-1635
Toll free: 800-633-6409
Phone: 541-474-3110
FAX: 541-474-3125

^ Back to top

Klamath County
Klamath Basin Senior Citizens Council
2045 Arthur St.
Mailing address: P.O. Box JE
Klamath Falls, OR 97602-1205
Phone: 541-883-7171
FAX: 541-883-7175
Klamath Falls SPD
714 Main Street, First Floor
Klamath Falls, OR 97601
Toll free (Voice/TTY): 888-283-9005
Voice/TTY: 541-883-5551
FAX: 541-883-5652

^ Back to top

Lake County
Lake County Seniors
11 North G Street
Lakeview, OR 97630
Phone: 541-947-4966
FAX: 541-947-6085
Lakeview SPD
108 E Street N
Lakeview, OR 97630
Toll free: 866-787-2900
Phone: 541-947-3172
Fax: 541-947-5076

^ Back to top

Lane County
Eugene AAA Lane Council of Governments
1015 Willamette, Suite 200
PO Box 11336
Eugene, OR 97440-3536
Toll free: 800-441-4038
Phone: 541-682-4498
FAX: 541-682-2484
TTY: 541-682-4567
E-mail, s&ds@lcog.org

Cottage Grove AAA Lane Council of Governments
37 N. 6th
Cottage Grove, OR 97424
Phone: 541-682-7800

^ Back to top

FAX: 541-682-7820
TTY: 541-682-7821
Seniors & People with Disabilities, LCOG - Florence
3180 Highway 101
Florence, OR 97439-0066
Phone: 541-902-9430
FAX: 541-902-2115

^ Back to top

Lincoln County
OR Cascades West Council of Governments (OCWCOG)
1400 Queen Avenue SE, Suite 206
Albany, OR 97322
Toll free: 800-638-0510
Phone: 541-967-8630
FAX: 541-967-6423
Toledo/Lincoln SSD OCWCOG
203 N. Main Street
Toledo, OR 97391
Information: 541-336-2289
Toll free: 800-282-6194
FAX: 541-336-1510
TTY: 541-336-8103
Toledo/Lincoln DSO
203 North Main
Toledo, OR 97391
Phone: 541-336-2289
FAX: 541-336-1517
TTY: 541-336-8103

^ Back to top

Linn County
Albany Senior Services Office -
OR Cascades West Council of Governments
1400 Queen Avenue SE, Ste 206
Albany, OR 97322
Toll free: 800-638-0510
Phone: 541-967-8630
FAX: 541-967-6423
Albany Disability Services Office
1400 Queen Ave SE, Suite 103
Albany, OR 97321
Toll free: 888-533-2233
Phone: 541-928-3636

FAX: 541-928-3729
TTY: 541-928-3670

^ Back to top

Malheur County
Malheur Council on Aging
842 SE First Avenue
PO Box 937
Ontario, OR 97914
Phone: 541-889-7651
FAX: 541-889-4940
Ontario/Malheur SPD
186 East Lane, Suite 4
Ontario, OR 97914-1849
Voice/TTY: 541-889-7553
FAX: 541-889-2485

^ Back to top

Marion County
(NWSDS) - North Salem Aging & Disability Office
3410 Cherry Ave NE
PO Box 12189
Salem, OR 97309-0189
Toll free: 800-469-8772
Phone: 503-304-3400
FAX: 503-304-3434
(NWSDS) South Salem Aging & Disability Office
3501 Fairview Industrial Drive SE
PO Box 12099
Salem, OR 97309-0099
Phone: 503-798-9060
FAX: 503-798-9065
TTY: 503-375-3584
(NWSDS) Woodburn Aging & Disability Office
1320 Meridian Drive
Woodburn, OR 97071-0297
Phone: 503-981-5138
FAX: 503-981-5145
TTY: 503-370-4307

^ Back to top

Morrow County
Community Action Program East Central OR
721 SE 3rd, Suite D

Pendleton, OR 97801
Toll free: 800-752-1139
Phone: 541-276-1926
FAX: 541-276-7541
Hermiston SPD
940 SE Columbia Drive, Suite E
Hermiston, OR 97838
Toll free: 888-374-8080
Phone: 541-567-2274
FAX: 541-567-4893
TTY: 541-564-2782

^ Back to top

Multnomah County
Branch 3515 - Multnomah County Aging and Disability Services
10615 SE Cherry Blossom Dr
Portland, OR 97216
Phone: 503-988-5480
FAX: 503-988-3490
TTY: 503-988-5436
Branch 2813 - Mid-area Aging and Disability Services Office and Mid-County YWCA
5139 N Lombard
Portland, OR 97203
Phone: 503-721-6777
TTY: 503-988-5436
FAX: 503-721-6781
Branch 3512 - IRCO Senior District Center
10615 SE Cherry Blossom Dr
Portland, OR 97216
Phone: 503-988-5480
FAX: 503-988-6039
TTY: 503-988-5436
Branch 3518 - East Multnomah Aging & Disability Services
600 NE 8th Street, Room 100
Gresham, OR 97030
Phone: 503-988-3840
FAX: 503-306-5676
TTY: 503-306-5678
Branch 3519 - East Multnomah DO - YWCA
600 NE 8th Street
Room 100
Gresham, OR 97030
Phone: 503-988-3840

FAX: 503-988-5676
TTY: 503-988-5678
Branch 2818 - Portland North/Northeast Aging Services Office
5325 NE Martin Luther King Boulevard
Building 322A, Main Floor
Portland OR 97211-3237
Phone: 503-988-5470
FAX: 503-988-5430
Branch 1412 - Portland Impact (OPI)
4610 SE Belmont Street, 2nd floor, Suite 102
Portland, OR 97215-1752
Phone: 503-988-3660
FAX: 503-988-3261
TTY: 503-988-6026
Branch 1413 - Adult Protective Services/ADS
4610 SE Belmont Street, Suite 206
Portland, OR 97215-1752
Phone: 503-988-4450
FAX: 503-988-4480
TTY: 503-988-4493
Branch 1418 - SE Portland ASO/DSO
4610 SE Belmont Street, Suite 200
Portland, OR 97215-1752
Phone: 503-988-3660
FAX: 503-988-3784
TTY: 503-988-6026
Branch 2518 - Portland West Aging Services Office
421 SW Oak St, Ste 175
Portland, OR 97204
Phone: 503-988-5460
FAX: 503-988-3560

^ Back to top

Polk County
Dallas Aging and Disability Services
260 NE Kings Valley Hwy
Dallas, OR 97338-0089
Toll free: 866-582-7458
Phone: 503-623-2301
FAX: 503-606-7601
TTY: 503-370-4307

^ Back to top

Sherman County - See Wasco County

^ Back to top

Tillamook County
Northwest Senior and Disability Services
(NWSDS)
5010 E Third Street
Tillamook, OR 97141
Toll free: 800-584-9712
Phone: 503-842-2770
FAX: 503-842-6290

^ Back to top

Umatilla County
Community Action Program East Central OR
721 SE 3rd., Suite D
Pendleton, OR 97801
Toll free: 800-752-1139
Phone: 541-276-1926
FAX: 541-276-7541
Hermiston SPD
940 SE Columbia Drive, Suite E
Hermiston, OR 97838
Toll free: 888-374-8080
Phone: 541-567-2274
FAX: 541-567-4893
TTY: 541-564-2782
Milton-Freewater SPD
303 N Columbia Street
Milton-Freewater, OR 97862
Phone: 541-938-4925
FAX: 541-938-4927
Pendleton SPD
1555 Southgate Place
Pendleton, OR 97801
Toll free: 800-442-4352
Phone: 541-278-4161
TTY: 541-278-1094
FAX: 541-278-0140

^ Back to top

Union County
Community Connection of Northeast OR, Inc.
104 Elm Street
La Grande, OR 97850-2621
Phone: 541-963-3186
FAX: 541-963-3187

La Grande SPD
1607 Gekeler Lane
La Grande, OR 97850
Toll free: 800-430-7231
Phone: 541-963-7276
FAX: 541-963-7698

^ Back to top

Wallowa County
Community Connection of Wallowa County
702 NW First
Enterprise, OR 97828
Phone: 541-426-3840
FAX: 541-426-6260
Enterprise SPD
104 Litch Street
PO Box 180
Enterprise, OR 97828
Phone: 541-426-3155
FAX: 541-426-3878
TTY: 541-426-3155

^ Back to top

Wasco County
Mid-Columbia COG
1113 Kelly Avenue
The Dalles, OR 97058
Phone: 541-298-4101
FAX: 541-298-2084
The Dalles SPD
3641 Klindt Drive
The Dalles, OR 97058
Toll free: 800-452-2333
Phone: 541-298-4114
FAX: 541-298-1251
TTY: 541-298-3270

^ Back to top

Washington County
Hillsboro SPD
133 SE Second Avenue
Hillsboro, OR 97123-4026
Phone: 503-640-3489
FAX: 503-640-6167

Tigard - SPD
11515 SW Durham Road, Suite E-5
Tigard, OR 97224
Phone: 503-968-2312
FAX: 503-624-8128
Beaverton - SPD
4805 SW Griffith Drive, Suite B
Beaverton, OR 97005-8722
Voice/TTY: 503-627-0362
FAX: 503-671-9076

^ Back to top

Wheeler County - See <u>Wasco County</u>

^ Back to top

Yamhill County
NorthWest Senior & Disability Services -
McMinnville Aging & Disability Services
300 SW Hill Road
McMinnville, OR 97128
Toll free: 866-333-7218
Phone: 503-472-9441
FAX: 503-472-4724

Caregiving: http://www.oregon.gov/DHS/spwpd/caregiving/home.shtml

- Overview
    - Who is a caregiver?
    - Successful caregiving
    - Types of caregiving
- Care of the caregiver
- Chronic pain - caregiver tips

- Communicating caregiving issues
- Native American caregiving
- National Family Caregiver Support Program
- Resources for caregivers
- Respite care (Lifespan Respite Care program)

Also see Long-term care

Overview

Explore the many issues facing caregivers today. Whether you're an informal caregiver caring for a relative, or a professional caregiver - all caregivers share certain experiences. This section deals with many of the issues facing caregivers today. You'll find information, resources and answers to your caregiving questions.

Who is a caregiver?

A caregiver is anyone who provides assistance to another person so that person can maintain an independent lifestyle. Family members and other informal caregivers are the backbone of Oregon's long-term care system.

For many people, caregiving isn't a job or a duty. It is doing what is right for a loved one. Caregiving is an unspoken promise that so many of us make in our relationships, to be there for our loved ones when they need us. Unfortunately, few people have the time, resources or ability to care for their aging or disabled loved one without any help. It is important as a caregiver to know your limits, take care of yourself, know your resources in the community, and understand the wants and needs of the person needing care.

Successful caregiving

Being a successful caregiver means finding a balance between providing the necessary care and encouraging the care receiver to be as independent as possible. Discussing the following questions with the person under your care may help you find the balance.

- How does she/he see herself in the role of the care receiver?
- What does she/he need from you?
- What can she/he do for herself?
- Does she/he know what to expect from you?
- Can you meet those expectations?
- What support is available in your family and community?

The caregiver is one of the most important people in the life of the care receiver. A caregiver doesn't have to be family or a loved one. There are numerous types of caregivers. Sometimes the best care plan includes a combination of caregiving types and caregivers.

Types of caregiving

There are two primary forms of caregiving: informal and formal.

Informal caregiving and long distance caregiving. Informal caregivers are usually family members, spouses, adult children and friends who provide unpaid assistance to an aging or disabled person. Most informal caregivers are women who provide assistance ranging from a few hours of shopping and cleaning to intensive 24-hour care. The care receivers are typically an aging parent or a spouse with a disability.

Long distance caregiving places additional burdens on a caregiver. Maybe you don't even consider yourself a caregiver because you live out of town and are away from the care receiver. You are still a caregiver. Do you call your loved one on a regular schedule due to her illness or disability? Do you spend your vacations visiting and helping the care receiver? You are not alone - approximately seven million Americans are involved in providing care for an aging relative or friend who lives at least an hour away. According to a 1997 survey co-sponsored by The National Council on the Aging and The Pew Charitable Trusts, the caregivers surveyed lived, on average, 300 miles away from their care recipient. Those who were the primary caregivers spent an average of 35 hours per month providing care.

If you are providing care from a distance, you probably have struggled with some of the following challenges:

- Maintaining effective communications with the care receiver
- Managing feelings of guilt or anger over the situation
- Attempting to balance your time with, and away, from the care receiver
- Locating resources in the care receiver's community.

All long distance caregivers face these challenges, and more. If you are feeling guilty or angry over the situation, try to understand why. Write down your feelings and try to find meaning in them. What is it about the situation that makes you feel anger or guilt? Is it something you can control? As a caregiver, the most important thing you can do is take care of yourself first.

Try to find a local support system for the care receiver. Check out what is available in the community and discuss the options. Offer ideas, but do not put a support system in place without the involvement of the care receiver.

Resources for Caregiving: http://www.oregon.gov/DHS/spwpd/caregiving/resources.shtml

Caregiver resources

The goal of caregiving is to help someone maintain an independent lifestyle as long as possible. What's the best way to achieve this? You can begin by being well-prepared and well-informed. DHS has several ways to help you.

- Oregon services and programs
- Other resources

Oregon Services and programs
Adult Day Services/Care

Adult day care can provide respite care as well as ongoing services. Learn more about this program. ADRC of Oregon

ADRC of Oregon is a comprehensive Web-based directory of local services for seniors and people with disabilities. The site will help all Oregonians find answers to questions about adult care facilities, Alzheimer's, end-of-life care, health care, care giving, nutrition, home repair, recreation, transportation and much more.

Oregon Lifespan Respite Care Program

Respite care services give families and other caregivers temporary relief from providing care for frail adults. Companionship, light assistance, recreational activities and security are provided in your home, out of the home in a group setting, or overnight in a residential setting. Respite care fosters a healthier quality of life for both the caregiver and care receiver.

The Oregon Lifespan Respite Care Program, part of DHS, helps counties develop and implement community-based lifespan respite care networks. The Lifespan networks help families and caregivers locate respite care services in their communities. DHS also has a list of other resources to help caregivers.

Oregon Home Care Commission (OHCC)

The Commission is responsible for ensuring the quality of home care services that are funded by the Department of Human Services for seniors and people with disabilities. The OHCC Registry and Referral System matches consumer-employers with available homecare workers. The Registry will assist employers to find and hire homecare workers by providing information about potential employees. The system can also assist with emergency and respite referrals.

Needs assessment and case management

When you or someone you care about needs more help than you have available, or if you are thinking about nursing home care, we can help you sort out the choices that may be available to you. We can also give you facts about care costs and help you plan so that you get the most for your money. Contact your DHS or Area Agency on Aging local office for help and more information.

Other resources

- AARP
- Administration on Aging web page for Elders & Caregivers
- Alzheimer's Disease Education & Referral Center
- Caregiver.com - online magazine
- Caregiving.com
- Family Caregiver Alliance
- National Alliance for Caregiving
- Nations Voice on Mental Illness (NAMI)
- National Family Caregiver Association (NFCA)
- NFCA - Tips & guides
- OHSU Caregiving Support
- Pain.com for information about chronic pain
- Rosalynn Carter Institute for Caregiving

Pennsylvania

Live in Pennsylvania: http://pa.gov/portal/server.pt/community/live/3000

With its low unemployment and crime, excellent schools, top-notch health care and affordable cost of living, it's no wonder Pennsylvania is such a great place to live, work and raise a family.

Whether you prefer bustling cities, vibrant small towns, or quiet, out-of-the-way communities, you'll feel right at home in the commonwealth.

Pennsylvania government works hard to ensure that its citizens are able to lead healthy, happy and prosperous lives. From paving roads to helping hard working families make ends meet, the commonwealth provides a wide range of services that have a direct impact on the day-to-day lives of its citizens.

Additional Resources

Apply for Benefits
Sign-up for health care, cash and energy assistance; food stamps and other social services at one convenient website. Learn more

Resource Guide
Find out more about health, welfare and other assistance programs provided by Pennsylvania. Learn more

Senior Citizens
Get information about programs and services for older adults through the Department of Aging. Learn more

Department of Aging:
http://www.aging.state.pa.us/portal/server.pt/community/department_of_aging_home/18206

Enhancing the quality of life of all older Pennsylvanians by empowering diverse communities, the family and the individual."

Older Adults' PACE and PACENET Prescription Benefits Protected

On Thursday, August 4, Governor Tom Corbett ceremonially signed House Bill 463, which ensures thousands of older Pennsylvanians enrolled in the PACE and PACENET programs will not lose their coverage.

More than 21,000 PACE and PACENET enrollees were in jeopardy of losing their benefits as a result of receiving a Social Security cost of living adjustment, or COLA. The COLA increased their income just enough to render the enrollees ineligible for program benefits. Those who no longer qualified for the program would have had to pay out-of-pocket monthly premiums and higher co-pays for their prescriptions.

The moratorium now extends until December 31, 2013.

Find out more about PACE/PACENET here.

Ways to Keep Healthy in the Heat

The Pennsylvania Department of Aging (PDA) encourages older adults to take the following precautionary efforts to minimize the dangers from excessive heat.

- Drink plenty of fluids
- Wear light weight and loose fitting clothing
- Stay in an air-conditioned setting if possible
- Minimize time spent outdoors and stay out of the sun whenever possible.
- Check on relatives and neighbors who may be susceptible to heat related conditions.
  - Move to a cool area and seek medical attention if symptoms of heat stroke or exhaustion develop.
  - Ensure pets have access to shaded and well-ventilated areas with sufficient amounts of water.

Your local Area Agency on Aging (AAA) can assist you in finding a cool location to seek relief from the heat.

YOU CAN HELP STOP ELDER ABUSE!

Anyone who believes an older adult is being abused, neglected, exploited or abandoned should contact the Department of Aging's elder abuse hotline at 1-800-490-8505. All calls are confidential. Contact also can be made to the local Area Agency on Aging (AAA).
Click Here

Please help us STOP the abuse of our elder citizens. Thank you for your help.

Click here for more information about the Shared Living Request for Information (RFI).

PLEASE NOTE:

*The RFI-DPW-ODP Shared Living deadline has been further extended until September 30, 2011.

Commonwealth of Pennsylvania
Department of Aging
555 Walnut Street, 5th Floor
Harrisburg, PA 17101-1919
Telephone: (717) 783-1550
Fax: (717) 783-6842
Email us at aging@pa.gov

Home and Community Based Services:
http://www.aging.state.pa.us/portal/server.pt/community/home_and_community_based_services/179
97

Services covering a wide range of needs are available allowing individuals to remain in their communities and homes. These services include home health care; personal care, providing assistance with bathing, dressing, eating, grooming, toileting, etc.; health support services such as housekeeping, shopping assistance, laundry and mending; respite care (caregiver relief); transportation and other routine household chores as necessary to maintain a consumer's health, safety and ability to remain in the home; home-delivered meals prepared at a central location and delivered to a person's home.

For a details on services in your local area, contact your local Area Agency on Aging

Home and Community Based Services:

Oral History Project

Direct Care Worker Training

Domiciliary Care (Dom Care)

Family Caregiver Support Program

Older Adult Day Services Center

Family Caregiver Support Program:
http://www.portal.state.pa.us/portal/server.pt?open=514&objID=616680&mode=2

When you are not feeling well, home is where you want to be, no matter what your age. The major focus of the Family Caregiver Support Program is to reinforce the care being given to older family members at home. The major benefit, therefore, is that it allows your caregivers to choose from available supportive services.

The package of benefits begins with an assessment to determine what benefits best meet the needs of your caregiver and you, the person receiving care.

Other benefits could also include:

- Counseling

- Education
- Financial information

Eligibility

Eligibility for Family Caregiver is based on your income and functional needs. Contact your county Area Agency on Aging for additional information on eligibility and to apply for the program.

Family Caregiver Supports Program takes a cost-sharing approach; income-eligible families may receive up to $200 per month to help with out-of-pocket expenses ranging from respite care to adult briefs. In addition, one-time grants of up to $2,000 may be given to qualified families to modify the home or purchase assistive devices to accommodate the frail relative. Such adaptations might include installing a stair climb or modifying a bathroom.

Learn More

- Pennsylvania's Family Caregiver Support Program Brochure

Contact

Your local Area Agency on Aging

Office of Long-Term Living
Bureau of Individual Support
717-787-8091

Domiciliary Care Services for Adults:
http://www.portal.state.pa.us/portal/server.pt?open=514&objID=616679&mode=2

The Domiciliary Care or "Dom Care" program was created as part of Act 70 of June 1978 by the Commonwealth of Pennsylvania to provide a homelike living arrangement in the community for adults age 18 and older who need assistance with activities of daily living and are unable to live independently. Dom Care providers open up their homes to individuals who need supervision, support and encouragement in a family-like setting.
Dom Care residents are matched to homes that best meet their special needs, preferences, and interests. Dom Care homes are smaller than the traditional personal care home in that home providers care for no more than three Dom Care residents. Unlike larger personal care homes, Dom Care homes are the individual provider's home. They are inspected annually to ensure they meet health and safety standards. If the home and provider passes this inspection, they become "Certified". For more information on these standards and the other state regulations governing the Dom Care program click on the following link:
PA Code Title 6, Aging, Chapter 21 Domiciliary Care
Who is a typical Dom Care resident?
Dom Care residents are adults age 18 or older, who cannot live independently, and generally are low in income. Most residents are either physically disabled, have demonstrated difficulties in social or personal situations that are usually associated with mental disability or mental retardation, or frail

elderly persons. They must be willing to live with a family. Persons with extreme behavior problems or substance additions are not appropriate for Dom Care.

Dom Care residents are not so functionally impaired as to need nursing home care and must be mobile or semi-mobile. Dom Care residents must be able to vacate the home in case of fire with minimal assistance. The local Area Agency on Aging will determine if a consumer is appropriate for Dom Care. To find your local Area Agency on Aging, click here.

Why become a Dom Care resident?

Residents in the program receive much more than room and board. Residents receive supervision with self-help skills such as personal hygiene and grooming, three nutritious meals a day, and housekeeping and laundry services. If the resident takes medications, the home provider makes sure they get the correct dosage at the right times. Because of the small, homelike setting, Dom Care residents are assured of caring and individualized attention. Most importantly, Dom Care residents become part of a stable, caring "family" and can enjoy a sense of belonging and independence.

Dom Care residents that receive Supplemental Security Income (SSI) are also eligible for a state supplement towards the cost of Dom Care and a personal needs allowance. Residents receive on-going care management and monitoring, and involvement with day program activities is strongly encouraged.

Who is a typical Dom Care home provider?

The success of the Dom Care program is dependent on nurturing individuals who are willing to open up their home and willing to provide the support and care a Dom Care resident requires. Dom Care providers come from all walks of life. Some are widows or older couples. Others are families with young children, but all are willing to open their homes to people in need.

Dom Care home provider applicants go through an extensive certification process to ensure that homes meet the health and safety requirements as stated in the regulations. The local Area Agency on Aging is responsible for certifiying Dom Care homes in their area. To find your local Area Agency on Aging, click here. Some of these health and safety requirements include:

- Be at least 21 years of age
- Must own or rent your home or apartment
- Live in the certified home with the consumer
- Show the results of a tuberculosis test or chest x-ray
- Hold current certification for both CPR and First Aid
- Have criminal history clearances
- Have satisfactory financial, medical, and personal references
- Work as a team member with care managers and consumers

How much does the Dom Care resident pay the provider?

Dom Care residents enter into a contract to pay the home provider on a monthly basis for the entirety of the Dom Care residential service. Per regulation 21.41(6), the Pennsylvania Department of Aging is responsible for determining the monthly dollar amount the resident pays the provider. This rate applies to all Dom Care consumers throughout the commonwealth. The rate usually increases every January 1 along with the annual increase in SSI. As of January 1, 2009, the monthly Dom Care payment for an individual is **$936.00** and **$1664.00** for an SSI couple who reside together in the Dom Care home.

Where do I go from here?

Prospective Dom Care home providers and consumers should contact the local Area Agency on Aging for more information on the program.

Additional Online Resources: (All files in Adobe pdf format)

The Department of Aging created Dom Care 101 as a basic guide for anyone in the Dom Care program.

The following forms may serve as an information source on the Dom Care program.

- General Guidelines for New Home Providers
- New Provider Checklist
- Sample Fire Drill Plan and Record
- Sample House Rules Agreement
- Sample Home Provider Medical Recommendation Form

Your Local Resources: Home & Community Care:

http://www.portal.state.pa.us/portal/server.pt/community/home___community_care/17959

Most older Pennsylvanians prefer to remain in their home and stay connected with their community as they age. Home and community-based care provides an older person with the programs and services to help them maintain their independence. Contact your local Area Agency on Aging or click on any of the following links to learn more about these programs. Also, the Long-Term Living section of this site provides even more information.

- Aging Waiver Program
- Adult Day Services
- Attendant Care Program
- OPTIONS Program
- Nutrition Services

Attendant Care Program:

http://www.portal.state.pa.us/portal/server.pt?open=514&objID=616550&mode=2

The Attendant Care Program provides in-home personal care services to help mentally alert, physically disabled older persons remain independent in their own homes.

The services are provided through the Area Agencies on Aging to consumers who are age 60 and over who were previously served by Department of Public Welfare's Attendant Care Program.
What kinds of services are provided?
Basic services include assisting a person to get in and out of a bed, wheelchair and/or motor vehicle; assisting a person with health maintenance activities such as, bathing and personal hygiene, dressing and grooming; and eating, including meal preparation and cleanup.
Ancillary services include shopping, laundry, cleaning, seasonal chores, assistance with transportation, letter writing, reading mail and escort; assistance with managing finances, planning activities and making decisions.
Additional information on the Attendant Care Program may be obtained from the Department of Public Welfare's Office of Long-Term Living.

Services for People with Disabilities:

http://www.portal.state.pa.us/portal/server.pt/community/disability_services/17954

Learn about the programs available in Pennsylvania for people with disabilities. Most of these services are available to people of all ages, but some are specifically for older adults. For more information, visit the Long Term Living in PA website.

Learn more about disability services for older Pennsylvanians:

- Attendant Care Program
  (A special program for those previously in the under 60 Attendant Care Program who are now over 60)
- Home and Community Based Services
- Blindness & Visual Services
- Deaf and Hard of Hearing
- Developmental Disabilities
- Vocational Rehabilitation
- Mental Health Services
- Other Services

Attendant Care Program:
http://www.portal.state.pa.us/portal/server.pt?open=514&objID=616423&mode=2

The Attendant Care Program provides in-home personal care services to help mentally-alert, physically-disabled older persons remain independent in their own homes.

The services are provided through the Area Agencies on Aging to consumers who are age 60 and over who were previously served by Department of Public Welfare's Attendant Care Program.
Basic Services
Basic services include assisting a person to get in and out of a bed, wheelchair and/or motor vehicle; assisting a person with health maintenance activities such as, bathing and personal hygiene, dressing and grooming; and eating, including meal preparation and cleanup.
Ancillary Services
Ancillary services include shopping, laundry, cleaning, seasonal chores, assistance with transportation, letter writing, reading mail and escort; assistance with managing finances, planning activities and making decisions.
Learn more about the Attendant Care Program
Additional information on the Attendant Care Program may be obtained from the Office of Long-Term Living.

Office of Long Term Living: http://www.portal.state.pa.us/portal/server.pt/community/office_of_long-term_living/19325

The majority of people will need assistance with daily activities, such as bathing, dressing and meal preparation, at some point in their lives, whether due to aging, injury, illness or disability. Knowing what types of services are needed, available and how to obtain them is not easy. Whether you need help now or are exploring future options for yourself or a loved one, services and supports available through the Pennsylvania Office of Long-Term Living can assist you.

The goal of this Web site is to provide you easy access to information about the services and supports available, across Pennsylvania, through the Office of Long-Term Living. Helpful information is available for those who provide care and for people interested in planning for future needs.

The Office of Long-Term Living helps Pennsylvanians find answers to these questions:

- What types of services and supports are available?
- Where can you find providers or caregivers?
- How do I become a provider of long-term living services?
- How will you pay for the services?

You may also call the toll-free Long-Term Care Helpline at 1-866-286-3636. Counselors will be able to provide information and refer you to the local agencies that can provide assistance with planning and arranging long term care and services.

Learn More

A-Z Directory of Services
Information for Families and Individuals
Information for Providers
Integrated Care for Dual Eligibles
Long-Term Living in Pennsylvania
Long Term Living Training Institute
Senior Care and Services Study Commission

Information for Families and Individuals:
http://www.portal.state.pa.us/portal/server.pt/community/information_for_families_and_individuals/19326

Adult Day Services

> Adult day services provide a protective environment for older adults who are not capable of full-time independent living.

> Alternatives to Nursing Homes
> The links on this page provide you with information on a range of options, services and funding sources for the Office of Long-Term Living's Home and Community-based Services.

> LIFE Program
> If you are an older Pennsylvanian, the Living Independence for the Elderly (LIFE) program offers all needed medical and supportive services to enable you to maintain your independence in your home as long as possible.

Support Services Waiver Information

Support Services Waiver -- or simply waiver -- is a shortened term for the Medicaid Home and Community Based Waiver Program. This program provides funding for supports and services to help you to live in your home and community. Waivers offer an array of services and benefits such as choice of qualified providers, due process and health and safety assurances.

Independent Enrollment Broker

The Independent Enrollment Broker provides enrollment services for applicants with physical disabilities who are 18-59 years of age applying for Attendant Care, COMMCARE, Independence, OBRA, and the 0192 (AIDS) Waivers and the Act 150 Attendant Care Program. Area Agencies on Aging (AAA) provide eligibility/enrollment services for applicants over age 60.

Rhode Island

Home: Residential Resources: Seniors and Elderly:

http://www.ri.gov/resident/?tags=seniors+and+elderly

For Residents

Aging and Disabilities Resource Center

> http://adrc.ohhs.ri.gov/
>
> The POINT provides information referrals and help getting started with programs and services for seniors adults with disabilities and their caregivers.
>
> View all tagged with: disabilitieshuman serviceslearnresident resourcesseniors and elderly
>
> G

Apartment Rental Information

> http://www.rhodeislandhousing.org/sp.cfm?pageid=422
>
> Rental apartment assistance for low-income senior citizens families and persons with disabilities provided by Rhode Island Housing.
>
> View all tagged with: housinglearnlow incomeresident resourcesseniors and elderly

Choosing a Nursing Home

> http://www.health.ri.gov/nursinghomes/
>
> Nursing home information for consumers provided by the Rhode Island Department of Health.
>
> View all tagged with: department of healthhealth careresident resourcesseniors and elderly
>
> G

Home and Community Care Program

> http://adrc.ohhs.ri.gov/livingathome/dea_home_care.php
>
> This program provides eligible seniors with several options to help them remain in the community and avoid or postpone being admitted to a nursing care facility or hospital.
>
> View all tagged with: health carehuman serviceslearnresident resourcesseniors and elderly
>
> G

Home Care Services

> http://www.dea.ri.gov/programs/home_care.php
>
> Home care information and resources provided by the Rhode Island Department of Elderly Affairs.
>
> View all tagged with: health carehuman servicesresident resourcesseniors and elderly
>
> G

Long Term Care Services

> http://www.dhs.ri.gov/Elders/LongTermCare/tabid/911/Default.aspx
>
> Long Term Care services consist of home and community based services and institutional care for elderly Rhode Islanders provided by the Rhode Island Department of Human Services.
>
> View all tagged with: health carehuman servicesresident resourcesseniors and elderly
>
> G

Medicare Premium Payment Program

> http://www.dhs.ri.gov/Elders/HealthMedicalServices/MedicarePremiumPaymentProgram/tabid/892/Default.aspx

The Medicare Premium Payment Program helps elderly and adults with disabilities pay all or some of the costs of MedicareÃ¯Â¿Â½s Part A and Part B premiums, deductibles and co-payments.

View all tagged with: <u>health care</u><u>human services</u><u>resident resources</u><u>seniors and elderly</u>

G

Reverse Mortgages for Elderly Homeowners

http://www.rhodeislandhousing.org/sp.cfm?pageid=627

Learn about how to apply for a reverse mortgage. Information from Rhode Island Housing.

View all tagged with: <u>housing</u><u>resident resources</u><u>seniors and elderly</u>

Rhode Island Association of Facilities & Services for the Aging

http://www.riafsa.org/

An association of non-profit facilities and services primarily for the elderly.

View all tagged with: <u>human services</u><u>resident resources</u><u>seniors and elderly</u>

P

Rhode Island Housing

http://www.rhodeislandhousing.org/

Rhode Island Housing helps everyday Rhode Islanders find homes they can afford.

View all tagged with: <u>government entity</u><u>housing</u><u>resident resources</u><u>seniors and elderly</u><u>state government</u>

RI Pharmaceutical Assistance to the Elderly (RIPAE)

http://www.dea.ri.gov/programs/prescription_assist.php

RIPAE is a program for low-income elderly Rhode Islanders that helps pay for prescription drugs.

View all tagged with: <u>health care</u><u>learn</u><u>resident resources</u><u>seniors and elderly</u>

G

Services for Elderly Rhode Islanders

http://www.dhs.ri.gov/DefaultPermissions/Elders/tabid/277/Default.aspx

Long-term care food stamps Medicare and assisted living programs available from the Department of Human Services.

DEA's Home and Community Care Program: http://adrc.ohhs.ri.gov/livingathome/dea_home_care.php

The DEA Home and Community Care Program provides eligible seniors with several innovative options to help them remain in the community and avoid premature institutionalization. These options are designed to assist the functionally impaired senior meet a wide variety of medical, environmental, and social needs.

Based on eligibility, Home and Community Care Programs may provide home health aide services, adult day services, **Meals on Wheels**, **Senior Companion**, Personal emergency response system, minor home modifications or minor assistive devices. If appropriate, placement in an assisted living facility may be made.

To be eligible for the **Home and Community Care Program**, a person must be 65 or older, a resident of Rhode Island, and be basically homebound (unable to leave home without considerable assistance).

For some persons on **Medical Assistance (Medicaid)**, services under the **Home and Community Care Program** are may be provided at no charge. Other Medicaid clients may have to make a contribution towards services.

For information call **462-0570.**

For persons meeting the guidelines for the **Rhode Island Pharmaceutical Assistance to the Elderly (RIPAE)** program, services are provided at a reduced rate. Currently, these annual income guidelines are $18,724 for a single person and $23,407 for a couple.

Each year these guidelines are changed to reflect the **Social Security cost-of-living adjustment (COLA)**.

DEA works with a network of regional case management agencies and other senior service organizations to develop care plans to help seniors remain in the least restrictive environment with maximum independence.

For more information about the **Home and Community Care Program, call 462-0570.**

The **Home Health Quality Initiative (HHQI)** is part of a national effort by the **Centers for Medicare and Medicaid Services (CMS)** to improve the quality of care for those who use home health care services provided by **Medicare**-certified suppliers. Go to **www.medicare.gov** or call **1-800-MEDICARE (1-800-633-4227) or 1-877-486-2048 (TTY)**, to get access to data intended to help seniors, family members, and caregivers find out about the quality of home care their loved ones are receiving.

Help with Living at Home: http://adrc.ohhs.ri.gov/livingathome/index.php

Adult Day Services

Aging & Disabled Care

Aging & Assisted Living Home & Community Based Care

Case Management

Community Living Options

DEA Home and Community Care Program

Emergency Response Systems

Food Assistance

Food Stamp Program

Friendly Visitor

Identification Cards

Modifying a Home to Make Life Easier

<u>Ocean State Center for Independent Living</u>

<u>Ombudsman Program</u>

<u>Respite Services</u>

<u>Senior Centers</u>

<u>Severely Disabled Home and Community Based Program</u>

<u>Transportation</u>

<u>Volunteering</u>

Independent Living: http://adrc.ohhs.ri.gov/wheretolive/ind_living.php

Rhode Island has two independent living organizations that provide information and services to disabled persons to enhance their independence.

Ocean State Center for Independent Living (OSCIL), 1944 Warwick Avenue, Warwick 02889 can be reached at 738-1013 (Voice) or 738-1015 (TTY).

People Actively Reaching Independence (PARI), 500 Prospect Street, Pawtucket 02860 can be reached at at 725-1966 (Voice/TTY).

The Office of Rehabilitation Services (ORS) in the Department of Human Services can also provide information on home modifications and assistive devices. Call 421-7005 (Voice) or 421-7016 (TTY).

TechACCESS of Rhode Island, 110 Jefferson Boulevard, Suite I, Warwick, RI 02889 enables persons with disabilities to try out computers, software, and other assistive and adaptive equipment. Call 463-0202 for an appointment or Information.

Relay Rhode Island can connect hearing-impaired Rhode Islanders with various government agencies and also assist them in completing the call. Their numbers are 1-800-745-5555 (English) and 1-800-855-2884 (Spanish).

Respite Services: http://adrc.ohhs.ri.gov/livingathome/respite_serv.php

Respite is temporary care given inside or outside the home for seniors who cannot entirely care for themselves. Respite provides relief to caregivers. **Respite Care Services**, 184 Broad Street, Providence 02903 offers two programs.

Subsidized Respite Program: This program provides relief to primary caregivers who live with someone 55 years or older, in need of personal care assistance. In-home respite, adult day services, and overnight stays in assisted living facilities are provided on a cost-sharing basis.

Homemaking Program: Homemakers are available for a reduced hourly rate to anyone 55 or older and handicapped or disabled adults of any age whose incomes are within the guidelines of the **RIPAE** program.

This program recruits, trains, and matches respite homemakers with eligible clients. Homemakers can provide assistance with home maintenance or companionship. Call at **421-7833**.

Help After a Hospital Stay: http://adrc.ohhs.ri.gov/hospital/index.php

Assistance in Getting Help
Home Health Care
Durable Medical Equipment
Skilled Nursing Facilities
Hospice Care

Paying for Care and Services: http://adrc.ohhs.ri.gov/paying/index.php

Medicare

Social Security

Supplemental Security Income

Prescription Assistance

Heating Assistance

Habilitation Home and Community Care Based Program

Home Equity Conversion Mortgage

Housing Authority Resource

Applying for Public Housing

Medicare Premium Payment Program

Tax Information

Department of Housing and Urban Development

Additional Assistance:

Where to Get Information: http://adrc.ohhs.ri.gov/assistance/index.php

Advocacy Groups
Senior Citizens Fire & Police Advocates
Alzheimer's Disease

National Family Caregiver Support

Brain Injury

Help for Veterans

Family Independence Program (FIP)

RI Commission on the Deaf & Hard of Hearing

Help for People with Disabilities

Help for Caregivers: http://adrc.ohhs.ri.gov/assistance/index.php

Caregiver Support

Adult Day Care

Help at Home

Respite Services

Caregiver Support: http://adrc.ohhs.ri.gov/caregivers/caregiver_support.php

If you're helping to care for an older person or a person with a disability, you know how important that job is and how demanding it can feel. What you many not know is that Rhode Island offers many services that can provide assistance to caregivers and make life better for you.

Caregiver support groups meet at senior centers, nursing homes and adult day centers across Rhode Island. To learn about groups in your area, please call:

• The Department of Elderly Affairs at 462-4000 or "The Point" at 462-4444.

Travelers Aid Society of Rhode Island offers a 24 hour Information and Referral Service and maintains an extensive listing of support groups and community resources. Please call:

• Travelers Aid at 521-2255 or 1-800-367-2700.

National organizations such as the Alzheimer's Association, American Cancer Society and the American Lung Association also maintain local chapters in the state and may provide assistance and support. These numbers are also contained within the business section of your local phone book.

Health Care: http://adrc.ohhs.ri.gov/healthcare/index.php

Finding a Doctor or Dentist
Assessing Level of Need
Finding Care for People with Disabilities
Choosing a Health Plan
Dental Services
Nursing Homes & Long Term Care
Geriatric Assessments
Health Centers
Hearing & Speech Services
Medical Assistance
Mental Health & Behavioral Health

South Carolina

Lieutenant Governor's Office on Aging: http://aging.sc.gov/Pages/default.aspx

Welcome to the Office on Aging

rograms within the Office on Aging
SCAccess - searchable database of services in South Carolina
Medicare and SHIP - health insurance options for the elderly
Ombudsman - for residents of long-term care facilites
BGTIME.org - an online community forum specially designed for senior citizens in South Carolina
Health and Safety - tips for maintaining a healthy lifestyle
Family Caregiver Support Program - offering help to caregivers
Alzheimer's Resource Coordination Center - helping individuals affected by Alzheimer's disease
Brochures - Several popular brochures are available for download

Family Caregiver Support Program:

http://aging.sc.gov/seniors/Pages/FamilyCaregiverSupportProgram.aspx

Offering Help to Caregivers Who Are:

- Unpaid family caregivers for a frail or disabled adults 60 or older
- Relative caregivers, 55 or older, responsible for raising a child related through blood, marriage or adoption
- Unpaid family caregivers for someone with Alzheimer's disease or a related neurological disorder
- Adults, 55 or older, who are an unpaid family caregivers for a child of any age with a disability

Services Available

- **Information** about local services and supports
- **Assistance** from a trained Family Caregiver Advocate to help caregivers assess needs and access support services
- **Counseling**, **support groups**, and **training**
- **Respite care** for caregivers
- Services are provided at no cost to qualifying participants and are federally funded under the Older Americans Act with state and local matching funds.

For information about the Family Caregiver Support Program and services in your area, call us at 1-800-868-9095 or contact the Family Caregiver Advocate at your Area Agency on Aging. The Family Caregiver brochure is also availble (small 100K pdf file).

Other Information:

Overview of the SC Family Caregiver Support Program (small 46KB pdf file)

Brochure: Family Caregiver Support Program (small 191KB pdf file)

Lieutenant Governor's Office on Aging

1301 Gervais Street, Suite 350

Columbia, South Carolina 29201

Phone: (803) 734-9900

Toll Free: (800) 868-9095

FAX: (803) 734-9887

Website: www.aging.sc.gov

Family Caregiver Support Overview:

http://aging.sc.gov/SiteCollectionDocuments/F/FCSPOverview107.pdf

Services To Be Provided

The program was established in 2002, through federal legislation to support unpaid family caregivers who provide most of the long term care in the United States. The State Unit on Aging works with Area Agencies on Aging and community and local service provider organizations to provide family caregiver support services including:

- Information on existing community resources and programs
- One-on-one counseling, support and assistance in gaining access to services
- Support groups
- Caregiver education and training
- Respite care to allow caregivers to take a short break from their caregiving responsibilities
- Supplemental services to complement the care provided by caregivers. These services may include incontinence supplies, chore or homemaker services, emergency response monitoring, nutritional supplements, assistive technology, transportation, or home modifications such as grab bars or wheelchair ramps.

CLIENT GROUPS TO BE SERVED
Two populations are targeted.
1. Adult family caregivers of any age caring for frail or disabled adults 60 years of age or older, and
2. Older individuals, 60 years or older, raising grandchildren who are not more than 18 years of age.

Priority for services is given to older individuals with greatest social and economic need, (with particular attention to low-income older individuals) and older individuals providing care and support to person with developmental disabilities.

METHOD OF SERVICE DELIVERY

Family caregivers across the state may contact the Family Caregiver Advocate at their Area Agency on Aging to obtain information, one-on-one assistance and support, and caregiver training. Eligible caregivers may also obtain a mini-grant, of approximately $500, to purchase respite and/or supplemental services and receive reimbursement later or they may access services through vouchers.

NUMBER OF CLIENTS TO BE SERVED

Funds should allow more than 15,000 unduplicated family caregivers to receive services through the Family Caregiver Support Program in fiscal year 2008. In addition to information, training, individual counseling, and support groups, it is expected that more than 1,600 caregivers will receive a grant to purchase respite services from the provider of their choice and that approximately 900 people will receive a small grant to purchase supplemental services.

GEOGRAPHIC IMPACT OF THE PROGRAM

Caregivers from all 46 counties will have access to services. Long distance caregivers from other states and countries who are coordinating services for family members in South Carolina may also receive information and assistance by contacting their Family Caregiver Advocate.

KEY OBJECTIVES

- Continue to serve as a resource for a portion of the estimated 416,214 unpaid family caregivers in South Carolina providing more than 446 million hours of care annually at a market value of $4,423 million dollars per year.
- Continue to improve the quality and availability of information to families and informal caregivers in South Carolina.
- Continue to provide counseling and support targeted to each individual caregiver.

Medicare and SHIP (State Health Insurance Program):

http://aging.sc.gov/seniors/medicare/Pages/index.aspx

Medicare Information

Medicare is insurance for the elderly and disabled. There are several parts to Medicare and many choices to be made by the consumer. To assist in these decisions, the state of South Carolina and the Federal government have put together a program call the **State Health Insurance Program (SHIP)** or alternatly known as the Insurance Counseling Assistance and Referrals for Elders program (I-CARE). What it means to consumers is there are people throughout the state who can provide health insurance counseling for Medicare, Medicare Supplement, Medicare Savings program, Medicare Advantage Plans and Senior Medicare Fraud programs.

If you would like help with Medicare information and Part D enrollment, contact the SHIP counselor for your area. For other areas of interest see the following:

Medicare Part A & B

As of October, 2007, the current addresses where directly billed Medicare beneficiaries must send their

Medicare Part B and/or A premium payments**Medicare Part D - Prescription Drug Coverage programs**

Help with Medicare Prescription Drug Coverage

Find out more about the Medicare Part D

Compare Medicare Prescription Drug Plans

"Choosing a Medigap Policy"

Medicare Supplemental/Medigap Plans - medium sized (550Kb) pdf file from the Federal website

Other Programs

QMB or SLMB Applications

Medicare Savings Programs - Get an application for

Extra Help or Low-Income Subsidy (LIS)

From the federal web site

Medicare

Federal Medicare Site

Medicare Fraud

Short primer on protecting yourself from fraud

National Consumer Protection Technical Resource Center

Non-profit national consumer protection technical resource

Office on Aging: http://aging.sc.gov/officeonaging/Pages/index.aspx

About the Office on Aging
Contact Information/Directory
Director's Pledge on Accountability and Transparency
Mission and Vision

Lt. Governor's Office on Aging Services

State Plan on Aging for 2009 - 2012 (very large 3.8MB pdf file)
The Older Americans Act requires that each state submit a State Plan on Aging in order to be eligible for federal funding. This plan provides a blueprint for how the Office on Aging will manage Older Americans Act programs, services and other activities.

Find out about The Great Central US ShakeOut eight state disaster preparedness drill on April 28th.

Accountability Reports
Lieutenant Governor's Office on Aging Accountability Report for fiscal year:

- 2007-2008 (medium 740K pdf file)

- 2006-2007 (medium 700K pdf file)

- 2005-2006 (medium 450K pdf file)

- 2004-2005 (medium 350K pdf file)

Agency Financial Details

Monthly reports on the cash and appropriation transactions for the agency.

Advisory Committees and Boards

Adult Protection Coordinating Council

Advisory Council on Aging - All welcome

ARCC Advisory Council - Alzheimers Resource Coordination Center Advisory Council

ElderCare Trust Advisory Board

CARE Commission - Advises the Lieutenant Governor on issues critical to the senior community

Silver Haired Legislature - Addressing issues for the older population

Memorandums (Informational and Program Instructions)

Memorandums #07-01

Program instructions for AAA Directors on the $2.9 million state supplemental funding (small 17KB file).

Lieutenant Governor's Transitions Orientation Manual

Orientation Manual

Department of Disabilities and Special Needs: http://ddsn.sc.gov/Pages/default.aspx

<u>WELCOME</u>

Welcome to the South Carolina Department of Disabilities and Special Needs (SCDDSN) Website. We are currently working to enhance our website by making it easier for you to navigate.

SCDDSN is the state agency that plans, develops, oversees and funds services for South Carolinians with severe, lifelong disabilities of intellectual disability, autism, traumatic brain injury and spinal cord injury and conditions related to each of these four disabilities. Our mission is to assist people with disabilities and their families in meeting needs, pursuing possibilities and achieving life goals, and to minimize the occurrence and reduce the severity of disabilities through prevention.

Consumer and Family Information: http://ddsn.sc.gov/CONSUMERS/Pages/default.aspx

The SC Department of Disabilities and Special Needs provides services for the severe, lifelong disabilities of intellectual disability and related disabilities, autism, traumatic brain injury, and spinal cord injury and related disabilities.

When you contact DDSN to determine if you are eligible for DDSN services, a list of questions will be asked to determine if you are likely to meet DDSN eligibility criteria. If your response clearly rules out eligibility, your Disabilities and Special Needs Board will refer you to more appropriate agencies/resources. If your response indicates you may be eligible, you will be provided with a list of service coordination providers. The provider you choose will help you through the eligibility process.

Please use the links below to provide you with more information on the various services and resources offered by DDSN, as well as information on how to acquire these services.

1. Applying for Services.
2. DDSN Divisions.
3. Medicaid Waiver Programs.
4. Finding a Qualified Service Provider.
5. Person Centered Services and its meanings.
6. Qualified Life Planners.
7. Early Intervention
8. SC Support and Advocacy Organizations.
9. Publications.
10. Opportunities to Participate in Research Studies
11. Find a Dentist
12. Family Relief From Caregiving.

Family Relief From Caregiving: http://ddsn.sc.gov/consumers/Pages/FamilyReliefFromCaregiving.aspx

CAREGIVER RELIEF PILOT PROJECT

March 2011 to August 2011

Aiken County Board of Disabilities/Tri-Development Center

Saturday - 9:00 AM to 4:30 PM at Vaucluse Road and North Augusta Satellite locations.

Initially providing services at one location each Saturday alternating locations. Possible expansion to both locations each Saturday depending on demand.

Babcock Center (in partnership with Richland/Lexington Disabilities and Special Needs Board)

Saturday and Sunday 9:00 AM to 4:00 PM - (two sessions each day 9:00 AM to 12:30 PM and 12:30 PM to 4:00 PM).

1st and 3rd weekend of the month – Adults 18 and over; 2nd and 4th weekend of the month - Children under the age of 18.

Bamberg County Disabilities and Special Needs Board

Monday through Friday – 2:00 PM to 5:00 PM and Saturday 8:00 AM to 5:00 PM.

Center hours will be flexible to accommodate needs in extenuating circumstances.

Charles Lea Center

Monday through Friday – 3:00 PM to 6:00 PM; Saturday 10:00 AM to 2:00 PM.

Times may change slightly due to adjusting to family/consumer needs. Hours may expand during summer months.

Greenville County Disabilities and Special Needs Board

Monday through Thursday – 4:00 PM to 8:00 PM and every 2nd and 4th Saturday 9:00 AM to 3:00 PM

York County Adult Day Care Services, Inc. – (Three Locations)

Fort Mill

Monday, Wednesday, and Thursday 3:00 PM to 6:00 PM; Tuesday and Friday 3:00 PM to 7:00 PM; Saturday 10:00 AM to 10:00 PM

Rock Hill

Monday and Wednesday 3:00 PM to 8:00 PM; Tuesday and Thursday 3:00 pm to 5:30 pm; Friday 3:00 PM to 9:00 PM; Saturday 10:00 AM – 9:00 PM

York

Tuesday and Thursday 3:00 PM to 8:00 PM; Friday 3:00 PM to 9:00 PM; Saturday 10:00 AM to 9:00 PM

Babcock WOW Program

Bamberg Caregiver Relief Program

Tri-Development Center - Saturday Activity Center Flyer

Greenville DSN - Caregiver Relief (FROG)

York County Adult Day Services - Group Caregiver Relief

How to Become a Qualified Provider : http://ddsn.sc.gov/providers/becomeqpl/Pages/default.aspx

Thank you for your interest in becoming a SC Department of Disabilities and Special Needs (DDSN) service provider.

DDSN is the state agency that provides services to South Carolinians with the severe lifelong disabilities of intellectual disability and related disabilities, autism, traumatic brain injury and spinal cord injury and similar disabilities.

We deliver DDSN services though a statewide network of local Disabilities and Special Needs (DSN) Boards and other qualified providers.

Many services available through DDSN can only be provided by organizations or agencies (service providers) who meet federal, state and DDSN requirements for quality and safety. Organizations or agencies that wish to provide these services to DDSN consumers must be approved for DDSN's Qualified Provider List (QPL). Applications for most services must be submitted through the SC Budget and Control Board's Materials Management Office (MMO).

Click here to view and obtain a copy of DDSN's current solicitation Request for Proposal # 5400003286. Within the form, you will find instructions on how to submit an application, and the quarterly deadlines for applications. Questions can be e-mailed to Mr. Chris Manos at CManos@mmo.sc.gov.

For Board Certified Behavior Analysts or those desiring to become a Qualified Provider of Behavior Supports or EIBI, click here.

If you have other questions about becoming a service provider, please contact Director, Intellectual Disability Division, SC Department of Disabilities and Special Needs, P.O. Box 4706, Columbia, SC 29240.

Thank you again for your inquiry.

South Dakota

Department of Human Services: http://dhs.sd.gov/

Disability Determination Services: http://dhs.sd.gov/dds/

Mission Statement
We are committed to providing accurate, impartial, and timely disability decisions for South Dakota citizens.

Who Are We?

Disability Determination Services (DDS) is the State Agency that makes the disability decisions for Social Security, according to federal guidelines. When Social Security added protection for the disabled in 1954, the Congress wrote into the law that the disability decision had to be made by a State Agency and not by a federal office. Social Security pays the State to run the office and make the decision. The DDS is responsible only for the medical eligibility portion of the disability claim. Social Security is responsible for the application process, any other eligibility criteria, and the calculation of benefits if awarded.

Adult Services and Aging: http://dss.sd.gov/elderlyservices/index.asp

The Division of Adult Services and Aging (ASA) provides home and community service options to individuals 60 years of age and older and 18 years of age and older with physical disabilities, regardless of income.

The focus of this division is to enable these South Dakotans to live independent, meaningful and dignified lives while maintaining close family and community ties.

ASA promotes in-home and community-based services to prevent or delay premature or inappropriate institutionalization. In-home services are available to those who need assistance with routine household tasks. Recipients of these services may be recovering from an illness or have physical limitations.

Specialists are available statewide to respond to inquiries or requests for long term services and support resources, either from the individual or on behalf of older adults or adults with physical disabilities

NEW: Aging and Disability Resource Connections (ADRC)

- ASA is in the process of implementing several changes to enhance the services and better help people access those services they need to remain in their own communities through the implementation of the Aging and Disability Resource Connections (ADRC). **LEARN MORE**.

ADRC: http://dss.sd.gov/elderlyservices/services/ADRC.asp

Introduction

A Grant from the Administration on Aging and the Centers for Medicare and Medicaid Services provided an opportunity for the Division of Adult Services and Aging to launch the state's first Aging and Disability Resource Connections (ADRC) in the community of Sioux Falls.

ADRCs provide objective information, assistance and access to long term services and support options for our consumers.

ADRCs in South Dakota are called **Aging and Disability Resource Connections** and enhance access to available public and private services to help individuals live as independently as possible within their local communities.

Part of implementing ADRCs is the development of an online, comprehensive and user-friendly database consisting of long term services and support resources available in South Dakota. This online database will be available to ADRC staff as they provide information and resources to South Dakotans over age 60 and to adults over age 18 with physical disabilities.

The first ADRC is in Sioux Falls and covers the below counties:

- Minnehaha
- McCook
- Lincoln
- Turner

Information from other providers across the state will be collected as the implementation process continues.

More Information for Consumers

- View ADRC brochure
- Call **1-877-660-0301** if you live in any one of the above counties and have questions about information and access to long term services and support options.

Training Information

- Provider Process Change

Inclusion/Exclusion Policy for Providers

The purpose of the inclusion/exclusion policy is to clearly define the types of entities, i.e., agencies, organizations, providers and
resources that are eligible for listing on the South Dakota Aging and Disability Resource Connections (ADRC) information and resource online database.

Please read the policy before submitting your information.

- <u>ADRC Database Inclusion/Exclusion Policy</u>

Request for Inclusion Form for Providers

By completing the <u>Request for Inclusion form</u>, you will be submitting information on the services your agency provides for consideration to be included in to the online resource database. **Please note the following before submitting your information.**

- If you operate multiple sites or provide multiple services, please fill out a separate form for each site and service (program) that will be listed (separately) in the database. Make duplicates of the form, as necessary.
- Complete the form in its entirety with accurate information.
- Be as detailed as possible in the "Description of Services" section.
- Please <u>review description examples</u> of what will be obtained from the inclusion form and then submitted in to the online database for consumer-use.
- **You can submit the form in various ways:**
  1. Print and mail the form to:
     1. South Dakota Department of Social Services
        Aging and Disability Resource Connections
        ATTN: Deb Petersen
        700 Governors Drive, Pierre, SD 57501
  2. Send via email by clicking the "send electronically" at the end of the form. The form will then be sent to the <u>ADRC@state.sd.us</u> email address.
  3. Fax the form to: 605-773-4085.
  4. Contact Deb Petersen at 605-773-3656 with questions.

The Request for Inclusion form submitted will be reviewed and a decision to include or exclude your agency will be emailed to you within 30 days from receipt of the form.

Resource Directory for the Elderly : http://dss.sd.gov/elderlyservices/resourcedirectory/

The following information assists older adults and their caregivers in finding local resources for needs like adult day services, in-home services, emergency contacts and transportation.

- <u>ASA Services</u>
- <u>Links and Resources</u>
- <u>Request Change Form</u>
- <u>Letter from ASA Division Director</u>
- <u>View Entire Directory</u>

| <u>Aurora</u> | <u>Day</u> | <u>Jackson</u> | <u>Perkins</u> |

Beadle	Deuel	Jerauld	Potter
Bennett	Dewey	Jones	Roberts
Bon Homme	Douglas	Kingsbury	Sanborn
Brookings	Edmunds	Lake	Shannon
Brown	Fall River	Lawrence	Spink
Brule	Faulk	Lincoln	Stanley
Buffalo	Grant	Lyman	Sully
Butte	Gregory	Marshall	Todd
Campbell	Haakon	McCook	Tripp
Charles Mix	Hamlin	McPherson	Turner
Clark	Hand	Meade	Union
Clay	Hanson	Mellette	Walworth
Codington	Harding	Miner	Yankton
Corson	Hughes	Minnehaha	Ziebach
Custer	Hutchinson	Moody	
Davison	Hyde	Pennington	

Senior Meals: http://dss.sd.gov/elderlyservices/services/seniormeals/locations.asp

Locations

If you are unable to find a location near you, please contact the Senior Nutrition Program at 605-773-3656.

Area IV Senior Citizens Planning Council (Aberdeen)

Sites: Aberdeen, Bowdle, Bristol, Britton, Claire City, Conde, Cresbard, Eden, Eureka, Faulkton, Frederick, Gettysburg, Groton, Hecla, Herreid, Hoven, Ipswich, Langford, McIntosh, McLaughlin, Mobridge, Mound City, New Effington, Onida, Pierpont, Pollock, Redfield, Roslyn, Selby, Seneca, Sisseton, Tulare, Veblen, Waubay, Webster, Wilmot

Address: 405 Eighth Ave. NW, Berkshire Plaza Suite 203A, Aberdeen, SD 57401-2705

Project Director: Rick Pesek
Phone: 605-229-4741
Fax: 605-229-4741
E-Mail: areaiv@nvc.net

Bennett County Senior Center (Martin)

Sites: Fort Pierre, Kadoka, Kyle, Martin, Murdo, Philip, Pierre

Address: 203 Main St., PO Box 636,Martin, SD 57551-0636
Project Director: Donna Noel
Phone: 605- 685-6642
Fax: 605-685-6980
E-Mail: bcseniors@gwtc.net

Senior Citizens Services (Sioux Falls)

Sites: Alcester, Beresford, Brandon, Bridgewater, Canton, Centerville, Chancellor, Chester, Dell Rapids, Garretson, Hartford, Hudson, Lennox, Montrose, Parker, Salem, Sioux Falls, Tea

Address: 2300 W 46th St, Sioux Falls, SD 57105-6528
Project Director: Gerald Beninga
Phone: 605- 336-6722
Fax: 605-336-7471
E-Mail: geraldbeninga@yahoo.com
Website: www.centerforactivegenerations.org

Huron Area Senior Center:

Sites: Highmore, Hitchcock, Huron, Wessington, Wessington Springs, Wolsey, Woonsocket

Address: 290 7th St. SW, Huron, SD 57350-2755
Project Director: Jim Hofer
Phone: (605) 352-6091
Fax: 353-9585
E-Mail: jhofer.hasc@midconetwork.com

Inter-Lakes Community Action Partnership (Brookings)

Sites: Arlington, Astoria, Badger, Brookings, Bruce, Bryant, Carpenter, Carthage, Clark, Clear Lake, Colman, DeSmet, Elkton, Estelline, Flandreau, Hayti, Hazel, Howard, LaBolt, Lake Norden, Lake Preston, Madison, Milbank, Oldham, Ramona, Raymond, Stockholm, Strandburg, Toronto, Volga, Watertown, White, Willow Lake

Address: 601 4th St., Suite 108, Brookings, SD 57006
or 111 N. Van Eps Ave., Madison, SD 57042-0268
Project Director: Kim Jones
Phone: Brookings -- (605) 692-6391 or FAX: 692-6392
Madison -- (605) 256-6518 or FAX: 256-2238
E-Mail: kjones@interlakescap.com

City of Mitchell

Sites: Emery, Ethan, Mitchell, Mt. Vernon, Parkston, Spencer, Tripp, Artesian

Address: 300 West 1st Ave., Mitchell, SD 57301
Project Director: Brenda Paradis
Phone: 605-995-8439
Fax: 605-995-8439
E-Mail: bparadis.rsvp@midconetwork.com

Spearfish/Sturgis Nutrition

Sites: Spearfish, Sturgis, Buffalo
Address: Hickory House, 430 Oriole Drive, Spearfish, SD 57783-3001
Project Director: Richard Laudanskas
Phone: 605-642-1277
Fax: 605-642-0620
E-Mail: rlaudanskas@4-evergreen.net

Rural Office of Community Service (ROCS)

Sites: Armour, Avon, Bonesteel, Burke, Chamberlain, Colome, Corsica, Delmont, Fairfax, Geddes, Gregory, Harrison, Kennebec, Kimball, Lake Andes, Menno, New Holland, North Sioux City, Platte, Plankinton, Presho, Pukwana, Reliance, Scotland, Springfield, Stickney, Tyndall, Vermillion, Wagner, White Lake, Winner

Address: 214 Main, Lake Andes, SD 57356-0070
Project Director: Shirley Soukup or Nancy Janak
Phone: 605-487-7635
Fax: 605- 487-7883
E-Mail: ssoukup@rocsinc.org or njanak@rocsinc.org

Miller Nutrition Project

Site: Miller
Address: 105 N. Broadway, Miller, SD 57362-1349
Project Director: Richard Palmer
Phone: 605-853-2869
E-Mail: manor@midconetwork.com

Western South Dakota Senior Services (Rapid City)

Sites: Belle Fourche, Bison, Custer, Dupree, Edgemont, Faith, Hill City, Hot Springs, Isabel, Keystone, Lemmon, Newell, New Underwood, Nisland, Rapid City, Timber Lake, Wall

Address: 303 N. Maple Ave., Rapid City, SD 57701-1538
Project Director: Marcia Murray
Phone: 605-394-6002
Fax: 605-394-6001
E-Mail: mmurray@rushmore.com

Yankton Area Senior Citizens

Sites: Tabor, Yankton
Address: 900 Whiting Drive, Yankton, SD 57078-5006
Project Director: Tamela Matuska
Phone: 605-665-1055
Fax: 605-260-4685
E-Mail: yscc@midconetwork.com
Website: www.yanktonseniorcenter.org

Homemaker Services: http://dss.sd.gov/elderlyservices/services/homemaker.asp

Homemaker Services may delay or prevent the need for care in an institution. This service makes it possible for older individuals to live in their own homes or to return to their homes by providing assistance in completing tasks they are unable to manage without assistance. This program is not designed to replace assistance provided by family and friends. Financial eligibility is based on income and resources. A cost share may be required.

Covered Services

A homemaker is assigned to provide basic household assistance, including:

- assistance with personal hygiene,
- essential shopping,
- laundry,
- light housekeeping,
- light meal preparation.

Non-Covered Services

A homemaker is not assigned to provide the following:

- washing outside windows,
- moving large furniture,
- shoveling snow,
- caring for a garden or yard,
- cleaning up before or after company,
- washing walls,
- caring for pets or house plants,
- painting,
- shampooing carpets,
- skilled nursing services,
- assisting with a bladder or bowel program,
- providing transportation, unless there is an emergency,
- other tasks not necessary to maintain a person in his or her home.

Hours of Service

An individual qualifying for services will receive services as approved in the individual care plan. These services are to be provided during normal working hours, 8:00 a.m. to 5:00 p.m., Monday through Friday.

Service Providers

The Division of Adult Services and Aging does not directly provide homemaker services, but contracts with local homemaker/home health agencies.

Other Funding Source

In addition to Homemaker Services, the Division of Adult Services and Aging has another funding source with specific eligibility requirements which can assist in the cost of payment for similar services.

- Title XIX Home and Community-Based Waiver

- Title XIX Personal Care

Medicare Part D: http://dss.sd.gov/medicarepartD/

Do You Need Help Paying Prescription Drug Costs?

Medicare offers prescription drug coverage for all people with Medicare. If you have Medicare and a limited income, you may also qualify for extra help with paying your prescription drug costs.

Medicare Prescription Drug Coverage will:

- Be available to all people with Medicare.
- Help people with Medicare pay for the prescriptions that they need.
- Provide low-cost drug coverage for those with limited income and assets.
- Pay for both brand name and generic drugs.
- Allow people with Medicare to choose between at least two Medicare prescription drug plans.
- Allow convenient access to local pharmacies.

Medicare will contract with private companies to provide prescription drug benefits. To receive Medicare Prescription Drug Coverage, you must select and enroll in a plan. Enrollment in a plan is voluntary.

Additional Information:

- County Listing of Where & When You Can Obtain Assistance
- Drug Plan Contacts for Exceptions and Appeals
- Information for Medical Providers
- Senior Health Information & Insurance Education (SHIINE)
- Using Medicare Prescription Drug Coverage Before Receiving A Drug Plan Card

Under "Public Assistance", "Food Stamp Manual", I founds these links...

2012 ELDERLY OR DISABLED

For food stamp purposes an "elderly or disabled member" means a member of a household who:

A. Definition of Elderly

People 60 and older are defined as elderly. This includes people who are 59 years old when they apply but who will become 60 on or before the last day of the month of application.

B. Definition of Disabled Identified Below:
   Individuals who meets one of the following criteria:

   o Eligible to receive or receiving SSI benefits, including presumptive SSI payments, or eligible under SSI 1619 B criteria
      - SDX or SVES verifies SSI benefits and individual must be receiving SSI benefit or approved to receive SSI benefits.
      - 1619B status is verified on the MEDX screen on the SDX when MED ELIG displays C
        ELIG and PAYMENT STATUS displays N01-NONPAY.
   o Receives SS disability or blindness payments.
      - Verified via BNDX or SVES.

- o Receives a disability retirement benefit from a local, state, or federal government agency and the disability is considered permanent according to criteria listed in Section 2013 below.
- o Receives federally or State-administered supplemental benefits provided the eligibility to receive the benefits is based on the SSI disability or blindness criteria. (South Dakota does not have disability based State general assistance benefits however someone
moving to South Dakota may have received this benefit from another State.)
- o Receives a disability annuity payment under the Railroad Retirement Act of 1974 and is
  - Is determined disabled under SSI criteria; or
  - Is eligible to receive Medicare by the Railroad Retirement Board.
- o Receives disability related medical assistance provided that the assistance is based upon disability or blindness criteria which are at least as stringent as those used under Title XVI of the Social Security Act. The disability based SD Medical Programs meeting the criteria are listed below. Eligibility for these programs is determined on the SS09 system:
  - DCP: Disabled Children's Program, 22 or 32
  - OTH: LTC assistance for hospitals 22 or 32
  - WPA or QUADS: Assistance Daily Living Services, 22 or 32
  - DAC: Disabled Adult Children, 22 or 32
  - PIC: Pickle, 22 or 32
  - MAWD: Working Disabled, 22 or 32
  - WSE: ASA Waiver Program, 16
  - DWW: Disabled Widow(er), 22 or 32
  - FSW: Family Support Waiver, 22 or 32
  - WSD: Waiver for Developmentally Disabled, 37 or 38
- o Receives federally or State-administered supplemental benefits under Section 212(a) of P.L. 93-66.
- o Veterans who receive VA benefits because they are rated a 100% service-connected or non-service connected disability or who, according to the VA, need regular aid and attendance or are permanently housebound.
- o Surviving spouses of deceased veterans who meet one of the following criteria according
to the VA:
  - need regular aid and attendance,
  - permanently housebound, or
  - receive or have been approved for benefits from the VA because of the veteran's
death and could be considered permanently disabled for Social Security purposes.
(Section 2013 defines social Security's criteria for permanent disability.)
- o Surviving children (any age) of a deceased veteran who the VA:
  - has determined are permanently incapable of self-support, or
  - has been approved for benefits because of the veteran's death and could be considered
permanently disabled for Social Security purposes. (See Section 2013.)

2013 SOCIAL SECURITY'S CRITERIA FOR DISABILITY

Any of the following 11 conditions determine, according to SSA, if a recipient is disabled:

- Permanent loss of use of both hands, both feet, or one hand and one foot.
- Amputation of leg at hip.
- Amputation of leg or foot because of diabetes mellitus or peripheral vascular diseases.
- Total deafness, not correctable by surgery or hearing aid.
- Statutory blindness, unless caused by cataracts or detached retina.
- IQ 59 or less, established after the person becomes 16 years old.
- Spinal cord or nerve root lesions resulting in paraplegia or quadriplegia.
- Multiple sclerosis in which there is damage to the nervous system caused by scattered areas of inflammation. The inflammation recurs and has progressed to varied interference with the function of the nervous system, including severe muscle weakness, paralysis, and vision and speech defects.
- Muscular dystrophy with irreversible wasting of the muscles, impairing the ability to use the arms or legs.
- Impaired renal function caused by chronic renal disease, resulting in severely reduced function which may require dialysis or kidney transplant.
- Amputation of a limb of a person at least 55 years old.

Some of these conditions are obvious and Benefits Specialists can determine their existence by observation. Others may require the opinion of a physician.

Note: Many of the people who would have one of the 11 conditions might already receive SSI or Social Security blindness or disability payments, or their disability is obvious (such as amputation of leg at hip). For example, a veteran's surviving spouse who also receives SSI already qualifies as disabled under paragraph 1. Benefits Specialists need not additionally prove Social Security permanent disability to classify the person as one of those receiving special treatment.

2014 SPECIAL PROVISIONS FOR ELDERLY OR DISABLED HOUSEHOLDS

Households containing an elderly or disabled person receive special treatment. The special provisions are:

- Separate household status - elderly individuals (and their spouses) who cannot prepare their own meals because they suffer from disabilities may be a separate household even if living and eating with others. Review Section 2231.A (7) for specifics.
- Non-citizen eligibility - elderly non-citizens who were lawfully residing in the US on 08-22-96, and continue to be lawful residents. Disabled individuals who are lawfully residing in the US. (Section 3220 L.)
- Income tests - households with elderly or disabled members are exempt from the gross income test.
- Medical deduction - Elderly or disabled members who have medical bills that exceed $35 a month are entitled to a medical deduction. Note: The $35 disregard is for the household, not the individual. All allowed medical expenses must be added together to determine if they are over $35.

- Excess shelter - households with elderly or disabled members receive an excess shelter deduction for the full monthly amount that exceeds 50% of the household's monthly income after the allowed deductions.
- Exemption from monthly reporting - if all adult household members are elderly or disabled and have no earned income, the household is exempt from monthly reporting.
- Resources - The resource limit is $3000 instead of $2000 if the household contains at least one elderly or disabled member. The resource limit is $2000 if the only elderly or disabled member in the household is disqualified (Section 5530).

2015 VERIFICATION

An elderly or disabled person who wants to claim separate household status must provide the information needed to determine if the person is elderly or disabled.

Tennessee

Department of Human Services: Adult Services: http://www.tn.gov/humanserv/Adult.html

Welcome to the Department of Human Services- Adult Services

Adult Day Care

Adult Protective Services

Child and Adult Child Care Food Program

Community Services Block Grant

Disability Determination Services

Family Assistance Service Centers

Home Energy Assistance

Families First

Food Stamps

Homemaker

Medicaid/TennCare

Vocational Rehabilitation

Social Services Block Grant

Weatherization

Disability Determination Services: http://www.tn.gov/humanserv/rehab/dds.html

The Tennessee Disability Determination Services (DDS) is a section within the Division of Rehabilitation Services of the Department of Human Services. The DDS operates by agreement between the State of Tennessee and the Social Security Administration to process Social Security and Supplemental Security Income disability claims. The DDS maintains effective working relationships with Social Security's Area Director's office, 30 district and branch offices, five Office of Hearings and Appeals (OHA) offices, medical and psychological associations, legislative offices, the legal community and other state and local organizations that serve the disabled. The DDS strives to provide all persons applying for disability benefits with an accurate decision, processing their claim promptly and providing assistance to the public in a courteous, helpful manner.

For more information on Social Security go to the following link: www.ssa.gov.

For a status on a pending disability claim, please contact our customer service line toll free at **1-800-342-1117**.

For more information:
Telephone: (615) 743-7300
Toll-Free, in Tennessee: 1-800-342-1117
TTY: (615) 253-1510
TTY: (Long Distance) 1-877-210-0008
Fax: (615) 253-2727
Fax (Long-Distance): 1-800-419-4290

Caregiving: http://www.tn.gov/comaging/caregiving.html

- **NATIONAL FAMILY CAREGIVER SUPPORT PROGRAM**

  General Information

  - **Are you a caregiver?**

  - **About the National Family Caregiver Support Program**

  - **Program Eligibility**

  - **What kind of help is available?**

  - **Contact Information**

  Are you a caregiver?
  Do you help an older family member:
  - Pay bills

- Do household chores such as:

  - Meal preparation

  - Laundry

  - Cleaning

- With medication

- Provide transportation

- Shop or run errands for a loved one

- With personal care such as:

  - Dressing

  - Toileting

  - Bathing

  - Feeding

- Arrange and coordinate outside services

If you said **YES**, to any of these you are probably a caregiver.

About the National Family Caregiver Support Program

The purpose of the program is to help families sustain their efforts to care for older relatives with chronic illness or disability in their homes. This program is available through the Commission and local Area Agencies on Aging and Disability.

The NFCSP was authorized under the Older Americans Act Amendment of 2000. Funding is provided by the U.S. Administration on Aging.

Program Eligibility

- -Adult family members (age 18 years or older) or other adult informal caregivers providing care to individuals 60 years of age and older.
- -Adult family members or other adult informal caregivers providing care to individuals any age with Alzheimer's disease and related disorders.
- -Grandparent and other relatives (not parents) 55 years of age and older providing care to children under the age of 18 years:
  - Lives with the child;

  - Is the primary caregiver of the child;

  - Has legal relationship to the child, such as legal custody or guardianship, or is raising

    the child informally

- -Grandparents and other relatives (not parents) 55 years of age and older providing care to adults, age 18 to 59 years, with disabilities.

What kind of help is available?

17. Information about available services
18. Assistance in gaining access to supportive services
19. Individual Counseling, Support Groups, Caregiver Training
20. Respite care for temporary relief, such as:
    - Personal care

    - Homemaker

    - Adult day care

    - In-home adult care

21. Supplemental services, such as:
    - Home delivered meals

    - Medical equipment/supplies

    - Minor home modification

    - Personal Response System

Availability of services may vary depending on service area.

Contact Information

Contact your local Area Agency on Aging and Disability's Information and Assistance Line for enrollment in the NFCSP or use the Statewide Toll Free Line, 1-866-836-6678.

Tennessee Commission on Aging and Disability: http://www.tn.gov/comaging/

Caregiver Resources: http://www.tn.gov/comaging/caregiving.html

- State of Tennessee Ombudsman

- The Center On Aging Life Series Booklets - University of Hawaii at Manoa

- Aging Parents and Elder Care

- Mental Health Issues and Needs of Older Adults

Options for Community Living: http://www.tn.gov/comaging/living.html

General Information

- **About the OPTIONS for Community Living Program**

- **Program Eligibility**

- **What kind of services is available?**

- **Contact Information**

About the OPTIONS for Community Living Program
OPTIONS for Community Living is a state-funded program. The program was created to provide the elderly and adults with disabilities home and community based services choices. This program is available through the local Area Agencies on Aging and Disability.

Program Eligibility
To be eligible for the OPTIONS program, an individual must:
- -Be a resident of Tennessee;
- -Be eighteen (18) years of age or older;
- -Must meet Activities of Daily Living (ADL) and Instrumental Activities of Daily Living (IADL) limitation requirements.

Consumers of OPTIONS services are adults with physical and/or cognitive disabilities (excluding individuals with mental retardation).
There is no income eligibility requirement for this program; however, there is a sliding fee scale based on income.

What kind of services is available?
The services funded through the State for OPTIONS include the following:
- -Homemaker services
- -Personal care
- -Home delivered meals

Contact Information
Contact your local Area Agency on Aging and Disability's Information and Assistance Line for enrollment in the OPTIONS for Community Living Program or use the Statewide Toll Free Line, 1-866-836-6678

Resources: http://www.tn.gov/comaging/resources.html

Important Links	
Administration on Aging	*Council on Aging of Greater Nashville*
Disability Info.gov	*Tennessee Vulnerable Adults Coalition*
Nursing Home Compare	*Health Information Tennessee*
Health Facilities Listings in Tennessee	*Tennessee Disability Training Network*
Mental Health Issues and Needs of Older Adults	*Tennessee Department of Health*
National Eldercare Locator	*Tennessee Osteoporosis Fact Sheet*
Tennessee Technology Access Project	*Department of Veterans Affairs*
Centers for Disease Control and Prevention	*Alzheimer's Association*

Council on Developmental Disabilities	*Department of Human Services*
National Organization on Disability	*Assisted Living Directory*
Find Your Legislator	*Rural Health Association of Tennessee*
Important Phone Numbers	
Contacting the Eldercare Locator	1-800-677-1116
Health Related Boards Complaint Hotline	1-800-852-2187
Home Health Agency Complaint Hotline	1-800-541-7367 (within Tennessee only)
TennCare Hotline	1-800-669-1851 or 741-4800 (Nashville area)
TennCare Mental Health and Substance Abuse Information Line	1-800-758-1638
Traumatic Brain Injury Hotline	1-800-882-0611
Adult Protective Services Hotline	1-888-APS-TENN or 1-888-277-8366
Food Stamp Hotline	1-800-342-1784
QMB (Qualified Medicare Beneficiary Hotline)	1-800-624-5547
Services for the Blind and Visually Impaired (In-State Only)	1-800-628-7818
Tennessee Council for the Hearing Impaired (In-State Only)	1-800-270-1349
Disability Determination Services (In-State Only)	1-800-342-1117
Osteoporosis Hotline:	1-888-734-BONE

Texas

Department of Aging and Disability Services (DADS): http://www.dads.state.tx.us/

Caregiver support: http://www.dads.state.tx.us/services/caregiver.html

Do you take care of an older or disabled family member? Do you take care of a grandchild? Do you need a break from caregiving? Do you have health or money worries because of your caregiving duties?

If you are 60 or older and you care for someone

Call 1-800-252-9240. Your local area agency on aging (AAA) may be able to help you:

- Find services in your area
- Help arrange for those services
- Provide short-term relief

If you care for someone 60 or older

Call 1-800-252-9240. Your local AAA may be able to help you:

- Find services in your area
- Help arrange for those services
- Provide short-term relief

If you care for a child

The National Family Caregiver Support Program provides support for the growing number of older people who care for children. This program can help grandparents or other relatives (age 55 and older) who are caring for a child age 18 or younger. Call 1-800-252-9240 to learn more.

If you get Medicaid

Some Medicaid programs pay for short-term relief for caregivers. This is called respite. Call your local DADS office to learn more. Click here to find your local DADS office.

If you have an intellectual or developmental disability

Your local mental retardation authority (MRA) may pay for short-term relief for caregivers. This is called respite. You can call them for more information. Click here to find your local MRA.

If you are a caregiver who needs some help

Even the most amazing caregivers need time and assistance! Take Time Texas challenges caregivers to take some time for themselves and reach for information, support and assistance. To encourage caregivers to take that time, the Texas Respite Coordination Center was created to offer caregivers and respite care providers services, resources and educational materials.

Where to call to receive DADS services and supports

Please click here to find your DADS local intake office, area agency on aging or mental retardation authority. You can search by city, county or ZIP code.

To learn more

Fact sheets about DADS programs that offer caregiver support services:

- Area Agencies on Aging (AAA)
- Community Based Alternatives (CBA)
- Community Living Assistance and Support Services (CLASS)
- Consolidated Waiver Program (CWP)
- Deaf Blind with Multiple Disabilities (DBMD)
- Home and Community–based Services (HCS)
- In-Home and Family Support Program - MR (IHFSP-MR)
- Medically Dependent Children Program (MDCP)
- Mental Retardation Authorities (MRA)
- Texas Home Living (TxHmL)

Other resources

- 211 Texas can provide information about local, state or federal services.
- Aging and Disability Resource Centers (ADRCs) — The ADRCs provide information about and help with state and federal benefits. They can also help you learn about local

programs and services. Anyone — individuals, family members, friends or professionals — can receive information tailored to their needs.

- Aging Texas Well provides information to help family members and other voluntary caregivers.

- Consumer Directed Services — If you want more control over who works for you in your own home, you can choose either Consumer Directed Services (CDS) or the Service Responsibility Option (SRO). You can only use CDS or SRO in some DADS programs.

- Explanation of Mental Retardation Services and Supports includes brief descriptions of DADS intellectual and developmental disability services and supports.

- Know Your Options (PDF) discusses the DADS Money Follows the Person (MFP) initiative that allows certain Texans who are eligible for Medicaid and living in nursing facilities to choose an appropriate community setting and receive community services and supports.

- Making Informed Choices: Community Living Options Information Process (PDF) — MRA staff can use this document to help explain options in the community to residents of state supported living centers.

- Making Informed Choices: Community Living Options Information Process for Legally Authorized Representatives of Residents in State Schools (PDF) — MRA staff can use to help explain options in the community to legally authorized representatives of state supported living center residents.

- Medicaid Estate Recovery Program — The state may file a claim against the estate of a deceased Medicaid recipient, age 55 and older, who applied for certain long-term care services on or after March 1, 2005. Claims include the cost of services, hospital care and prescription drugs supported by Medicaid under certain programs.

- Yourtexasbenefits.com — This website offers you easy and secure online access to Texas Health and Human Services

Commission (HHSC) benefits including Medicaid, SNAP food benefits, Temporary Assistance for Needy Families, Children's Health Insurance Program (CHIP), and

Making your home accessible

Do you need your house changed so you can get around better? Do you need a ramp to your front door? Does your bathroom need grab bars or a wider door?

About making your home accessible

Ramps, grab bars or wider doorways make life easier and safer for you. DADS can help with some of these changes. However, we can't pay for major changes, such as:

- Adding a new structure
- Adding more space
- Remodeling
- Regular maintenance

The Texas Department of Housing and Community Affairs can help Texans with home repairs and weatherization.

Where to call to receive DADS services and supports

Please click here to find your DADS local intake office, area agency on aging or mental retardation authority. You can search by city, county or ZIP code.

To learn more

Fact sheets about DADS programs that can help make your home more accessible:

- Area Agencies on Aging (AAA)
- Community Attendant Services (CAS)
- Community Based Alternatives (CBA)
- Community Living Assistance and Support Services (CLASS)
- Consolidated Waiver Program (CWP)

- Deaf Blind with Multiple Disabilities (DBMD)
- Family Care (FC)
- Home and Community-based Services (HCS)
- In-Home and Family Support Program (IHFSP)
- In-Home and Family Support Services– MR (IHFSP-MR)
- Medically Dependent Children Program (MDCP)
- Primary Home Care (PHC)
- Texas Home Living (TxHmL)

In Home Family Support and Services: http://www.dads.state.tx.us/services/faqs-fact/ifs.html

In-Home and Family Support Program

This program provides direct grant benefits to people who have physical disabilities and or their families to help them purchase services that enable them live in the community. Eligible people choose and purchase services that help them to remain in their own homes.

Services

- Attendant care, home health services, home health aide services, homemaker services, chore services that provide assistance with training, routine body functions, dressing, preparing and consuming food, and ambulating.
- Counseling and training programs that help provide proper care of an individual with a disability.
- Medical, surgical, therapeutic, diagnostic and other health services related to a person's disability.
- Other disability related services prior-approved by DADS.
- Pre-approved transportation and room and board cost incurred by person with physical disability or his family during evaluation or treatment.
- Purchase or lease of special equipment or architectural modifications of a home to facilitate the care, treatment therapy or general living conditions of a person with a disability.
- Respite care
- Transportation services

Financial eligibility requirements

Financial eligibility is determined by the Texas Department of Aging and Disability Services.

Other eligibility requirements

- Be age 4 or older.
- Have a physical disability which substantially limits the person's ability to function independently.
- Co-payment schedule begins at 105 percent of the state median income for household size.

Availability

Services are available statewide in every county; however, there are long interest lists in all areas.

How to apply for services

Contact your local DADS office.

To learn more

- In-Home and Family Support Services provider website
- Access and Intake Community Options Manual (PDF format)
- DADS Reference Guide

Help for Texans: Personal Care: http://www.dads.state.tx.us/services/personalcare.html

Personal care

Do you live in your own home? Do you need help with everyday tasks such as bathing, dressing, shopping or cooking? Do you need someone to help you with chores or taking care of your home? Do you need help eating or do you need meals delivered to you?

About personal care

DADS can offer help with the following types of personal care:

- Attendant services
- Housekeeping or chores
- Meals

Attendant services

Sometimes all you need is a little help so you can stay in your own home. DADS can find someone to help you with your everyday tasks — bathing, dressing, shopping, cooking and others. We call this attendant services.

Housekeeping or chores

You will feel better if your house and clothes are clean and you have food to eat. If you are physically limited, DADS can find someone to help you with chores in your home such as dusting, vacuuming or bed making.

Meals

DADS offers several programs that can help make sure you get healthy meals.

- **Group meals** — Group meals are often available at local community or senior centers.
- **Help eating** — If you have certain physical limitations, DADS can find someone to help you eat.
- **Help preparing meals**—DADS can get someone to come to your home and cook for you. This service is often part of a program that provides help with other chores.
- **Meals delivered to your home** — Volunteers bring noontime meals to people in their homes. This is usually during the work week. In some places it is called Meals-on-Wheels.

Where to call to receive DADS services and supports

Please click here to find your DADS local intake office, area agency on aging or mental retardation authority. You can search by city, county or ZIP code.

To learn more

Fact sheets about DADS programs that can help with personal care services:

- Area Agencies on Aging (AAA)
- Community Attendant Services (CAS)
- Community Based Alternatives (CBA)
- Community Living Assistance and Support Services (CLASS)
- Consolidated Waiver Program (CWP)
- Consumer-Managed Personal Attendant Services (CMPAS)

- Day Activity and Health Services (DAHS)
- Deaf Blind with Multiple Disabilities (DBMD)
- Emergency Response Services (ERS)
- Family Care (FC)
- Home and Community–based Services (HCS)
- Home-delivered Meals (HDM)
- In-Home and Family Support Program (IHFSP)
- In-Home and Family Support Program - MR (IHFSP-MR)
- Medically Dependent Children Program (MDCP)
- Primary Home Care (PHC)
- Special Services to Persons with Disabilities (SSPD)
- Special Services to Persons with Disabilities 24-hour Shared Attendant (SSPD-SAC)
- Texas Home Living (TxHmL)

Other resources

- 211 Texas can provide information about local, state or federal services.
- Aging and Disability Resource Centers (ADRCs) — The ADRCs provide information about and help with state and federal benefits. They can also help you learn about local programs and services. Anyone — individuals, family members, friends or professionals — can receive information tailored to their needs.
- Consumer Directed Services — If you want more control over who works for you in your own home, you can choose either Consumer Directed Services (CDS) or the Service Responsibility Option (SRO). You can only use CDS or SRO in some DADS programs.
- Medicaid Estate Recovery Program — The state may file a claim against the estate of a deceased Medicaid recipient, age 55 and older, who applied for certain long-term care services on or after March 1, 2005. Claims include the cost of services, hospital care and prescription drugs supported by Medicaid under certain programs.
- Searchable list of home health agencies website allows you to search for home health care by city, county, area code or ZIP code.
- Yourtexasbenefits.com — This website offers you easy and secure online access to Texas Health and Human Services Commission (HHSC) benefits including Medicaid, SNAP food benefits, Temporary Assistance for Needy Families, Children's Health Insurance Program (CHIP), and nursing home care and other services for people who are elderly or have disabilities.

Utah

Seniors: http://www.utah.gov/seniors/

Information for Seniors

Information for older individuals including topics such as nutrition, care services, available benefits, employment, and recreation.

Learn More > >

Information for Caregivers

Information and resources for caregivers - a family member, friend, or neighbor who helps care for an elderly individual or person with a disability who lives at home.

Learn More > >

General Information

Information for students, teachers, researchers, media, and consumers who are interested in general issues and statistics related to seniors.

Learn More > >

Utah's 211

Seniors

- Information for Seniors
- Information for Caregivers
- General Information

Quick Links

- Financial
- Housing and Living Arrangements
- Health, Medical, and Safety
- Legal Issues
- Caregiver Support

Related Online Services

- Occupational & Professional Licensee Lookup
- Renew Vehicle Registration
- Utah Job Search

- Veteran Services
- Utah State Parks
- Find a Legislator

Information For Senior Caregivers: http://www.utah.gov/seniors/caregiver.html

The following links provide access to information on topics of interest, such as living arrangements, health, and transportation, to those who care for seniors.

- Benefits
- Financial
- Legal Issues
- Housing and Living Arrangements
- Health, Medical and Safety
- Transportation
- Lifestyle
- Education
- General Information

Utah's 211

Seniors

- Information for Seniors
- Information for Caregivers
- General Information

Quick Links

- Financial
- Housing and Living Arrangements
- Health, Medical, and Safety
- Legal Issues
- Caregiver Support

Related Online Services

- Occupational & Professional Licensee Lookup
- Renew Vehicle Registration
- Utah Job Search
- Veteran Services
- Utah State Parks
- Find a Legislator

Senior Living and Housing Arrangements: http://www.utah.gov/seniors/seniorshousing.html

Some of the following are blatantly commercial websites, which is both unfortunate, and interesting that such are on the <u>official</u> Utah.gov website...

- Senior Living Finder
- Licensed Utah Nursing and Assisted Living Facilities
- Home Care or Hospice Agency Locator
- General Information on Health Facilities, Questions to Ask, etc.
- Encyclopedia of Senior Living Options
- Senior Community Housing
- Locate and Choose a Nursing Home
- Guide to Retirement Communities
- Helpful Aids and Advice for Independent Living
- Medical Emergency Response Information
- Verify that Your Contractor is Licensed
- Weatherization Assistance

Aging and Adult Services: http://www.hsdaas.utah.gov/caregiver_support.htm

Are You a Caregiver for Someone 60 or Older?

You are a Caregiver if you are...

- Performing tasks to help with shopping, errands, transportation, bills, or home repairs.
- Providing personal care such as bathing, laundry, toileting or dressing.
- Changing roles and beginning to think of your care receiver as depending on you for making decisions for them.
- Seeking assistance and formal services of others to stay with or provide care for your care receiver.
- Considering changes in your work or living arrangements: relocating or adjusting your work schedule to allow you more time with your care receiver.

- Considering long term care placement: trying to make a decision about a nursing home and how involved to be day-by-day.
- Coping with loss and dealing with difficult adjustments in your relationship.

Caregiving can be costly...

- Your relationship with your family may suffer. Your family and friends may feel left out.
- Your physical and mental health may be compromised.
- Your job may not receive all the attention it should.
- Your social life is diminished.
- You may feel you never have a moment to yourself.
- Your coping methods are becoming destructive: overeating, smoking, and drinking.
- Guilt is the most common feeling.

Utah Caregiver Support Program

Purpose

1. To provide information, assistance, support, caregiver training, and counseling to:

   - caregivers of adults 60 years or older;
   - caregivers 60 years of age who are caring for persons with mental retardation and related developmental disabilities; and
   - grandparents or older individuals who are relative caregivers of a child not more than 18 years of age.

To provide respite and supplemental services to caregivers of adults 60 years or older who are unable to perform at least two <u>activities of daily living</u> without substantial human assistance, including verbal reminding, physical cueing, or supervision.

Eligibility

Services are provided to family or informal caregivers.

Priority shall be given to caregivers providing care and support to individuals, 60 years of age or older, who are in greatest social and economic need (with particular attention to low-income older individuals) providing care and support to persons with mental retardation and related developmental disabilities.

Respite and supplemental services are determined by using the Division of Aging and Adult Services approved assessment tool.

For information on services and activities in your area, please contact your nearest <u>Area Agency on Aging.</u>

Area Agency on Aging: http://www.hsdaas.utah.gov/pdf/utah_area_agencies_on_aging.pdf

DIVISION OF AGING AND ADULT SERVICES

UTAH DEPARTMENT OF HUMAN SERVICES

195 North 1950 West, Salt Lake City, Utah 84116
PHONE: 801-538-3910

TOLL FREE: 1-877-424-4640

FAX: 801-538-4395

Website: hsdaas.utah.gov

Director: Assistant Director: OAA Assistant Director: APS

Nels Holmgren Michael S. Styles (vacant)
E-mail: nholmgren@utah.gov mstyles@utah.gov

AREA AGENCIES ON AGING January 27, 2011

Bear River Area Agency on Aging
Box Elder, Cache, Rich

Michelle Benson, Aging Svcs. Dir.

170 North Main
Logan, UT 84321
Phone: 435-752-7242 or
1-877-772-7242
Fax: 435-752-6962
E-Mail: michelleb@brag.utah.gov
Website: www.brag.utah.gov

Davis County Health Dept., Family Health and Senior Services Division
Davis

Sally Kershisnik, Director of Family
Health and Senior Services
22 South State St -Clearfield UT 84015
PO Box 618 - Farmington UT 84025-0618
Phone: 801-525-5000
Fax: 801-525-5061
E-Mail: skershis@daviscountyutah.gov
Website: www.daviscountyutah.gov

Five-County Area Agency on Aging

Beaver, Garfield, Iron, Kane, Washington

Carrie Schonlaw, Director
1070 West 1600 South, Bldg. B
(P. O. Box 1550, ZIP 84771-1550)
St. George, UT 84770
Phone: 435-673-3548
Fax: 435-673-3540
E-Mail: cschonlaw@fivecounty.utah.gov

Mountainland Dept. of Aging and Family Services
Summit, Utah, Wasatch

Scott McBeth, Director
586 East 800 North
Orem, UT 84097-4146
Phone: 801-229-3800
Fax: 801-229-3671

Website: www.mountainland.org
E-Mail: smcbeth@mountainland.org

Salt Lake County Aging Services

Salt Lake

Sarah Brenna, Director
2001 South State, #S1500
Salt Lake City, UT 84190-2300
Phone: 801-468-2454
Fax: 801-468-2852
E-Mail: sbrenna@slco.org
Website: www.aging.slco.org

San Juan County Area Agency on Aging

San Juan

Tammy Gallegos, Director
117 South Main (P. O. Box 9)
Monticello, UT 84535-0009
Phone: 435-587-3225
Fax: 435-587-2447
E-Mail: tgallegos@sanjuancounty.org

Six-County Area Agency on Aging

Juab, Millard, Piute, Sanpete, Sevier, Wayne

Scott Christensen, Director
250 North Main
(P. O. Box 820)
Richfield, UT 84701
Phone: 435-893-0700
Toll free: 1-888-899-4447
Fax: 435-893-0701
E-Mail:
schristensen5@ sixcounty.com

Southeastern Utah AAA

Carbon, Emery, Grand

Maughan Guymon, Director
Technical Assistance Center
375 South Carbon Avenue
(P. O. Box 1106)
Price, UT 84501
Phone: 435-637-4268 or 5444
Fax: 435-637-5448
E-Mail: mguymon@seualg.utah.gov

Tooele Co. Div. of Aging and Adult Services

Tooele

Josh Maher, (435) 843-4125
59 East Vine Street
Tooele, UT 84074

Phone: 435-843-4110
Fax: 435-882-6971
E-Mail: jmaher@co.tooele.ut.us
Uintah Basin Area Agency on Aging
Daggett, Duchesne
Louise Warburton, Director
330 East 100 South
Roosevelt, UT 84066
Phone: 435-722-4518
Fax: 435-722-4890

E-Mail: louisew@ubaog.org

Council on Aging - Golden Age Center – (Uintah County PSA)
Uintah County
Louise Martin, Director
155 South 100 West
Vernal, UT 84078
Phone: 435-789-2169
Fax: 435-789-2171
E-Mail: lmartin@co.uintah.ut.us
Weber Area Agency on Aging
Morgan, Weber
Kelly VanNoy, Director
237 26th Street, Suite 320
Ogden, UT 84401
Phone: 801-625-3770
Fax: 801-778-6830
E-Mail: kellyv@weberhs.org

In Home Services: http://www.hsdaas.utah.gov/ss_in_home_services.htm

Alternatives Program

The Alternatives Program offers in-home services to persons to enable these individuals to remain in their own home for as long as possible. If these services were not available, these seniors who have health, mobility or functional limitations would not be able to continue living in their current living arrangements. The program offers a wide variety of in-home services available to adults based on an assessment of their needs.

The individual receives a comprehensive assessment by a case manager and, at times, a registered nurse, examining the client's physical, mental, social and financial status. The case manager works closely with the individual, their family, and other social and health agencies to identify service needs and the funding resources available to meet those needs.

The case manager develops and manages a comprehensive care plan of services designed to maintain the individual at home based on the assessment. Services are monitored monthly by the case manager to re-evaluate the individual's needs.

Services that may be Available

Case Management: Assessment, development of a care plan, coordination and monitoring of formal and informal services.

Homemaker Services: Assistance with supplemental homemaking activities.

Chore Services: Workers assist with minor home repair and maintenance necessary to protect the health and safety of the individual. Typical chore services include shoveling snow off walkways, clearing trash out of a yard, replacing locks, and minor plumbing repairs such as unclogging a drain.

Supportive Maintenance: Assistance with personal care needs.

Adult Day Care: Socialization, recreation and cultural activities provided in a supervised setting.

Personal Emergency Response System: An automatic telephone dialing service worn by the individual to contact family or other medical personnel in an emergency situation.

Respite Care: Short-term services to relieve persons who care for a homebound individual.

Eligibility

To be eligible to participate in the program a person must:

- Be 18 years or older
- Be at risk of nursing home placement
- Have health and personal needs which can be adequately met in the community within established cost limits
- Have low income and minimal assets

Cost

Financial eligibility for the Alternatives Program is determined by the Area Agency on Aging case manager. Individuals who qualify for the program may be required to pay a small fee based on a sliding fee schedule. Donations are always appreciated.

Examples of Services Available

- Adult Day Care
- Residential and Nursing Facility over night stays
- Home Health Aides
- Homemaking
- Home Modification
- Rented and purchased equipment
- Senior Companion
- Personal Emergency Response Systems

Application or Referral

Please contact your nearest Area Agency on Aging for more information.

Medicaid Aging Waiver Program

The purpose of this program is to provide an option for people 65 and older who have medical problems to live outside of an institution. The goal is to assist seniors who meet nursing home admission requirements but wish to remain in a home setting, to do so in a safe manner. It is different from regular Medicaid because it allows special income deductions to meet their living expenses, exempts income from spouse even if they are living with them, and has a separate formula for calculation of assets. Clients receive all of the standard Medicaid benefits as well as the additional benefits of the Aging Walver. Medicaid will recover only the cost of actual care provided from the estate of the client. Medicaid does not take the entire estate.

A client must be age 65 or older, be a resident of the State of Utah and meet both financial and medical eligibility. The core service provided by the Aging Waiver is Case Management. A Case Manager will work with the applicant throughout this process and, if the client is accepted for this program, the Case Manager will be involved in the client's plan of care as long as they remain at home with services. The role of the Case Manager is to assist with accessing community resources, authorizing use of Medicaid services, assuring quality of services provided and assuring that the health and safety needs of client are able to be met in a home setting.

In addition to Case Management, other Waiver Services that the client may qualify for include:

- Personal Care Services (Home Health Aide or Personal Care Attendant)
- Homemaking Services (may include cleaning, laundry, shopping, meal preparation, errands, assistance with medical appointments)
- Chore Services
- Non-medical Transportation
- Emergency Response System
- Medication Reminder System
- Adult Day Care Services
- In Home Caregiver Respite (limited)
- Nursing Home Overnight Caregiver Respite (limited)
- Home-delivered Meals
- Companion Services
- Medical Equipment (on a limited basis)
- Home Modification (on a limited basis)
- Assistance with Caregiver Training
- Medical Card for Medications and Medical Expenses

The Aging Waiver is administered through the Department of Health Care Financing. They contract with the State Division of Aging and Adult Services for the daily operation of the program. There is a Case Management Agency for every area of the State of Utah. For information on how to inquire further about this program, please contact your local Area Agency on Aging or the State Division of Aging at 1-801-538-3910.

Services for People With Disabilities: http://www.dspd.utah.gov/#

We promote opportunities and provide support for persons with disabilities to lead self-determined lives. We oversee home and community-based services for more than 4,000 people who have disabilities. Support includes community living, day services, supported employment services, and support for people with disabilities and their families.

We also provide services to about 250 people at the Utah State Developmental Center (USDC), a state operated Intermediate Care Facility for people with Intellectual Disabilities (ICF/ID).

Services Overview: http://www.dspd.utah.gov/servicesoverview.htm

The Division of Services for People with Disabilities provides several services to the public ranging from Housing assistance to companion services. Please click below to learn about the different services.

- Companion Services
- Extended Community Living Support
- Host Home Support
- Professional Parent
- Community Living Residential Transportation
- Supported Living (Hourly)
- Chore and Homemaker Services
- Supported Living Natural Support
- Family Training/Brain Injury
- Family Assistance and Support -DD/MR
- Respite Care Support
- Senior Support
- Site and Non-Site Support - Children
- Site and Non-Site Training
- Day Training Transportation
- Supported Employment Services (Hourly)
- Support Coordination

For additional information, see Division Directive 1.2 (Eligibility and Intake) and Administrative Rule R539-1 (Eligibility).

The Division will work with the person to decide which services a person is eligible to receive.

Vermont

(A large number of programs, but where to start is the question...)

Agency of Human Services: http://humanservices.vermont.gov/

Department For Children and Families: Essential Person Program:
http://dcf.vermont.gov/esd/essential_person

ESD

- About Us
- Contact Us
- Rules
- Statistics

Programs & Services

- 3SquaresVT
- Emergency Assistance
- Essential Person
- Farm to Family
  - Fuel Assistance
    - Crisis Fuel Assistance
- Health Insurance
- Long-Term Care
- Phone Assistance
- Reach Up

Essential Person Program in Vermont

The official State website for the Essential Person program in Vermont.

The Essential Person Program helps you stay in your home by contributing to the cost of having someone live with you to provide essential care.

Who is eligible?

People who are blind, have a disability, or are 65 or older AND meet the income guidelines.

How do I apply?

1. Click here to go to our online application.Or call our Benefits Service Center at 1-800-479-6151 to request a paper application.
2. If you are age 60 and older and need help applying, call the Senior Helpline at 1-800-642-5119.

How does it work?

You can choose to receive monthly cash assistance through direct deposit or an EBT (electronic benefit transfer) card called Vermont Express. Click here to learn more about how the card works and where it can be used.

Right To A Timely Decision.
Learn about your right to a timely decision on an application.

Division of Disability and Aging Services: Older Vermonters and Family Caregiving Services:
http://www.ddas.vermont.gov/ddas-programs/programs-oaa/programs-oaa-default-page

Older Vermonters and Family Caregiver Services (Older Americans Act)

The Older Americans Act (OAA) provides funding for a range of programs that offer services and opportunities for older Vermonters to remain as independent as possible and to be active and contributing members of their community.

The OAA also provides a range of services to family caregivers to support them to continue in this essential role. The Older Americans Act focuses on improving the lives of older adults and family caregivers in areas of income, housing, nutrition, health, employment, retirement, and social and community services.

- **Services**

- **Eligibility**

- **Providers of Services**

- **Program Contacts**

- **Policies & Guidelines**

- **Publications**

- **Manuals**

- **Forms**

Services Include

- Case Management

- Dementia Respite

- Senior Food and Nutrition Programs

- Health Promotion and Disease Prevention

- Information, Referral and Assistance Services

- Legal Assistance

- National Family Caregiver Support Program (NFCSP)

- Senior Community Services Employment Program (SCSEP)

Return to Program Informational Menu

Eligibility

- Older adults age 60 and over

- Family caregivers (of any age) of older adults

- Older relative caregivers of children under age 18

Return to Program Informational Menu

Providers of Services

- **Area Agencies on Aging**
  Area Agencies on Aging provide support to people 60 and older in their efforts to remain active, healthy, financially secure, and in control of their own lives.

If you do not know which of these agencies provides services in your area, call the *Senior Helpline* at *1-800-642-5119* for assistance.

Return to Program Informational Menu

Program Contacts

- Community Development Unit
  Phone: (802) 241-4534
- Case Management
  Kathy Rainville
  Phone: (802) 786-5052
- Dementia Respite, and National Family Caregiver Support Program (NFCSP)
  Maria Mireault, Dementia Project Director
  Phone: (802) 241-3738
- Nutrition Programs (Food and Nutrition), and Health Promotion & Disease Prevention
  Mary Woodruff
  Phone: (802) 241-2930

Return to Program Informational Menu

Policies & Guidelines

- **Revised Case Management Standards & Certification Procedures for Older American Act and Choices for Care** - June 2009

- **Case Manager Training Process** - 2009

- **Case Management Reference Manual and Study Guide** (June 2007) (Updated October 2008)
  This study guide should help you prepare for the Case Management Certification Exam. It is not intended to be a training guide to become a Case Manager. It should be used in addition to the core training and orientation you have completed through your agency.

- **AAA Funding Formula** (April 2006)
  How the Numbers Change - An Overview of Data Sources

- **Area Agency on Aging (AAA) Time Study**

  FFY08 AAA Time Study Instructions and Spreadsheet

  - AAA Time Study Instructions FFY2008
  - AAA Time Study Form

  NAPIS Reporting Instructions and Spreadsheet

  - NAPIS Reporting Procedures Updated November 2010
  - NAPIS Templates for AAA's FFY 2009
  - Napis Reporting Requirements (November 2004)
    Reporting Requirements For Title III and VII of the Older Americans Act (Not including LTC Ombudsman Program) For FY '05 and Subsequent Years
  - NAPIS Template for AAAs for FFY2007

Return to Program Informational Menu

Publications

- **DAIL-DDAS Service Codes and Rates**
  Service Codes and Rates for all DAIL-DDAS services, includes Choices for Care, Adult Day services, Traumatic Brain Injury and Developmental Disabilities Services, Children's Personal Care and High Technology Home Care, and services for Older Vermonters.

- **Nursing Home Diversion Project Proposal Abstract**

- **Nursing Home Diversion Project Grant Attachment B-Narrative (Sept 2007)**

- **FFY09 Food Stamp Outreach Time Study Results - October 1-31, 2008**

- **FFY08 Food Stamp Outreach**

  Time Study Results - October 1-31, 2007

  - Central Vermont Council on Aging (CVCOA)
  - Champlain Valley Agency on Aging (CVAA)
  - Council on Aging for Southeastern Vermont (COASEV)
  - Northeast Kingdom Council on Aging (NEKCOA)

- Southwestern Vermont Council on Aging (SVCOA)
- Statewide Results
- Data Summary

- **2007 US Administration on Aging Vermont's Senior Center Earmark Project Final Report (April 26, 2007)**

- **2007 US Administration on Aging Vermont's Senior Center Earmark Project Grantee Final Report Excerpts (April 25, 2007)**

- **2007 Vermont's Senior Center Earmark Project Grantee Final Report Excerpts (April 27, 2007)**

- **Vermont's Senior Center Earmark Project Evaluation of Project Outcomes Executive Summary Final Report (April 23, 2007)**

- **Vermont's Senior Center Earmark Project Evaluation of Project Outcomes Summary Final Report - Appendices Included (April 23, 2007)**

- **US Administration on Aging (AOA) Strategic Action Plan FY 2007 - 2012 (April 2007)**
  AoA's previous Strategic Action Plan provided a framework for modernizing the role of the Aging Services Network in long-term care. This modernization strategy was designed to strengthen the Network's role in advancing systemic changes in long-term care at the state and community-level. This Strategic Action Plan for 2007-2012 continues the focus on modernizing the Aging Services Network's role in long-term care, and gives particular attention to implementing the new provisions contained in the Older Americans Act Amendments of 2006.

- **Updated - Area Agency on Aging - Area Agency Plan Instruction FFY10-Final (March 2009)**
  Complete instructions for submission of Area Plans (narrative, budget, signed assurances and waiver requests) to the Department of Aging and Independent Living.

- **Area Agency on Aging - Area Agency Plan Instructions FFY2007 to 2010 (January 2006)**
  Complete instructions for submission of Area Plans (narrative, budget, signed assurances and waiver requests) to the Department of Aging and Independent Living.

- **Napis State Program Report** (2006)
  Annual state program report to the Administration on Aging, describing services provided by Area Agencies on Aging and the people served.

National Family Caregiver Support Program: http://www.ddas.vermont.gov/ddas-programs/programs-oaa/programs-oaa-nfcsp

National Family Caregiver Support Program (NFCSP)

The National Family Caregiver Support Program was established as a result of the increased awareness of the contribution and the commitment of family caregivers and other non-relative caregivers. It recognizes the individuality of caregivers, the diversity of their caregiving situations and the range of their needs. The program is designed to provide unpaid caregivers with the assistance they need, when they need it, so they may continue in their caregiving roles.

The National Family Caregiver Support Program is supported by Older Americans Act Title III E funding and administered by the Vermont Department of Disabilities, Aging and Independent Living and local Area Agencies on Aging.

- **Services**

- **Eligibility**

- **Applying for Services**

- **Providers of Services**

- **Program Contacts**

- **Publications**

- **Forms**

- **Legislation, Statutes and Regulations**

- **Other Resources**

Services Include

- **Information** for caregivers about available services.

- **Assistance** for caregivers in gaining access to services and resources available within their community.

- **Individual counseling, support groups and training** to help caregivers gain knowledge, make decisions and solve problems relating to their caregiving roles.

- **Respite Care** to temporarily relieve caregivers from their caregiving responsibilities. Funds can be used
  to pay for services such as Adult Day, in-home caregiving, overnight and weekend respite.

- **Supplemental services**, on a limited basis, to complement care provided by caregivers. Examples of supplemental services are legal assistance, financial consultation and home safety interventions.

Return to Program Informational Menu

Eligibility

Family Caregivers and Non-Relative Caregivers of Older Adults

- Respite and supplemental services are limited to care recipients aged 60 or older who are unable to perform two or more activities of daily living (ie., bathing, dressing, mobility etc.) without assistance, or who have a cognitive impairment and require supervision.

- Priority is given to older individuals with the greatest social or economic need.

- There is no minimum age requirement for the informal caregiver.

Family Caregivers of Children Age 18 or Younger

- Family caregivers are age 60 or older and are a grandparent, step-grandparent or other older caregiver related to the child by blood or marriage.

- The family caregiver resides with, and is the primary caregiver of a child because the biological or adoptive parents are unable or unwilling to serve as the primary caregiver.

- The family caregiver has a legal relationship to the child or is raising the child informally.

Return to Program Informational Menu

Applying for Services

For more information about the National Family Caregivers Support Program services available in your area, please call the local Area Agency on Aging.

The table below lists the Area Agencies on Aging phone numbers. For additional contact information for any of the agencies listed click on the Agency name.

Area Agencies on Aging Contact Information

Agency Name	Contact Phone Number
Central Vermont Council on Aging	(802) 479-0531
Champlain Valley Agency on Aging	(802) 865-0360
Senior Solutions-Council on Aging	(802) 885-2655
Northeast Kingdom Council on Aging	(802) 748-5182
Southwestern Vermont Council on Aging	(802) 786-5991

If you do not know which of these agencies provides services in your area, call the *Senior Helpline* at *1-800-642-5119* for assistance.

Return to Program Informational Menu

Providers of Services

Services are coordinated through Vermont's Area Agencies on Aging. Service providers vary depending on the needs of the family caregiver.

- Area Agencies on Aging

Return to Program Informational Menu

Program Contacts

Maria Mireault, Program Director
Division of Disability and Aging Services
103 South Main Street
Weeks Building
Waterbury, VT 05671-1601
Phone: (802) 241-3738
E-mail: maria.mireault@ahs.state.vt.us

Attendant Services Program: http://www.ddas.vermont.gov/ddas-programs/programs-asp-default-page

Attendant Services Program

The Attendant Services Program supports independent living for adults with disabilities who need physical assistance with daily activities. This is a "Consumer Directed Personal Care" Program. Program participants hire, train, supervise, and schedule their personal care attendant(s). The program participant is the employer, and the attendant's hourly wage is funded by the program.

- **Services**

- **Eligibility**

- **Applying for Services**

- **Providers of Services**

- **Program Contacts**

- **Policies and Guidelines**

- **Publications**

- **Forms**

- **Boards and Committees**

- **Legislation, Statutes and Regulations**

Services Include

Attendant Services Program offers the following services:

- **Activities of Daily Living (ADLs)**
  Assistance with daily living activities such as dressing, bathing, grooming, toileting, transferring, mobility, range of motion exercises, positioning and eating.

- **Instrumental Activities of Daily Living (IADLs)**
  Assistance with instrumental activities such as meal preparation, medication management, care of adaptive and health equipment, management of finances and mail, shopping, and cleaning.

Return to Program Informational Menu

Eligibility

To be eligible for Attendant Services Program the person must:

- Be a Vermont Resident

- Be at least 18 years old, and

- Have a disability and need physical assistance with instrumental and daily living activities in order to live in their homes;

    1. General Fund Personal Services
       Have a disability.
       Need physical assistance with at least one activity of daily living or meal preparation.
       Have Medicaid.
    2. General Fund PDAC - Participant Directed Attendant Care
       Have a permanent and severe disability.
       Need physical assistance with at least two activities of daily living, and be able to direct your own personal care services. Apply and be found ineligible for services from other Medicaid-funded personal care or attendant care programs.
    3. Medicaid PDAC - Participant Directed Attendant Care
       Have a permanent and severe disability.
       Need physical assistance with at least two activities of daily living, and be able to direct

own personal care services.
Be willing to hire an attendant other than a spouse or civil union partner; and
Have Medicaid.

Return to Program Informational Menu

Applying for Services

Complete an Attendant Service Program Application.

Attendant Services Program and Patient Share Frequently Asked Questions (FAQ's)

Applications are available at;

- Any office of the Department of Disabilities, Aging, and Independent Living, including regional offices of Vocational Rehabilitation.

- Local Home Health Agency.

- Rehabilitation center, nursing homes, and hospital discharge units.

- On the web at Attendant Service Program Forms - Attendant Service Program Application

Return to Program Informational Menu

Provider of Services

The list below gives a brief description of Attendant Services Program service providers.

- The participant in the program (or a designee under Personal Services) hires, trains, supervises and schedules his or her personal care attendant.

- The participant is the employer. There is no cost to the participant. The program pays an hourly wage to the attendants.

- Any legal worker may be employed except a spouse or civil union partner under the Medicaid PDAC program.

- An attendant who has a substantiated history of abuse, neglect or exploitation will not be paid under this program.

Return to Program Informational Menu

Program Contacts

For information about Attendant Services Program:

- Attendant Services Program: (802) 241-2196

Return to Program Informational Menu

Policies and Guidelines

Listing of Attendant Services Program Policies and Guidelines:

- **Attendant Services Program Employer Handbook**
  Informational handbook to assist in all aspects of Attendant Services Program (ASP); intent of ASP, roles and responsibilities, employer eligibility/certification, employer consider, services/covered activities, and more.

Return to Program Informational Menu

Publications

Attendant Services Program Publications:

- **Attendant Service Consumer Directed Brochure**
  Informational brochure containing helpful information about the Attendant Services Program.

  ASP Consumer Directed Brochure - Text Only

- **Information for Attendants Brochure**
  Information brochure containing information for attendants working for ASP

  Information Attendants Brochure - Text Only

- **Consumer Satisfaction Survey Reports**

  o LTC Consumer Satisfaction Survey - 2008
  o LTC Consumer Satisfaction Survey - 2007
  o LTC Consumer Satisfaction Survey - 2006

Return to Program Informational Menu

Forms

Attendant Services Program Forms:

- **Attendant Service Application**

- **Attendant Services Time Sheet**

- **Employer Certification (October 2005)**

- **Independent Living Assessment (2009)** Full ILA

DDAS Dementia Respite Program: http://www.ddas.vermont.gov/ddas-programs/programs-dementia-respite-default-page

Dementia Respite Program

Caregiving for a person with memory loss can be both stressful and rewarding. Taking a break from caregiving responsibilities can help caregivers maintain the stamina needed to be successful caregivers. If you are caring for someone with memory loss, a Dementia Respite Grant could help you get a well-deserved time off.

The Dementia Respite Program is supported by State and Federal funds administered by the Vermont Department of Disabilities, Aging and Independent Living and locally by Area Agencies on Aging.

Additional services and funding may also be available through the National Family Caregiver Support Program. The National Family Caregiver Support Program was established as a result of the increased awareness of the contribution and the commitment of family caregivers and other non-relative caregivers. It recognizes the individuality of caregivers, the diversity of their caregiving situations and the range of their needs. The program is designed to provide unpaid caregivers with the assistance they need, when they need it, so they may continue in their caregiving roles. For more information about this program: National Family Caregiver Support Program.

- **Services**

- **Eligibility**

- **Applying for Services**

- **Providers of Services**

- **Program Contacts**

- **Publications**

- **Forms**

- **Boards and Committees**

- **Other Resources**

Services Include

Dementia Respite Grants can be used for a range of services that give family caregivers a break from their caregiving responsibilities. For example, the grant can be used to pay for in-home caregiving services so the family caregiver can attend support groups or participate in other wellness activities. Some family caregivers use the funds to assist with payment of Adult Day services for their loved one so the family caregiver can continue working outside the home. Others use the Dementia Respite Grant to hire someone to help with chores when the responsibilities of caregiving and maintaining a household becomes too difficult for them.

Return to Program Informational Menu

Eligibility

A Dementia Respite Grant is a limited amount of funding available on a yearly basis, to a family member or other unpaid primary caregiver who is providing day-to-day care in the home, for a Vermont resident who has been diagnosed with Alzheimer's Disease or other type of dementia and meets certain financial criteria. Priority is given to those who are ineligible for other programs and who anticipate needing out-of-home placement if they do not receive respite services.

Return to Program Informational Menu

Applying for Services

For more information about the program or to apply for the Dementia Respite Grant, please call the Area Agency on Aging serving your loved one's community.

The table below lists the Area Agencies on Aging phone numbers. For additional contact information for any of the agencies listed click on the Agency name.

Area Agencies on Aging Contact Information

Agency Name	Contact Phone Number
Central Vermont Council on Aging	(802) 479-0531
Champlain Valley Agency on Aging	(802) 865-0360
Council on Aging of Southeastern Vermont	(802) 885-2655
Northeast Kingdom Council on Aging	(802) 748-5182
Southwestern Vermont Council on Aging	(802) 786-5991

If you do not know which of these agencies provides services in your area, call the **Senior Helpline** at **1-800-642-5119** for assistance.

Return to Program Informational Menu

Providers of Services

Services are coordinated through Vermont's Area Agencies on Aging. Service providers vary depending on the needs of the individual with dementia and the family caregiver.

- Area Agencies on Aging
  Area Agencies on Aging provide support to people 60 and older in their efforts to remain active, healthy, financially secure, and in control of their own lives.

Return to Program Informational Menu

Program Contacts

Maria Mireault, Dementia Project Director
Division of Disability and Aging Services
103 South Main Street
Weeks Building
Waterbury, VT 05671-1601
Phone: (802) 241-3738
E-mail: maria.mireault@ahs.state.vt.us

Return to Program Informational Menu

Publications

- Vermont State Plan on Dementia - Full Report (2009)

- **VT State Plan on Dementia-Executive Summary** (2009)

- **Developmental Services Resource Guide on Aging and Dementia** (2008)

    Section IV: Additional Reading - For the items in this section that a website resource link is not available the content has been provided below.

    - Fact Sheet: Aging-Older Adults and Their Aging Caregivers
    - Fact Sheet: Aging and Intellectual Disabilities
    - Fact Sheet: Dementia and Intellectual Disabilities
    - Fact Sheet: For the Caregiver for the Person with Intellectual/Developmental Disability and Alzheimer's Disease: Information and Resources
    - PCAD Project: Protocol for Recording Baseline Behavior Information for Person with Down Syndrome

- Administration on Aging Alzheimer's Disease Demonstration Grant to States (2007)
  Evaluation of State Programs to Provide Supportive, Educational and Direct Service Interventions for Caregivers of People with Alzheimer's Disease or a Related Disorder

- **Alzheimer's/Dementia Respite Program (2001)**
  There is an increasing awareness that Alzheimer's/dementia care requires a comprehensive system of care and support for the person with dementia as well as all those who care for them. This report supports that awareness and looks for ways to provide funding.

- **Dementia Care: Building the Capacity in Vermont (2000)**
  Vermont is poised to take full advantage of the Administration on Aging's FY2000 Alzheimer's Disease Demonstration grant. Read about our plans in this report on Dementia Care.

Virginia

Information for Senior Citizens: http://portal.virginia.gov/residents/citizens_families/seniors/

- **INFORMATION FOR SENIOR CITIZENS**

A network of 25 local agencies, called **Area Agencies on Aging or AAAs**, provides most of the services for seniors in Virginia communities. Each AAA in Virginia serves a specific territory of counties and cities that share common geographic, demographic, and economic boundaries.

List of Area Agencies on Aging

- **QUICK LINKS**
  - Virginia's Senior Alert System
  - Seniors' News from the Virginia Department for the Aging
  - Virginia Department of Aging
    Help Virginians find the information and services they need to lead healthy and independent lives as they grow older.
  - Commonwealth Council on Aging
  - Virginia Public Guardian and Conservator Advisory Board
  - Commonwealth Alzheimer's Disease and Related Disorders Commission
  - Virginia Easy Access
    For seniors and adults with disabilities and the providers that support them.
  - Adult Day Care Centers (ADCC)
    Find out the Assisted Living Facilities in Virginia.
  - Adult Protective Services (APS)
    Learn more about the Adult Protective Services from the Department of Social Services.
  - SeniorNavigator
    Virginia's Resource for Health and Aging.
  - Virginia Center on Aging
    Study, research, information and resource facility for the Commonwealth of Virginia utilizing the full capabilities of faculty, staff, libraries, laboratories and clinics for the benefit of older Virginians and the expansion of knowledge pertaining to the aged and to the aging process.
  - Virginia Retirement System
  - Virginia GrandDriver
    Educates seniors and those who care about them about how to drive safely, stay mobile and remain independent for as long as possible.
  - Senior Connections
    The Capital Area Agency on Aging is dedicated to helping seniors maintain quality of life and independence as they age.
  - The Senior List
    Senior Care Services.

- o Senior Services of Southeastern Virginia
  Supports and enriches the lives of older southeastern Virginians in and their families through advocacy, education, information and comprehensive services.
- o Virginia's Association of Area Agencies on Aging
  Dedicated to helping older persons to live with dignity and choices in their homes and communities for as long as possible, and to enhance elder rights.

Department for the Aging: http://www.vda.virginia.gov/aaalist.asp

List of Area Agencies on Aging

View a map of Virginia to locate the AAA that serves your community.

Note: Links to web sites produced by organizations other than the Virginia Department for the Aging (VDA) are provided for your convenience. When you select one of these links, you will leave VDA's web site. VDA is not responsible for the content of linked web pages, and does not endorse products or services that may be offered on the linked pages. Also, the privacy policies of these sites may differ from the privacy policy followed by the Department for the Aging. Please report incorrect or outdated links to VDA's Web Designer.

Alexandria Office of Aging and Adult Services

MaryAnn Griffin, Director
2525 Mount Vernon Avenue, Unit 5
Alexandria, VA 22301-1159

Phone: 703-746-5999
TDD: 703-836-1493
Fax: 703-746-5975

E-mail: MaryAnn.Griffin@alexandriava.gov
Web site: http://alexandriava.gov/humanservices/info/default.aspx?id=8016
Local Areas Served: City of Alexandria.

Appalachian Agency for Senior Citizens

Regina Sayers, Director
216 College Ridge Road, Wardell Industrial Park
P.O. Box 765
Cedar Bluff, VA 24609-0765

Toll-Free: 1-800-656-2272

Phone: 276-964-4915
TTY: 276-964-5765
Fax: 276-963-0130

E-mail: aasc@aasc.org
Web site: http://www.aasc.org
Local Areas Served: Counties of Buchanan, Dickenson, Russell and Tazewell.

Arlington Agency on Aging

Terri Lynch, Director
c/o Department Of Human Services
2100 Washington Boulevard, 4th floor
Arlington, VA 22204

Phone: 703-228-1700
TTY: 703-228-1788
Fax: 703-228-1148

E-mail: arlaaa@arlingtonva.us
Web site: http://www.arlingtonva.us/aging
Local Areas Served: County of Arlington.

Bay Aging

Kathy Vesley, President
5306 Old Virginia Street
P.O. Box 610
Urbanna, VA 23175-0610

Toll-Free: 1-866-758-2386
Phone: 804-758-2386
Fax: 804-758-5773

E-mail: kvesley@bayaging.org
Web site: http://www.bayaging.org
Local Areas Served: Counties of, Essex, Gloucester, King and Queen, King William, Lancaster, Mathews, Middlesex, Northumberland, Richmond and Westmoreland.

Top of page

Central Virginia Area Agency on Aging, Inc.

Brenda Lipscomb, Acting Director
501 12th Street
Lynchburg, VA 24504

PO Box 1390
Lynchburg, VA 24505

Phone: 434-385-9070
Fax: 434-385-9209

E-mail: cvaaa@cvaaa.com
Web site: http://www.cvaaa.com
Local Areas Served: Counties of Amherst, Appomattox, Bedford and Campbell. Cities of Bedford and Lynchburg.

Crater District Area Agency on Aging

David L. Sadowski, Sr. Executive Director
23 Seyler Drive
Petersburg, VA 23805-9243

Phone: 804-732-7020
Fax: 804-732-7232

E-mail: director@cdaaa.org
Web site: http://www.cdaaa.org
Local Areas Served: Counties of Dinwiddie, Greensville, Prince George, Surry and Sussex. Cities of Colonial Heights, Emporia, Hopewell and Petersburg.

District Three Senior Services

Mike Guy, Executive Director
4453 Lee Highway
Marion, VA 24354-4269

Toll-Free: 1-800-541-0933
Phone: 276-783-8157 or 276-783-8158
Fax: 276-783-3003

E-mail: district-three@smyth.net
Web site: http://www.district-three.org

Local Areas Served: Counties of Bland, Carroll, Grayson, Smyth, Washington and Wythe. Cities of Bristol and Galax.

Eastern Shore Agency on Aging

Diane Musso, Executive Director
Community Action Agency, Inc.
(Street Address)
5432A Bayside Road
Exmore, VA 23350
(Mailing Address)
P.O. Box 415
Belle Haven, VA 23306-0415

Toll-Free: 1-800-452-5977
Phone: 757-442-9652
Fax: 757-442-9303

E-mail: esaaa@aol.com
Local Areas Served: Counties of Accomack and Northampton.

Top of page

Fairfax Area Agency on Aging

Sharon Lynn, Director
12011 Government Center Parkway, Suite 708
Fairfax, VA 22035-1104

Toll-Free: 1-866-503-0217
Phone: 703-324-5411
TTY: 703-449-1186
Fax: 703-449-8689

E-mail: fairfax_aaa@fairfaxcounty.gov
Web site: http://www.fairfaxcounty.gov/dfs/oldcradultservices/
Local Areas Served: County of Fairfax. Cities of Fairfax and Falls Church.

Jefferson Area Board For Aging

Gordon Walker, Chief Executive Officer
674 Hillsdale Drive, Suite 9
Charlottesville, VA 22901-1799

Phone: 434-817-5222
Fax: 434-817-5230

E-mail: info@jabacares.org
Web site: http://www.jabacares.org
Local Areas Served: Albemarle County (see Senior Center contact info above); Fluvanna Co. Senior Center Phone:(434) 842-3693; Greene Co. Senior Center Phone: (434) 985-2869; Louisa Co. Senior Center Phone: (540) 967-4433; and Nelson Co. Senior Center Phone: (434) 263-7155. City of Charlottesville Senior Center see contact info above.

Lake Country Area Agency on Aging

Gwen Hinzman, President/CEO
1105 West Danville Street
South Hill, VA 23970-3501

Toll-Free: 1-800-252-4464
Phone: 434-447-7661
Fax: 434-447-4074

E-mail: ghinzman@lcaaa.org
Web site: http://www.lcaaa.org
Local Areas Served: Counties of Brunswick, Halifax and Mecklenburg.

LOA Area Agency on Aging, Inc.

Susan Williams, Executive Director
706 Campbell Avenue, SW
P.O. Box 14205
Roanoke, VA 24038-4205

Phone: 540-345-0451
Fax: 540-981-1487

E-mail: info@loaa.org
Web site: http://www.loaa.org
Local Areas Served: Alleghany County (540) 962-0465; Botetourt County:(540) 966-1094 & (540) 882-2892; Craig County: (540) 864-6031. Cities of Covington, Roanoke (see contact info shown above) and Salem.

Top of page

Loudoun County Area Agency on Aging

Lynn A. Reid, Ph.D., Director
215 Depot Court SE, 2nd Floor
Leesburg, VA 20175-3017

Phone: 703-777-0257
Fax: 703-771-5161

E-mail: aaa@loudoun.gov
Web site: http://www.loudoun.gov/aaa
Local Areas Served: County of Loudoun.

Mountain Empire Older Citizens, Inc.

Marilyn Pace Maxwell, Executive Director
1501 3rd Avenue East
P.O. Box 888
Big Stone Gap, VA 24219-0888

Toll-Free: 1-800-252-6362
Phone: 276-523-4202
Fax: 276-523-4208

E-mail: meoc@meoc.org
Web site: http://www.meoc.org
Local Areas Served: Counties of Lee, Scott and Wise. City of Norton.

New River Valley Agency on Aging

Tina King, Executive Director
141 East Main Street, Suite 500
Pulaski, VA 24301-5029

Toll-Free: 1-866-260-4417
Phone: 540-980-7720
Fax: 540-980-7724

E-mail: nrvaoa@nrvaoa.org
Web site: http://www.nrvaoa.org
Local Areas Served: Counties of Floyd, Giles, Montgomery and Pulaski. City of Radford.

Peninsula Agency on Aging, Inc.

William Massey, Executive Director
739 Thimble Shoals Boulevard, Executive Center
Building 1000, Suite 1006
Newport News, VA 23606-3585

Phone: 757-873-0541
Fax: 757-873-1437

E-mail: information@paainc.org
Web site: http://www.paainc.org
Local Areas Served: Counties of James City and York. Cities of Hampton, Newport News, Poquoson and Williamsburg.

Top of page

Piedmont Senior Resources Area Agency on Aging, Inc.

Ronald Dunn, Executive Director
939 Inverness Road
P.O. Box 398
Burkeville, VA 23922

Toll-Free: 1-800-995-6918
Phone: 434-767-5588
Fax: 434-767-2529

E-mail: psraaa@embarqmail.com
Local Areas Served: Counties of Amelia, Buckingham, Charlotte, Cumberland, Lunenburg, Nottoway, and Prince Edward.

Prince William Area Agency on Aging

Courtney Tierney, Director
5 County Complex, Suite 240
Woodbridge, VA 22192-9200

Phone: 703-792-6400
Fax: 703-792-4734
TDD: 703-792-6444

E-mail: ctierney@pwcgov.org
Web site: http://www.pwcgov.org/aoa
Local Areas Served: County of Prince William. Cities of Manassas and Manassas Park.

Rappahannock Area Agency on Aging, Inc.

Jim Schaefer, Executive Director
171 Warrenton Road
Fredericksburg, VA 22405-1343

Toll-Free: 1-800-262-4012 (Virginia only)
Phone: 540-371-3375
Fax: 540-371-3384

E-mail: info@raaa16.org
Web site: http://www.raaa16.org
Local Areas Served: Counties of Caroline, King George, Spotsylvania and Stafford. City of Fredericksburg.

Rappahannock-Rapidan Community Services Board and Area Agency on Aging

Brian D. Duncan, Executive Director
15361 Bradford Road
P.O. Box 1568
Culpeper, VA 22701-1568

Phone: 540-825-3100
Fax: 540-825-6245
TDD: 540-825-7391

E-mail: rrcsb@rrcsb.org
Web site: http://www.rrcsb.org
Local Areas Served: Counties of Culpeper, Fauquier, Madison, Orange and Rappahannock.

Top of page

Senior Connections, The Capital Area Agency on Aging, Inc.

Thelma Bland Watson Ph.D., Executive Director
24 East Cary Street
Richmond, VA 23219-3796

Toll-Free: 1-800-989-2286
Phone: 804-343-3000
Fax: 804-649-2258

E-mail: twatson@youraaa.org
Web site: http://www.seniorconnections-va.org
Local Areas Served: Counties of Charles City, Chesterfield, Goochland, Hanover, Henrico, New Kent and Powhatan. City of Richmond.

Senior Services of Southeastern Virginia

John Skirven, Executive Director
Interstate Corporate Center, Bldg. 5
6350 Center Drive, Suite 101
Norfolk, VA 23502-4101

Phone: 757-461-9481 (for cities of Chesapeake, Norfolk, Portsmouth and Virginia Beach)
Fax: 757-461-1068

E-mail: services@ssseva.org
Web site: http://www.ssseva.org
Local Areas Served: Isle of Wight County (757) 357-4050; Southampton County (757) 653-2105; and cities of Chesapeake*, Franklin (757) 569-8206; Norfolk*, Portsmouth*, Suffolk (757) 934-1661; and Virginia Beach*.

Shenandoah Area Agency on Aging, Inc.

Helen Cockrell, Executive Director
207 Mosby Lane
Front Royal, VA 22630-3029

Toll-Free: 1-800-883-4122
Phone: 540-635-7141
Fax: 540-636-7810

E-mail: saaa@shenandoahaaa.com
Web site: http://www.shenandoahaaa.com
Local Areas Served: Counties of Clarke, Frederick, Page, Shenandoah and Warren. City of Winchester.

Southern Area Agency on Aging, Inc.

Teresa Carter Fontaine, Executive Director
204 Cleveland Avenue
Martinsville, VA 24112-2020

Toll-Free: 1-800-468-4571
Phone: 276-632-6442
Fax: 276-632-6252

E-mail: saaa@southernaaa.org
Web site: http://www.southernaaa.org
Local Areas Served: Counties of Franklin, Henry, Patrick and Pittsylvania. Cities of Danville and Martinsville.

Valley Program for Aging Services, Inc.

Paul Lavigne, Executive Director
325 Pine Avenue
P.O. Box 817
Waynesboro, VA 22980-0603

Toll-Free: 1-800-868-8727
Phone: 540-949-7141
Fax: 540-949-7143

E-mail: paul@vpas.info
Web site: http://valleyprogramforagingservices.com
Local Areas Served: Counties of Augusta, Bath, Highland, Rockbridge and Rockingham. Cities of Buena Vista, Harrisonburg, Lexington, Staunton and Waynesboro.

Information for Service Providers: http://www.vda.virginia.gov/service_menu.asp

Service Programs

- Adult Day Care

- Care Coordination

- Care Coordination for Elderly Virginians (CCEVP)

- Checking

- Chore

- Chronic Disease Self-Management (CDSMP) and Diabetes Self-Management

- Communication, Referral, Information and Assistance (CRIA)

- Community Living Program (CLP)

- Congregate Nutrition

- Disease Prevention and Health Promotion

- Elder Abuse Prevention

- Emergency

- Employment - Title III

- Employment - Title V

- Fan Care and Summer Cooling

- Guardianship

- Health Education and Screening

- Home Delivered Nutrition

- Home Health

- Homemaker

- I.D. Discount

- Legal Assistance

- Local Contact Agency (LCA) Staff Information for Money Follows the Person (MFP)

- Long-Term Care Coordinating Activities

- Long-Term Care Ombudsman

- Money Management

- Personal Care

- Preparation and Administration of the Area Plan

- Public Information / Education

- Residential Repair and Renovation

- Respite Care

- Senior Farmers' Market Nutrition Program (SFMNP)

- Socialization and Recreation

- Transportation

- Virginia Insurance Counseling and Assistance Program (VICAP)

- Volunteer

Caregiving: http://www.vda.virginia.gov/caregiving.asp

Caregiving

Caring for a loved one at home can range from providing only minimal help to giving assistance 24 hours a day. The care recipient may need help only with some everyday activities, such as eating, bathing, dressing, or using the toilet, or they may need professional nursing care or other medical help. In all instances, caregiving requires a big commitment on the part of the caregiver.

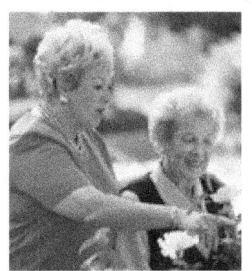

Caregivers must be able to handle both the physical and emotional aspects of caring for another person. The following are some factors that caregivers need to consider in deciding whether to be (or continue to be) a caregiver:

Environment

The safety of the care recipient must be assured in every area of the home to which they have access. Special physical needs of the care recipient (use of a mobility aid, such as a cane or wheelchair) are especially important to consider so that accidents and injuries can be avoided.

Medical care

The need for medical care will vary depending upon the health of the care recipient, but it is recommended that emergency medical care be be accessible at all times. Caregivers should consider their ability to physically assist the care recipient (lifting, bathing, walking, turning in bed, etc.,) as well as perform such tasks as changing dressings or administering medication.

Finances

Consideration must be given as to how products, equipment, alterations to the home and outside assistance (day care, nursing care, etc.) will be paid for (insurance, financial aid services, savings, etc.)

Capabilities

Caregivers should consider whether they have the time, aptitude and attitude necessary to be a caregiver. Assistance should be sought from others (relatives, neighbors, friends, or organizations) whenever possible to provide the caregiver with some respite from their duties.

Emotional Needs

The caregiver must take into account not only the emotional needs of the care recipient (need for privacy, companionship, etc.), but also his or her own emotional needs, and the needs of others who may be providing care and/or living with the care recipient (spouse, children, etc.)

Many caregivers say that they get a great deal of satisfaction from their role, even though their job may be difficult. All caregivers should also periodically reassess their situation to be sure that the level of care being provided is appropriate for both the care recipient and themselves.

For more information on caregiving, visit our <u>Links</u> page and look under the subject heading "Caregiving". You can also <u>contact</u> us for more information or assistance.

Links: http://www.vda.virginia.gov/links.asp

CHANGE TEXT SIZE:

Links

The Virginia Department for the Aging (VDA) provides links to other web sites for your convenience. Links are arranged in alphabetical order by subject.

When you select one of the links on this page, **you will leave VDA's web site.**

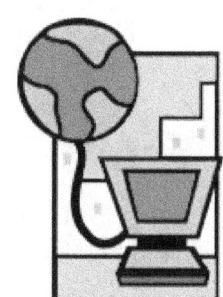

VDA is not responsible for the content of linked web pages, and does not endorse products or services that may be offered on the linked pages. Also, the privacy policies of these sites may differ from the <u>privacy</u> policy followed by the Virginia Department for the Aging. Please report incorrect or outdated links to <u>VDA's Web Designer</u>.

Try using the "Find on This Page" function (found under the "Edit" menu) of your web browser to search this page for your topic. We also direct your attention to the "Search VDA" function near the top of this page, for searching this web site.

Abuse and Neglect

<u>National Center on Elder Abuse</u>

<u>Virginia Coalition for the Prevention of Elder Abuse</u>

<u>Virginia Department of Social Services - Adult Protective Services</u>

Area Agencies on Aging (AAAs)

<u>Find the AAA that serves your local area</u>

<u>List of all Area Agencies on Aging (in alphabetical order)</u>

<u>Virginia Association of Area Agencies on Aging (V4A)</u>

Aging - General Information

AARP

Age in Action Newsletter from VCU's Center on Aging

American Geriatrics Society, The

Children of Aging Parents

EasyAccess Virginia

Eldercare Locator Service

General Aging Resources - Demographics, Laws, Associations, Medicare Info

National Association of Senior Move Managers (NASMM)

National Council on the Aging (NCOA)

National Institute on Aging

SeniorNavigator

U.S. Administration on Aging (AoA)

U.S. Department of Health and Human Services

U.S. Social Security Administration

U.S. Veterans Affairs Department

Virginia Retirement System
- administers benefits for Virginia's current and retired public employees

Top of page

Alzheimer's Disease and Related Disorders

For information on Alzheimer's Disease services in your area, please visit SeniorNavigator or EasyAccess, listed above in the Aging section.

Alzheimer's Association (Virginia Chapters)

AlzPossible - Virginia's New Virtual Center on Alzheimer's Disease

Alzheimer's Association (National Chapter)

Alzheimer's Disease Education and Referral Center (ADEAR)

Alzheimer's Family Day Center

Normal Pressure Hydrocephalus (NPH) Net at the Medical College of VCU

UVa's Memory Commons

VCU Parkinson's Disease Center

Caregiving

Full Circle of Care

National Family Caregivers Association

National Private Duty [Homecare] Association (NPDA)
- National voice for organizations that provide private duty home care services and an advocate for services which benefit the consumers for whom they care.

Respite Services

City and Town Information (U.S.)

City and Town Info
- Demographics, property data and resources for U.S. cities and towns.

Cooling Assistance

Dominion Virginia Power
- FanCare and EnergyShare Programs

Virginia Department of Social Services
- Energy Assistance Program

Top of page

Commonwealth of Virginia

Commonwealth Calendar

Home Page for the Commonwealth of Virginia

List of State Agency Web Sites

Virginia Retirement System
- administers benefits for Virginia's current and retired public employees

Complaints

Better Business Bureau

Virginia Attorney General's Office

Virginia Department of Professional and Occupational Regulation

U.S. Federal Citizen Information Center

Dementia - see "Alzheimer's Disease and Related Disorders"

Demographics - Aging-Related:

Aging Programs and Gerontology:

U.S. Administration on Aging

Census Data

University of Virginia's Weldon Cooper Center for Public Service

U.S. Bureau of the Census

Virginia Employment Commission

City and Town Information

City and Town Info
- Demographics, property data and resources for U.S. cities and towns.

Health Statistics

Statistical Resources on the Web - Health

U.S. Center for Disease Control and Prevention

U.S. Center for Health Statistics

U.S. Agency for Healthcare Research and Quality

Virginia Dept. of Health - District and Local Health Dept. Offices

Virginia Center for Health Statistics

Virginia Department for Health Professions

Public Assistance Programs:

Centers for Medicare and Medicaid Services

Virginia Department of Medical Assistance Services

Search Engines for Government Information:

U.S. Federal Statistics

Virginia Residential/Care Options for Senior Citizens:

Virginia Bureau of Insurance - Continuing Care Retirement Centers

Virginia Health Information

Top of page

Disabilities / Handicapping Conditions

American Foundation for the Blind (AFB)

Virginia Voice

Digital Television

DTV Transition 2009

Disaster Preparedness - See "Emergency Response"

Driving - Mature Driver Safety

American Automobile Association (AAA) - MidAtlantic Region

Virginia GrandDriver

Virginia Department of Motor Vehicles' Highway Safety web site

Virginia Department of Motor Vehicles' Mature Driver Safety

Elder Education

Project 2025: Enhanced Access to Legal Assistance for Older Adults in Virginia

The State Council on Higher Education for Virginia (SCHEV)'s list of Public Colleges and Universities

The Virginia Center on Aging at Virginia Commonwealth University

Elderhostel

Elderhostel at Virginia Commonwealth University

Emergency Response

American Red Cross

Federal Administration on Aging

Federal Emergency Management Agency (FEMA)

Virginia Department of Emergency Management

Virginia Department of Health's Emergency Preparedness and Response Programs

Virginia Senior Alert - a service of Virginia State Police to help locate missing senior adults

Fraud

Better Business Bureau

Virginia Attorney General's Office

Virginia Department of Professional and Occupational Regulation

U.S. Federal Citizen Information Center

GrandDriver

Virginia GrandDriver

Grandparenting - see "Kinship Care"

Top of page

Health and Wellness - also see "Nutrition"

Centers for Disease Control and Prevention (CDC)

Centers for Medicare and Medicaid Services (CMS)

National Association for Continence

National Hospice and Palliative Care Organization

National Institutes of Health (NIH)

National Institute of Mental Health (NIMH)

National Stroke Association

Sexuality Information and Education Council of the U.S.

U.S. Department of Health and Human Services (HHS)

- Find & Compare Hospitals
- Find & Compare Home Health Providers
- Find Health Care Providers

Heating Assistance

Dominion Virginia Power
- EnergyShare Program

Virginia Department of Social Services
- Energy Assistance Program

Home Care

MySeniorCare
- An online resource connecting families with a nationwide network of pre-screened, qualified senior care providers, covering home care, senior housing, and hospice.

Homecare Online - the National Association for Home Care and Hospice

Home Care Provider Directory
- A nationwide directory of Home Care providers. Seniors and their families can learn about Home Care options and request information from Home Care providers.

Home Health Compare
- This tool provides you with information on how well the home health agencies in your area care for their patients.

National Private Duty Association (NPDA)
- National voice for organizations that provide private duty home care services and an advocate for services which benefit the consumers for whom they care.

Virginia Association for Home Care and Hospice
- Dedicated to representing the home care interests and needs of providers, consumers and policy makers in the Commonwealth of Virginia through advocacy, education and networking.

Hospice Care

Medicare's Hospice Benefits web page

Virginia Association for Hospices

Housing

U.S. Department of Housing and Urban Development (HUD)

National Association of Senior Move Managers (NASMM)

Virginia Department of Housing and Community Development

Virginia Housing Development Authority

Top of page

Identity Theft

Federal Trade Commission

Virginia Attorney General's Office

Virginia Department of Agriculture and Consumer Affairs'

- Office of Consumer Affairs

Virginia State Corporation Commission's Bureau of Financial Institutions

Virginia State Corporation Commission's Bureau of Insurance

Insurance

National Association of Insurance Commissioners (NAIC)

The Virginia Long-term Care Partnership (.pdf)

Virginia State Corporation Commission's Bureau of Insurance

Kinship Care

AARP

Brookdale Foundation, The

Generations United

Grandsplace

VDA's Kinship Care Page

Legal Issues and Services

American Bar Association's (ABA's) "Find Legal Help.org"

Association for Conflict Resolution, The

Center for Social Gerontology, The

Equal Employment Opportunity Commission

Employee Benefits Security Administration (DOL)

Pension Benefit Guaranty Corporation

Project 2025: Enhanced Access to Legal Assistance for Older Adults in Virginia

VaLegalAid.org

Virginia Legal Aid Society

Long-Term Care

Creditation for Health Organizations

Assisted Living Source
- Nationwide directory of Senior Housing with a special emphasis on Assisted Living. Seniors and their families can learn about senior housing options and request information.

Home Health Compare
- This tool provides you with information on how well the home health agencies in your area care for their patients.

The Joint Commission

Long-Term Care Insurance Rate Guide

Medicare's Hospice Benefits web page

National Association of Professional Geriatric Care Managers

Virginia Association for Hospices

Virginia Association of Non-Profit Long-Term Care Homes for the Aging

Virginia Department of Social Services Assisted Living Facility Info page

Virginia Health Information

Top of page

Long-Term Care Ombudsman Program

Office of the State Long Term Care Ombudsman

Mediation Services

Association for Conflict Resolution, The

Center for Social Gerontology, The

Medicare

Medicare Prescription Drug Plan Finder

Medicare.gov

Medicare Rights Center

Medicaid

Medicaid

Medication

Extra Help with Medicare Prescription Drug Costs

FreeMedicineFoundation.com

Generic Drugs: The Unadvertised Brand (brought to you by Blue Cross Blue Shield)

Health Assistance Partnership (HAP)

Needymeds.com (help with the cost of medicine)

Ten/Twenty Prescription Program

U.S. Food and Drug Administration on Generic Drugs

Virginia Health Care Foundation list of drug discount programs

Moving

National Association of Senior Move Managers (NASMM)
- Non-profit, professional association of organizations dedicated to helping older adults and their families with the physical and emotional aspects of moving, to maximize the dignity and autonomy of older adults as they transition from one living environment to another.

Normal Pressure Hydrocephalus (NPH)

Normal Pressure Hydrocephalus (NPH) at VCU Aging Brain Center

Top of page

Nursing Homes

Joint Commission on Accreditation for Health Organizations

Medicare's Nursing Home Comparison page

National League for Nursing Accrediting Commission, Inc.

Virginia Department of Health - Division of Long Term Care

Virginia Association of Non-Profit Long-Term Care Homes for the Aging

Virginia Health Information

Nutrition

healthfinder®

Nutrition.gov

U.S. Department of Health and Human Services (HHS) Home Page

U.S. Food and Drug Administration

Virginia Cooperative Extension

Olmstead Plan

One Community - Virginia's Olmstead Initiative

Money Follows the Person - Assisting individuals to transition from long-term care into communities.

Prescription Drug Assistance - see "Medication"

Retirement

Employee Benefits Security Administration (at US DOL)

Pension Benefit Guaranty Corporation

U.S. Social Security Administration

U.S. Veterans Affairs Department

Virginia Retirement System
- administers benefits for Virginia's current and retired public employees

Telephone Discounts

Lifeline and Link-Up help ensure everyone has access to telephone service

Statistics - see "Demographics

Transportation Fund for the Elderly and Disabled

Virginia Department of Taxation - Voluntary Contributions

For good or ill (or obfuscation), Virginia as you can tell seems to have more links than most states. Hopefully you will be able to find what you need amongst them. Never be afraid to ask for what you need however. You would be amazed at how much some people know concerning how to get what you truly are looking for from all the available resources of your state. Anyway, here's some more disabled specific...

Resources For the Disabled: http://portal.virginia.gov/residents/citizens_families/disabled/

- **RESOURCES FOR THE DISABLED**

  The Americans with Disabilities Act (ADA) of 1990 was enacted to ensure that all qualified individuals with disabilities enjoy the same opportunities that are available to persons without disabilities. It guarantees equal opportunity for individuals with disabilities in public accommodations, employment, transportation, state and local government services, and telecommunications.

  The U.S. Department of Justice's ADA Home Page
  Information and technical assistance on the Americans with Disabilities Act.

- **QUICK LINKS**
    - Americans with Disabilities Act (ADA)
      The Americans with Disabilities Act (ADA) of 1990 was enacted to ensure that all qualified individuals with disabilities enjoy the same opportunities that are available to persons without disabilities.
    - Woodrow Wilson Rehabilitation Center
      Provide training and therapy to people with disabilities to enable them to re-enter the work force and live more independently.
    - Virginia Easy Access
      For seniors and adults with disabilities and the providers that support them.
    - Department for the Blind and Vision Impaired
      Provide quality services to assist Virginia's citizens who are blind, deaf, blind or vision impaired in achieving their maximum level of employment, education, and personal independence.

- ○ Department of Rehabilitative Services
  Provide and advocate for the highest quality services that empower individuals with disabilities to maximize their employment, independence and full inclusion into society.
- ○ Department of the Deaf and Hard of Hearing
  The Virginia Department for the Deaf and Hard of Hearing (VDDHH) works to reduce the communication barriers between persons who are deaf or hard of hearing and their families and the professionals who serve them.
- ○ Assistive Technology Loan Fund Authority
  Facilitates favorable credit financing of assistive technology for Virginians with disabilities.
- ○ Virginia Assistive Technology System
  Develop a statewide comprehensive system of assistive technology (AT), and to assist Virginians with disabilities in accessing assistive and information technology (IT) devices and services.
- ○ VIDD - Together We Can
  The Virginia project to assist children and youth who are deaf blind.
- ○ Board for People with Disabilities
  Enrich the lives of Virginians with disabilities by providing a VOICE for their concerns.
- ○ Partnership for People with Disabilities
  To partner with people with disabilities and others to build communities where all people can live, learn, work and play

Virginia Easy Access: http://www.easyaccess.virginia.gov/

Welcome to

Virginia Easy Access

For seniors and adults with disabilities and the providers that support them

A public private partnership with the Commonwealth of Virginia, SeniorNavigator, and 2-1-1 Virginia

Your secure and confidential connection to community resources

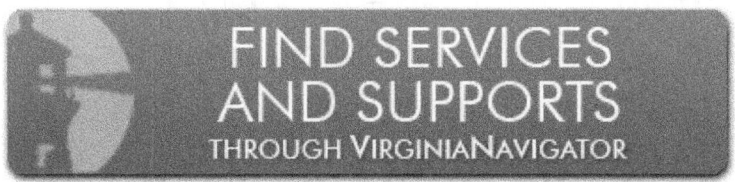

Virginia Navigator: http://www.srnav.org/virginianavigator/IndexEasyNav.aspx

Washington, D.C.

DC Office on Aging: http://dcoa.dc.gov/DC/DCOA

DC Office on Aging

Office Hours
Monday - Friday, 8:30 am - 5 pm

How to Reach Us
441 4th Street, NW, Suite 900 South
Washington, DC 20001
dcoa@dc.gov

Phone: (202) 724-5622
Phone 2: (202) 724-5626
Fax: (202) 727-4979
TTY: (202) 724-8925

FOIA Information
Agency Performance

Website: http://www.dcoa.dc.gov

Lead Agency Service Providers: http://dcoa.dc.gov/DC/DCOA/Our+Programs/Lead+Agencies

Lead Agency Service Providers:

The Office on Aging funds comprehensive service-delivery organizations and designates them "*Lead Agencies*." These agencies plan and deliver direct services to the District's elderly residents and their caregivers. Each ward has one or more Lead Agencies that provide services to seniors in the ward.

Wards 1 & 4
Barney Neighborhood House Senior Program
5656A Third Street, NE
Washington, DC 20011

(202) 939-9020

Ward 2
Emmaus Services for the Aging
1426 9th Street, NW
Washington, DC 20001
(202) 745-1200

Wards 2 & 3 (Georgetown-Foggy Bottom)
IONA Senior Services
4125 Albermarle Street, NW
Washington, DC 20016
(202) 966-1055

Ward 5
Seabury Ward 5 Aging Services
2900 Newton Street, NE
Washington, DC 20018
(202) 529-8701

Ward 6
Family Matters Aging Services
900 G Street, NE, 4th Floor
Washington, DC 20002
(202) 547-7502

Ward 7
East River Family Strengthening Collaborative
3917 Minnesota Avenue, NE
Washington, DC 20019
(202) 534-4880

Ward 8
Access Housing Inc., Senior Program
4301 9th Street, SE
Washington, DC 20032
(202) 562-6860

Senior Services Network: http://dcoa.dc.gov/DC/DCOA/Our+Programs/Senior+Service+Network

Senior Service Network

The Office on Aging is the District of Columbia's Agency on Aging that oversees direct services to persons 60 and older through a Senior Service Network. Within the Senior Service Network are seven community-based agencies, funded by the Office on Aging, to provide nutritious and tasty meals, social and recreational activities, as well as information on staying well. However, seniors are required to become registered participants in order to use the services. In-house, the Office on Aging operates two direct services programs: the Senior Employment and Training Program and the Information and Assistance Unit. The Office on Aging also oversees two nursing homes within the District. Other services provided through the community agencies include: Adult Day Care; Adult Education; Emergency Shelter; Health Insurance Counseling; In-Home Relief; Legal Services; and Transportation.

Community Based Agencies:
Barney Neighborhood House Senior Program
5656– A Third Street, NE, DC 20011
Service Area: Wards 1 and 4
(202) 939-9020 Fax: (202) 939-5755

Iona Senior Services
4125 Albemarle Street, NW, DC 20016
Service Area: Ward 3, and parts of 2
(202) 966-1055 Fax: (202) 895-0244

Emmaus Services for the Aging
1426 9th Street, NW, DC 20001
Service Area: Ward 2
(202) 745-1200 Fax: (202) 745-1246

Seabury Ward 5 Aging Services
2900 Newton Street, NE, DC 20018
Service Area: Ward 5
(202) 529-8701 Fax: (202) 832-0127

Family Matters Aging Services Ward 6
900 G Street, NE, 4th Floor
Washington, DC 20018
(202) 547-7502

East River Family Strengthening Collaborative
3917 Minnesota Ave. NE, DC 20019
Service Area: Ward 7
(202) 534-4880 Fax: (202) 388-7691

Access Housing Inc. Senior Program
4301 9th St. SE, DC 20032
Service Area: Ward 8
(202) 562-6860 Fax: (202) 562-7825

Office on Aging Based Programs:
Information and Assistance
Information and Assistance operates Monday through Friday, 8:30am -5:00pm, excluding holidays. Seniors, family members, caregivers and others may call (202) 724-5626 to inquire about or access

services that are available to seniors in the District of Columbia. Walk-ins are welcome.

Job Training and Employment Program
The Older Workers Employment and Training Program (OWETP) assists District residents 55 years of age and older with finding jobs. The older worker gains additional income, an expanded support system and personal growth. The employment and training program may be contacted by calling (202) 724-3662.

DC Office on Aging Nursing Homes
Washington Center for Aging Services
2601 18th Street, NE
Washington, DC 20018
In July 2010, the District/Office on Aging entered a long-term ground lease with Stoddard Baptist Foundation to operate and manage the Washington Center for Aging Services (WCAS). The decision to move forward with this new public-private partnership does not change the fact that the District still owns the facility. WCAS will continue to be a Medicare/Medicaid certified facility with 259-beds that provides skilled and intermediate nursing care residents 60 years of age and older. The facility will also continue to provide geriatric day care services (adult day care) called "Center Care", an Alzheimer's special care unit, and offer respite care or short-term relief for caregivers, based on availability. According to the Centers for Medicare & Medicaid Services (CMS), the nursing home is a four-star facility. For more information about this facility, please call the Nursing Home Administrator at (202) 541-6200

JB Johnson Nursing Center
901 First Street, NW
Washington, DC 20001

In December of 2010, the District/Office on Aging entered a long-term ground lease with Vital Management Team (VMT) to operate and manage JB Johnson Nursing Center (JBJ). JB Johnson, a 230-bed Medicare/Medicaid certified facility, will continue to be a District-owned nursing facility. It will also continue to provide skilled and intermediate nursing care to residents as young as 18 years of age. According to the Centers for Medicare & Medicaid Services (CMS), the nursing home has a 3 out of 5 star rating. For additional information, please call the Nursing Home Administrator at (202) 535-1100.

Adult Day Care Services

A listing of senior service network providers of adult day care programs for the elderly.

Adult Education

A listing of senior service network providers of adult education services for the elderly.

Advocacy and Ombudsman Service

A listing of senior service network providers of advocacy and ombudsman services for the elderly.

Case Management

A listing of senior service network providers of case management services for the elderly.

Emergency and Group Housing

A listing of senior service network providers of emergency and group housing for the elderly.

Employment and Job Training

A listing of senior service network providers of employment and job training services for the elderly.

Group (Congregate) Meals

A listing of senior service network providers of meal and nutrition services for the elderly.

Health Care In Home Support

A listing of senior service network providers of in-home health care and support for the elderly.

Legal Assistance

A listing of senior service network providers of legal assistance for the elderly.

Most Frequently Requested Phone Numbers

A listing of DC Government frequently requested telephone numbers

Recreation and Socialization

A listing of senior service network providers of recreation and socialization services for the elderly.

Transportation

A listing of senior service network providers of transportation services for the elderly.

Wellness Programs

A listing of senior service network providers of wellness programs for the elderly.

Health Care in Home Support:

http://dcoa.dc.gov/DC/DCOA/Our+Programs/Senior+Service+Network/Health+Care+In+Home+Support

Health care and in-home support services are provided to help seniors in the community maintain their independence and avoid premature institutionalization. Call for further information.

AL-CARE
1234 Massachusetts Avenue, Suite C, NW, DC 20005
202/638-2382 Fax: 202/638-3169

DC Caregivers' Institute
1234 Massachusetts Avenue, NW, Suite C-1002, DC 20005
202/464-1513 Fax: 202/638-3169

EMMAUS Services for the Aging
1426 9th St. NW, DC 20001
202/745-1200 Fax: 202/745-1246

Family Matters of Greater Washington Weekend Alzheimer's Program (Weekend Respite)
1901 Evarts St. NE, DC 20018 (Model Cities)
202/635-1900 Fax: 202/635-1477

Family Matters of Greater Washington
Heavy Housecleaning
1509 16th Street, NW, DC 20001
202/289-1510 Ext. 1180 Fax: 202/518-8928

George Washington University Health Insurance Counseling
2136 Pennsylvania Avenue, NW, DC 20052
202/739-0668 Fax: 202/293-4043

Home Care Partners
1234 Massachusetts Avenue, NW, Suite C-1002, DC 20005
202/638-2382 Fax: 202/638-31692

Interfaith Caregivers Program (S.O.M.E.)
2812 Pennsylvania Avenue, SE, DC 20020-3855
202/581-8000 Ext 3 Fax: 202/582-7112

UDC - Institute of Gerontology Respite Aide Program
4200 Connecticut Avenue, NW, Building 32, Rm. 203, DC 20008 **202/274-6623 Fax: 202/274-6605**

Washington Center for Aging Services (Respite)
2601 18th Street, NE, DC 20018
202/541-6200 Fax: 202/541-6188

Caregiver Support: http://dcoa.dc.gov/DC/DCOA/Our+Programs/Caregiver+Support

DC Caregivers' Institute

The District of Columbia Caregivers' Institute (DCCI), a service of the DCOA/ADRC, supports unpaid caregivers residing in the District of Columbia including caregivers of (1) older, vulnerable DC residents; (2) persons with dementia; (3) older grandparents of disabled adults; (4) older grandparents care for grand children. The Institute is designed to act as a one-stop resource to help caregivers make critical decisions, develop and implement a caregiver support plan, advocate for themselves and their loved one, and participate in activities designed for personal rejuvenation. The Institute offers information and assistance, telephone support groups, educational seminars, caregiver case management, peer support and reimbursement for caregiving-related expenses.

Lifespan Respite Information
DCOA is committed to supporting caregivers for persons of all ages. By contacting the DCOA/ADRC, caregivers can find out about services designed to help them get a break from their responsibilities. Caring for someone can be very hard work. Caregivers get exhausted, stressed and even sick if they don't make time for themselves. A temporary break from the daily routine of assisting someone else helps the caregiver maintain mental stability and physical wellbeing.

Additional Services
In addition, DCOA funds caregiver support activities offered by agencies throughout the city. Whether you need adult day services, caregiving supplies or weekend care for an Alzheimer's patient, resources are available. Contact us for referrals to caregiver services offered by agencies in your community and throughout the city.

Senior Services Network: http://dcoa.dc.gov/DC/DCOA/Find+Services/Senior+Service+Network

Senior Service Network

The Office on Aging is the District of Columbia's Agency on Aging that oversees direct services to persons 60 and older through a Senior Service Network. Within the Senior Service Network are seven community-based agencies, funded by the Office on Aging, to provide nutritious and tasty meals, social and recreational activities, as well as information on staying well. However, seniors are required to become registered participants in order to use the services. In-house, the Office on Aging operates two direct services programs: the Senior Employment and Training Program and the Information and Assistance Unit. The Office on Aging also oversees two nursing homes within the District. Other services provided through the community agencies include: Adult Day Care; Adult Education; Emergency Shelter; Health Insurance Counseling; In-Home Relief; Legal Services; and Transportation.

Community Based Agencies:
Barney Neighborhood House Senior Program
5656– A Third Street, NE, DC 20011
Service Area: Wards 1 and 4
(202) 939-9020 Fax: (202) 939-5755

Iona Senior Services
4125 Albemarle Street, NW, DC 20016
Service Area: Ward 3, and parts of 2
(202) 966-1055 Fax: (202) 895-0244

Emmaus Services for the Aging
1426 9th Street, NW, DC 20001
Service Area: Ward 2
(202) 745-1200 Fax: (202) 745-1246

Seabury Ward 5 Aging Services
2900 Newton Street, NE, DC 20018
Service Area: Ward 5
(202) 529-8701 Fax: (202) 832-0127

Family Matters Aging Services Ward 6
900 G Street, NE, 4th Floor
Washington, DC 20018
(202) 547-7502

East River Family Strengthening Collaborative
3917 Minnesota Ave. NE, DC 20019
Service Area: Ward 7
(202) 534-4880 Fax: (202) 388-7691

Access Housing Inc. Senior Program
4301 9th St. SE, DC 20032
Service Area: Ward 8
(202) 562-6860 Fax: (202) 562-7825

In chasing after disabled resources, I found that they seem to end up at the previously listed resources...

Washington

Public Health and Safety: http://access.wa.gov/living/publicsafety.aspx

- Adult Abuse and Prevention - *DSHS*

- Adult/Senior Services & Information - *DSHS*

- Applying for Medicaid - *DSHS*

- Assisted Living Options - *DSHS*

- Caregiver Resources - *DSHS*

- Certified Professional Guardian Program - *AOC*

- Compare Nursing Home Quality Measures - *HHS*

- Residential Care Services - *DSHS*

Related Topics

- American Red Cross
- Emergency Resource Guide
- State Agency News Releases
- Washington Insurance Blog

Related Agencies

- Department of Social and Health Services(DSHS)
- Administrative Office of the Courts(AOC)
- Home Care Referral Registry(HCRR)

Department of Social and Health Services: http://www.aasa.dshs.wa.gov/pubinfo/

Adult/Senior Services & Information

There are a variety of different programs, services, and resources to help an adult who needs care.

Getting Started

- What You Need to Know

How to Find...

- In-home Care Services

- Assisted Living Options (Adult Family Homes, Boarding Homes or Nursing Homes)
- Local Services
- Services Outside of Washington State
- Information about your Personal CARE Assessment

Paying for Care

- Medicare
- Medicaid
- Finding Benefits
- Other Insurance Programs
- Prescription Drugs
- Finding State or Federal Benefits
- Veteran's Benefits

Health Information

- Alzheimer's and Other Illnesses
- Falls and Prevention
- Healthy Aging
  - Physical Activity
  - Good Nutrition
  - Keeping Your Mind Active
  - Maintaining Social Connections
  - Volunteering
  - Important Health Check Ups
- Flu Information and Resources

Planning for Your Future

- Why Plan Ahead?
- Financial Planning
- Legal Planning & Advance Directives

Services that help an adult remain at home:

http://www.aasa.dshs.wa.gov/pubinfo/services/servicetypes.htm

Services that help an adult remain at home

Did You Know ?

It's never too late to make simple lifestyle changes and stay independent longer. Learn more.

The following is a sample of the many services and resources available to help adults remain at home. Learn more about:

- Hiring an aide to help with personal care, meals, or housekeeping
- Hiring skilled nursing or other professional care
- Community resources (e.g. Meals on Wheels, transportation services)
- Home modification/Assistive Technology
- Hospice and respite care

Hiring an Aide

Learn More About

who to contact to find out more about these services.

People that need help with such things as preparing meals, personal care (e.g. bathing, dressing), and housekeeping have several options for hiring help. See "Hiring Skilled Nursing Care" below if skilled nursing or other professional care is needed.

Adults receiving Medicaid and eligible to hire an aide (Individual Provider) can use the Home Care Referral Registry to get a list of prescreened Individual Providers in their area. Visit the Referral Registry on-line or call 1-800-970-5456 for more information.

AARP has an entire section on providing care at home – including an article Help Wanted: Tips for Hiring a Home-Care Worker.

« Back to top

Home care agencies

Home care agencies recruit, train, pay, supervise, and are responsible for the care provided by the aide they send to your home. These agencies are licensed by Washington State. Use The National Association of Home Care and Hospice locator to find a home care agency in your area or contact your local Senior Information and Assistance office.

Private hires

You can also find, hire, train, pay, and supervise an aide yourself. Learn more from the Family Caregiver Alliance's fact sheet hiring in-home help . (PDF)

Volunteer chore services

Volunteer chore services exists for low income adults who can't afford to pay for in-home services but do not qualify for other state assistance. Volunteers can help with things like household chores, shopping, moving, minor home repair, yard care, personal care, and transportation.

Faith in Action volunteers

Faith in Action volunteers give their time to help neighbors with long-term health needs by providing simple assistance. Find out if free services are available in your area.

« Back to top

Hiring Skilled Nursing Care

Learn More About

who to contact to find out more about these services.

Home health care agencies

People that need skilled nursing care (e.g. wound care, giving injections) often get it from a home health agency. Home health agencies recruit, supervise, and pay the person and assume responsibility for the care provided. Home health care through an agency must be authorized by a doctor. Home health care agencies are licensed by Washington State. Learn more from *A Home Health Care Primer* from the National Family Caregivers Association (PDF).

Use The National Association of Home Care and Hospice locator to find a home health agency in your area or contact your local Senior Information and Assistance office.

You can also hire a nurse or therapist directly. In this case, you are responsible for finding, hiring, supervising, and paying the person. Learn more from the Family Caregiver Alliance's fact sheet hiring in-home help . (PDF)

Adults receiving state-funds (Medicaid) to pay for long term care services may also be eligible for the Nurse Delegation Program. With Nurse Delegation, a caregiver may be trained to help with certain nursing type care tasks in your home or a boarding or adult family home. Learn more about Nurse Delegation.

To find a home health agency in your area:

- Use Medicare's Home Health Care website run by Medicare. This on-line tool provides you with information on how well the home health agencies in your area care for their patients.
- Use The National Association of Home Care and Hospice locator to find a home health agency in your area.
- Contact your local Senior Information and Assistance office.

« Back to top

Community Resources

Learn More About

who to contact to find out more about these services.

Adult day care

Adult day care is a daytime program for an adult who needs some level of care but doesn't need the level of care provided by an RN or rehabilitative therapist. Services in most adult day care programs include help with personal care, social services and activities, education, routine health monitoring, general therapeutic activities, a nutritious meal and snacks, coordination of transportation, first aid, and emergency care.

Adult day health

Adult day health is a daytime program for an adult who needs skilled nursing care or a licensed rehabilitative therapist. An adult day health center provides skilled nursing services, rehabilitative therapy such as physical therapy, occupational therapy or speech-language therapy, brief psychological and/or counseling services and all of the services listed for adult day care above.

Companion services

Routine visits or phone calls are made to people who live alone or are not able to leave their home. Some companion services may also include help with transportation of shopping.

Home delivered meals

Nutritious meals are delivered to people who have difficulty leaving their home. Another option for meals for seniors is in a group setting at many senior center.

Senior centers

Senior centers are facilities in a community where older people can meet, share a meal, get services, and take part in recreational activities.

Transportation

Transportation is provided for someone who no longer can drive or has access to a car.

« Back to top

Home Modification / Assistive Technology

Learn More About

who to contact to find out more about these services.

Environmental modifications

Modifications are added into the home that help an adult with a medical or disabling condition adapt to his/her changing needs safely (e.g. ramps, a grab-bar in the shower or near a toilet, or widened doorways for a wheelchair).

Learn more about different types of assistive technology and how to find them.

- ABLEDATA
- National Public Website on Assistive Technology

Personal Emergency Response System (PERS)

An adult is given an electronic device to summon help in an emergency. The device is connected to a phone or the adult may also wear a portable "help" button. When activated, staff at a response center call 911 or take whatever action has been asked for ahead of time.

« Back to top

Hospice Care and Respite Care

Learn More About

who to contact to find out more about these services.

Hospice care

Hospice care involves a team of professionals and volunteers who provide medical, psychological, and spiritual care to a dying person and his or her family. Hospice care is normally provided in the person's home but is also available in other care settings, including a hospital. Hospice staff are available 24 hours a day to help care for the dying person, ensure he or she is comfortable and free from pain, and provide counseling and support for the person and his or her family. Learn more from the Hospice Association of America's publication All About Hospice: A Consumer's Guide.

Use The National Association of Home Care and Hospice locator to find a hospice agency in your area or contact your local Senior Information and Assistance office.

Learn more about caring for someone close to you who is dying in The National Institute on Aging's booklet End of Life: Helping with Comfort and Care (PDF).

Respite care

Respite care is when another person or facility temporarily takes care of a frail adult so the person caring for them at home can have a break. Respite care can be arranged through the Family Caregiver Support Program (FCSP), home health agencies, adult family homes, boarding homes, adult day health or adult day care, nursing facilities, or family, friends, and volunteers.

Agencies that Help: http://www.aasa.dshs.wa.gov/pubinfo/help/agencies.htm#FCSP

Agencies That Help

- Area Agency on Aging (AAA)
  - Senior Information and Assistance

- - Aging and Disability Resource Centers
  - Family Caregiver Support Program
- Home and Community Services (HCS)
  - Adult Protective Services
- Long-term Care Ombudsman

Area Agency on Aging (AAA)

AAAs were established under the Federal Older Americans Act in 1973 to help older adults (60 or older) remain in their home. AAAs are located throughout the United States and are available in every county within Washington State.

AAA's help older adults plan and find additional care, services, or programs. Help can range from getting services for a frail adult so he/she can remain at home to providing access to activities and socialization through programs like senior centers. They also provide support and services to the family or friends helping to care for older adults. Read the AAA mission statement.

Why would you contact them?

AAA offices are a tremendous resource and one of the best places to start for any adult over 60 who needs or wants additional support or services. Your local AAA staff are experts on what services and supports are available where you live. AAA staff can help assess the current situation and plan for what is needed. They are also a valuable resource for family or friends who are providing care to an aging adult and need information, support, and/or respite services. Find the local AAA office.

« Back to top

Senior Information & Assistance (I & A)

I & A is a **free** information and referral service for adults age 60 and older and for family and friends helping care for the older adult.

Why would you contact them?

Contact them any time you have a question or concern about getting help for an adult sixty or older or for anyone providing unpaid care for that adult. Local offices throughout Washington State can help you:

- plan, find and get more care, services, or programs (e.g. transportation, meals, housekeeping, personal care);
- explore options for paying for long term care and review eligibility for benefits;
- figure out health care insurance and prescription drug options;
- get a listing of local adult housing and assisted living; and
- sort through legal issues (e.g. setting up advance directives, living wills) or make referrals for legal advice.

Find the local I & A office.

« Back to top

Aging and Disability Resource Centers (ADRCs)

Aging and Disability Resource Centers offer free long-term care information, referral, and assistance for people of all ages.

Why would you contact them?

Contact them any time you have a question or concern about getting help for anyone needing long-term care or for anyone providing unpaid care for an adult. ADCRs can help you:

- plan, find and get more care, services, or programs (e.g. transportation, meals, housekeeping, personal care);
- explore options for paying for long term care and review eligibility for benefits;
- figure out health care insurance and prescription drug options;
- get a listing of local adult housing and assisted living; and
- sort through legal issues (e.g. setting up advance directives, living wills) or make referrals for legal advice.

Pierce County is the pilot site as Washington's first Aging and Disability Resource Center.

« Back to top

Quick Link

Find the telephone number for your local Family Caregiver Support Program.

Family Caregiver Support Program (FCSP)

The Family Caregiver Support Program is a service available to unpaid caregivers of adults needing care and living in Washington State. There are local Family Caregiver Support Program offices throughout the state staffed with caring and knowledgeable people who can help you:

- Find local resources/services.
- Find caregiver support groups and counseling.
- Get training on specific caregiving topics.
- Get respite care if you need a break.
- Talk through specific issues you are having and offer practical information and caregiving suggestions.

Generally, these services are offered free or at low cost. Certain eligibility requirements may apply and availability varies from community to community.

Find the telephone number for your local Family Caregiver Support Program.

Why would you contact them?

Providing unpaid care to a family member or friend can be emotionally and physically draining and can be an isolating time. Staff with the FCSP program can provide information, support, and services that can be a lifesaving resource. Find the local FCSP.

« Back to top

Home and Community Services (HCS)

Home and Community Services is part of the Aging and Disability Services Administration, an agency within the Department of Health and Social Services (DSHS). At the local level, HCS staff help adults who need care services but may need state funds (Medicaid) to help pay for them. Learn more about applying for Medicaid.

If the person is eligible for Medicaid, an HCS case manager will work with the adult to decide what additional care is needed and develop a care plan based on his/her needs. Your local HCS staff are experts on the services and support available where you live. Read the HCS mission statement and the ADSA mission statement.

Why would you contact them?

HCS offices are a tremendous resource and the best place to start for an adult who may need help paying for long term care due to a medical or disabling condition. Find a local HCS office.

« Back to top

Adult Protective Services

APS protects vulnerable adults by investigating allegations of abuse, neglect, abandonment, and financial exploitation when the person lives in their own home. APS conducts an investigation at no charge and without regard to the income of the alleged victim. Some protective services may be provided without cost. Learn more about what happens when you call APS.

Why would you contact them?

Contact them any time you suspect a vulnerable adult living in his/her own home may be being harmed. Learn more about vulnerable adult abuse and prevention. Find your local APS office.

« Back to top

Long-Term Care Ombudsman

The Washington State Long-Term Care Ombudsman Program protects and promotes quality of life for people living in licensed, long-term adult care facilities (e.g. adult family home, boarding home, nursing home). An ombudsman:

- Advocates for the rights of clients in adult care facilities;
- Works with clients, families and facility staff to meet the needs and concerns of the people living there; and
- Provides a way to get complaints and concerns heard and resolved.

The following people can use the Ombudsman Program:

- residents living in a care facility and his/her relatives or friends;
- administrators and staff of an adult family home, boarding home or nursing home.

Why would you contact them?

A local ombudsman is an excellent resource for information and help and is a trusted resource in mediating complaints or concerns you may have about anyone living in an adult care facility. Call them if there is a problem you can't resolve or you need another knowledgeable resource that works in the long-term care community. Find your local ombudsman office.

Who to Call to Find Local Services: http://www.aasa.dshs.wa.gov/pubinfo/services/default.htm

Who to Call to Find Local Services

Learn More About

The types of services that help an adult remain at home.

Finding other places to live and get care if the adult can no longer live at home.

Ways to stay independent as long as possible.

The types of care (services and programs) available for an adult is different in each community. Who to contact to know what services and programs are available locally depends on where the person who needs the care lives, how old he/she is, and whether or not state funding is needed to help pay for care.

For people 60 and Older

Senior Information and Assistance (I & A) is a free information and referral service for adults 60 and over and for family and friends helping care for the older adult.

Find your local I & A office. Learn more about what your local I & A office can do for you.

For People Under 60

If the person is between the ages of 18 and 59, contact your local Home & Community Service Office (HCS) for assistance. Learn more about what your local HCS office can do for you.

For Adults Who Need Medicaid or Other State Funding

If you think state funding (Medicaid) may be needed to help pay for are services, contact your local Home and Community Services (HCS) office.

For People Living with a Developmental Disability

If the person needing care is an adult living with a developmental disability, see the Division of Developmental Disabilities Local Offices (DDD) for the phone number and location of the nearest local office or DDD Services for a list of services that may be available.

Caregiver Resources: http://www.aasa.dshs.wa.gov/caregiving/

Caregiver Resources

If you are helping care for a family member or friend, you are not alone! More than 600,000 Washington State citizens provide care to an adult who needs help with care. Below are a variety of ways to find some information, resources, and people that can help.

Caregiver Support is a Phone Call Away

Talk to caring people for practical caregiving information and help finding local resources/services.

Contact your local Family Caregiver Support Program.

- **Talk to Knowledgeable and Caring People**
  The Family Caregiver Support Program is a service available to unpaid caregivers of adults who need care. Staff at local offices throughout Washington can give you practical information and advice and connect you to local resources/services that meet your needs. Services are free or low cost. Contact your local Family Caregiver Support Program.
- **Find Information on the Internet**
  Look through and click on the topics of interest below for a variety of links to helpful information and resources.

The Year of the Family Caregiver

The U.S. Administration on Aging is proud to sponsor a yearlong celebration to commemorate the 10th anniversary of the National Family Caregiver Support Program and spotlight the important role of family caregivers. Washington State's Family Caregiver Support Program began a year before the national program. Find out more about the Year of the Family Caregiver or Washington State's Family Caregiver Support Program.

Help Caring For a...

- Person with Alzheimer's Disease or Other Dementia

- Mom and Dad
- Adult Who Lives Far Away (Long Distance Caregiving)
- Relative's Child (Kinship Care)
- Person with Developmental Disabilities

Taking Care of Yourself

- The Importance of Self Care
- Caregiver Support Groups
- Managing Stress
- Depression
- Respite Care
- Caregiver Training

Providing Day-To-Day Care

- Basics of Providing Care
- How A Disease Impacts Care
- Prescription Medications (help paying for, factsheets etc.)
- Working with Doctors
- Driving
- Incontinence

General Information

- Becoming a Paid Caregiver
- TCARE® Personal Caregiver Survey

Aging & Disability Services Administration (ADSA): http://www.aasa.dshs.wa.gov/

Adult/Senior Services & Information

Find in-home services, residential care (assisted living, nursing home), resources to pay for care, possible state and federal benefits, legal and financial planning, and aging health information.

- In-home Care Services
- Assisted Living Options
- Find Local Services

- Apply for Medicaid
- Alzheimer's and Other Illnesses
- Flu Information and Resources
- ...more Services & Information topics

Caregiver Resources

Resources, services, programs, and helpful information for people caring for an adult who needs long-term care.

- Dementia Care
- Mom and Dad
- Support and Self Care

- Becoming a Paid Caregiver
- Long Distance Caregiving
- Providing Day to Day Care
- ...more Caregiver topics

Abuse & Prevention

How to report abuse if you suspect a vulnerable adult is being harmed, signs to look for, abuse prevention tips, and information for mandatory reporters.

General Public

- Report Abuse – General Public
- Types and Signs of Abuse
- Tips to Help Prevent Abuse
- ...more General Public topics

Mandatory Reporters

- Who are mandatory reporters?
- Report Abuse – Mandatory Reporters
- Mandatory reporter Training
- ...more Mandatory Reporter topics

Developmental Disability Eligibility & Services

Eligibility, services, programs, and resources for children and adults with developmental disabilities, their families, and caregivers and service providers.

- Services
- Eligibility
- Autism Awareness
- ...more Developmental Disabilities topics

Professionals & Providers

Information for Business Partners, Vendors, Contractors and other interested parties.

- Adult Family Home Providers
- Boarding Home Providers

- <u>Nursing Home Professionals</u>
- <u>Residential Care Services</u>
- <u>Training Requirements & Classes</u>
- <u>ProviderOne Project</u>

- <u>Nurse Delegation Program</u>
- <u>Nursing Assistant Program</u>
- <u>Family Caregiver Assessment and Planning</u>
- <u>Employment Opportunities</u>
- <u>...more Professional & Provider topics</u>

West Virginia

Bureau of Senior Services: http://www.wvseniorservices.gov/

Welcome to WVSeniorServices.gov

Welcome to the West Virginia Bureau of Senior Services' website. The information we offer is tailored to those who are seeking to locate programs and services for themselves or their loved ones and also for professionals who may be looking for up-to-date information relating to the field of aging.

We hope that you find our website easy to navigate and useful. If you have any trouble locating what you are looking for, please let us know — one of our experienced staff is just a phone call or e-mail away.

We are very proud of the senior programs and services that are offered throughout the state of West Virginia — from transportation to meals to exercise classes to in-home services. Our site areas (Getting Answers, Staying Healthy, Help At Home, Staying Safe, Special Events and Document Center) are designed to help you find these programs and services quickly and easily.

As our nation's aging population grows, about 27,000 West Virginia Baby Boomers will turn 60 every year. The Bureau of Senior Services will continue to focus on the changing needs of older West Virginians and to lead the way with programs that promote health, dignity and independence.

Quick Links to Provider Listings

- County Aging Providers (Senior Centers)
- Case Management Agencies
- Homemaker Agencies
- Personal Care Agencies

- **West Virginia Bureau of Senior Services**
  Mailing address:
  1900 Kanawha Blvd. East
  Charleston, WV 25305
- Location:
  Town Center Mall, 3rd level
  Charleston, WV
- Phone: (304) 558-3317, (877) 987-3646
  Fax: (304) 558-5609

County Aging Providers:
http://www.wvseniorservices.gov/GettingAnswers/OverviewofAgingProgramsInWestVirginia/CountyAgingProvidersSeniorCenters/CountyAgingProviders/tabid/113/Default.aspx

County Aging Providers

Barbour County Senior Center, Inc.
PO Box 146 (101 Church St.)
Philippi, WV 26416
Telephone: 304-457-4545
Fax: 304-457-2017
Email: bcsc@bcscwv.org
Website: www.bcscwv.org
Brenda Wilmoth, Director

Berkeley Senior Services
217 North High Street
Martinsburg, WV 25401
Telephone: 304-263-8873
Fax: 304-263-6598
Email: bssdir@berkeleyseniorservices.org
Website: www.berkeleyseniorservices.org
Linda Holtzapple, Director

Bi-County Nutrition (Doddridge and Harrison
nutrition)
416 1/2 Ohio Avenue
Nutter Fort, WV 26301
Telephone: 304-622-4075
Fax: 304-622-4675
Email: bicountyseniors@yahoo.com
Wanda Carrico, Director

Boone County Community Organization
PO Box 247 (347 Kenmore Dr., Suite 1-A)
Madison, WV 25130
Telephone: 304-949-3673; 304-369-0451
Fax: 304-949-3673
Email: bcco.jeaster@suddenlinkmail.com
Judy Easter, Director

Braxton County Senior Citizens Center, Inc.
33 Senior Center Drive
Sutton, WV 26601
Telephone: 304-765-4090; 304-765-4091; 304-765-4092; 888-654-9321
Fax: 304-765-4095
Email: dirbcscc@frontier.com
Mary Chapman, Director

Brooke County Committee on Aging (also
nutrition provider for Hancock)

948 Main Street
Follansbee, WV 26037
Telephone: 304-527-3410
Fax: 304-527-4278
Email: brookejoy@aol.com
Joy Crawford, Director

**Cabell County Community Services
Organization, Inc.**
724 10th Avenue
Huntington, WV 25701
Telephone: 304-529-4952
Fax: 304-525-2061
Email: cccsoinc@cccso.com
Website: www.cccso.com
Robert E. Roswall, Director

Calhoun County Committee on Aging, Inc.
PO Box 434 (#3 Market St.)
Grantsville, WV 26147
Telephone: 304-354-7822; 304-354-7017
Fax: 304-354-6859
Email: rpoling@cccoa-wv.org
Rick Poling, Executive Director

Clay County Development Corp. (IIIB only, no
nutrition)
PO Box 455 (174 Main St.)
Clay, WV 25043
Telephone: 304-587-2468
Fax 304-587-2856
Email: claycountyseniorcenter@hotmail.com
Website: www.claycountyseniorcenter.com
Pamela Taylor, Director

Doddridge County Senior Citizens, Inc. (IIIB
only, no nutrition)
PO Box 432 (403 West Main Street)
West Union, WV 26456
Telephone: 304-873-2061
Fax 304-873-1769
Email: dcscoffice@gmail.com
Marvin "Smokey" Travis, Director

Fayette County Office (administered by Putnam
Aging Services)

PO Box 770 (108 Lewis St.)
Oak Hill, WV 25901
Telephone: 304-465-8484
Fax: 304-465-8607
Email: jszamiela@yahoo.com
Janet Zamiela, Director

Council of Senior Citizens of Gilmer County, Inc.
720 North Lewis Street
Glenville, WV 26351
Telephone: 304-462-5761
Fax: 304-462-8239
Email: gilmerseniors@yahoo.com
Sallie Mathess, Director

Grant County Commission on Aging
111 Virginia Avenue
Petersburg, WV 26847
Telephone: 304-257-1666
Fax: 304-257-9145
Email: gccoafs@frontier.com
Website: www.grantcountycoa.com
Darlene Keplinger, Director

Greenbrier County Committee on Aging
PO Box 556 (1003 Greenbrier St.)
Rupert, WV 25984
Telephone: 304-392-5138
Fax: 304-392-5969
Email: gcca@suddenlinkmail.com
John Wyman, Director

Hampshire County Committee on Aging
PO Box 41 (School St. & Birch Ln.)
Romney, WV 26757
Telephone: 304-822-4097 (TDD); 304-822-4030;
304-822-4499
Fax: 304-822-7322
Email: aginginhamp@hardynet.com
Website: www.aginginhampshire.us
Sandra Viselli, Director

Committee for Hancock County Senior Citizens
(IIIB only, no nutrition)
PO Box 1284 (647 Gas Valley Road)
New Cumberland, WV 26047-1284
Telephone: 304-564-3801

Fax: 304-387-2693
Email: emknabenshue@hancocksrsvs.org
Website: www.hancocksrsvs.org
Mark Knabenshue, Director

Hardy County Committee on Aging
PO Box 632 (409 Spring Ave.)
Moorefield, WV 26836
Telephone: 304-530-2256; 800-538-2256
Fax: 304-530-6989
Email: hccoa1@hardynet.com
Phyllis Helmick, Director

Harrison County Senior Citizens, Inc. (IIIB only, no nutrition)
500 West Main Street
Clarksburg, WV 26301
Telephone: 304-623-6795
Fax: 304-623-6798
Email: hcsc@clarksburg.com
Website:
http://members.iolinc.net/seniorcenter/
Cindy Freeman, Director

Jackson County Commission on Aging, Inc.
PO Box 617 (121 So. Court St.)
Ripley, WV 25271
Telephone: 304-372-2406
Fax: 304-372-9243
Email: jccoawv@hotmail.com
Website: www.jccoawv.org
Gerry Dunbar, Director

Jefferson County Council on Aging
103 West 5th Street
Ranson, WV 25438
Telephone: 304-725-4044
Fax: 304-725-9500
Email: jccoadirector@frontiernet.net
Amy Wellman, Acting Director

Kanawha Valley Senior Services (IIIB only, no nutrition)
2428 Kanawha Boulevard, East
Charleston, WV 25311
Telephone: 304-348-0707
Fax: 304-348-6432
Email: stephv@kvss.org, lharrison@kvss.org

Website: www.kvss.org
Director - Vacant

Lewis County Senior Citizens Center, Inc.
171 West 2nd Street
Weston, WV 26452
Telephone: 304-269-5738, 1-800-695-4594
Fax: 304-269-7329
Email: dinahlynnmills@aol.com
Website: www.lcseniorcenter.org
Dinah Mills, Director

Lincoln County Opportunity Co., Inc.
360 Main Street
Hamlin, WV 25523
Telephone: 304-824-3448
Fax: 304-824-7662
Email: lcoc@zoominternet.net
Website: www.lincolncountyopportunity.com
Alice Tomblin, Director

PRIDE in Logan County, Inc.
PO Box 1346 (699 Stratton St.)
Logan, WV 25601
Telephone: 304-752-6868
Fax: 304-752-1047
Website: www.prideinlogan.com
Email: vicky@prideinlogan.com
Vicky Browning, Aging Program Director
Email: reggie@prideinlogan.com
Reggie Jones, Executive Director

Marion County Senior Citizens, Inc.
105 Maplewood Drive
Fairmont, WV 26554
Telephone: 304-366-8779; 304-366-3186
Fax: 304-366-3186
Email: debbie@marionseniors.org
Website: www.marionseniors.org
Debbie Harvey, Director

Marshall County Committee on Aging (IIIB only,
no nutrition)
805 5th Street
Moundsville, WV 26041
Telephone: 304-845-8200
Fax: 304-845-8239
Email: jhoward@wvdsl.net

Website: www.mcseniorcenter.com
Joyce Howard, Director

Mason County Action Group, Inc.
101 2nd Street
Point Pleasant, WV 25550
Telephone: 304-675-2369
Fax: 304-675-2069
Email: masonseniors@aol.com
Website: www.masonseniors.com
Renae Riffle, Executive Director

McDowell County Commission on Aging
725 Stewart Street
Welch, WV 24801
Telephone: 304-436-6588
Fax: 304-436-2006
Email: mcoa@citlink.net
Lisa Sanderson, Interim Director

CASE Commission on Aging (Mercer IIIB only,
no nutrition)
PO Box 1507 - 600 Trent Street
Princeton, WV 24740
Telephone: 304-425-7111
Fax: 304-487-8801
Email: swolfe@casewv.org
Sandy Wolfe, Director

**Mercer Community Action of South Eastern
WV** (CASE) (nutrition only)
307 Federal Street, Suite 323
Bluefield, WV 24701
Telephone: 304-324-8397; 304-323-2365
Fax: 304-327-6683
Email: ohubbard@casewv.org
Website: www.casewv.org
Oraetta Hubbard, Director

**Aging and Family Services of Mineral County,
Inc.**
1 South Main Street
Keyser, WV 26726-3127
Telephone: 304-788-5467
Fax: 304-788-6363
Email: smallery@wvaging.com
Website: www.wvaging.com
R. Scott Mallery, Director

Coalfield Community Action Partnership, Inc.
(Mingo)
PO Box 1406 (815 Alderson St.)
Williamson, WV 25661
Telephone: 304-235-1701
Fax: 304-235-1706
Email: tsalmons@coalfieldcap.org
Tim Salmons, Director

Senior Monongalians, Inc.
P. O. Box 653
(5000 Greenbag Rd., Suite 7, Mountaineer Mall)
Morgantown, WV 26507-0653
Telephone: 304-296-9812
Fax: 304-296-3917
Email: brobinson@seniormons.org
Website: www.seniormons.org
Betsy Robinson, Director

Monroe County Council on Aging
PO Box 149 (Route 219)
Lindside, WV 24951
Telephone: 304-753-4384
Fax: 304-753-9886
Email: mccoa24951@yahoo.com
Mike Will, Director

Senior Life Services of Morgan County
187 South Green Street, Suite 5
Berkeley Springs, WV 25411
Telephone: 304-258-3096
Fax: 304-258-3190
Email: slsmc1@hotmail.com
Website: www.slsmc.org
Joel Tuttle, Director

Nicholas Community Action Partnership, Inc.
1205 Broad Street
Summersville, WV 26651
Telephone: 304-872-1162
Fax: 304-872-5796
Email: djarroll@hotmail.com
Dave Jarroll, Director

Family Service - Upper Ohio Valley (also nutrition in Marshall and Wetzel)
51 11th Street

Wheeling, WV 26003
Telephone: 304-232-6730; 1-800-631-1954
Fax: 304-233-7237
Email: lwineman@ovrh.org
Website: www.familyserviceuov.org
Lonnie Wineman, Director; June Leindecker, Nutrition Director

Pendleton Senior and Family Services, Inc.
PO Box 9 (231 Mill Rd.)
Franklin, WV 26807
Telephone: 304-358-2421
Fax: 304-358-2422
Email: pendletonseniorcenter@frontier.com
Carolyn Wells, Director

Pleasants County Senior Citizens Center (IIIB, no nutrition)
209 2nd Street
St. Marys, WV 26170
Telephone: 304-684-9243
Fax: 304-684-9382
Email: pcscmt@frontiernet.net
Marie Taylor, Director

Pleasants Senior Nutrition (nutrition only)
Post Office Box 576 (219 2nd St.)
St. Marys, WV 26170
Telephone: 304-684-9319
Fax: 304-684-9319
Email: seniornutrition@creeds.net
David Hoyt, Director

Pocahontas County Senior Programs
PO Box 89 (State Route 219N, HC69, Box 7)
Marlinton, WV 24954
Telephone: 304-799-6337
Fax: 304-799-4972
Email: pocahontascoseniors@gmail.com
John R. Simmons, Director

Preston County Senior Citizens, Inc.
PO Box 10 (108 Senior Center Drive)
Kingwood, WV 26537
Telephone: 304-329-0464; 800-661-7556
Fax: 304-329-2584
Email: prestonseniors@atlanticbb.net
Sidney Murphy, Director

Putnam Aging Program, Inc. (also nutrition in Clay, Fayette and Kanawha)
694 Winfield Road
St. Albans, WV 25177-1554
Telephone: 304-755-2385
Fax: 304-755-2389
Email: jarthur@putnamaging.com
Website: www.putnamaging.com
Joyce McCormick-Arthur, Interim Director

Raleigh County Commission on Aging
1614 S. Kanawha St.
Beckley, WV 25801-5917
Telephone: 304-255-1397
Fax: 304-252-9360; 304-255-2881
Email: rccoa@raleighseniors.org
Website: www.raleighseniors.org
Jack Tanner, Director

The Committee on Aging for Randolph County, Inc.
PO Box 727 (5th St. & Railroad Av.)
Elkins, WV 26241
Telephone: 304-636-4747
Fax: 304-637-4991
Email: randolphcountyseniorcenter@yahoo.com
Website: www.randolphcountyseniorcenter.com
Rebecca Poe, Director

Ritchie County Integrated Family Services
PO Box 195 (S. Court St. & Edgeview Ln.)
Harrisville, WV 26362
Telephone: 304-643-4941
Fax: 304-643-4936
Email: rcseniors@zoominternet.net
Lee Jones, Director

Roane County Committee on Aging, Inc.
811 Madison Avenue
Spencer, WV 25276
Telephone: 304-927-1997
Fax: 304-927-2273
Email: cricks@rccoawv.org
Website: www.rccoawv.org
Chuck Ricks, Director

Summers County Council on Aging
120 2nd Avenue
Hinton, WV 25951
Telephone: 304-466-4019
Fax: 304-466-1890
Email: sccoalg@suddenlinkmail.com
Website: www.summersseniors.com
Mr. Lin Goins, Director

Taylor County Senior Citizens, Inc.
Route 2 Box 514 (US Rt. 119 & US Rt. 250)
Grafton, WV 26354
Telephone: 304-265-4555
Fax: 304-265-6083
Email: taylorcscfm@aol.com
Frank Mayle, Director

Tucker County Senior Citizens, Inc.
206 3rd Street
Parsons, WV 26287
Telephone: 304-478-2423
Fax: 304-478-4828
Email: tcsc@frontiernet.net;
rdnestor@hotmail.com
Roxanne Tuesing, Director

Council of Senior Tyler Countians, Inc.
PO Box 68 (504 Cherry St.)
Middlebourne, WV 26149
Telephone: 304-758-4919
Fax: 304-758-4680
Email: amy.cstcwv@frontier.com
Amy Haught, Executive Director

Upshur County Senior Citizens Opportunity Center, Inc.
28 North Kanawha Street
Buckhannon, WV 26201
Telephone: 304-472-0528
Fax: 304-472-6424
Email: acook@upwvsc.org
Website: www.upwvsc.org
Allen Cook, Director

Wayne County Community Services Organization, Inc.
3609 Hughes Street

Huntington, WV 25704
Telephone: 304-429-0070
Fax: 304-429-0026
Email: rmeredith@wccso.org
Sr. Center – 1300 Norfolk Avenue, Wayne
25570; 304-272-6060, 304-272-6068
Website: www.wccso.org
Rose Meredith, Director

Webster County Commission of Senior Citizens
148 Court Square
Webster Springs, WV 26288
Telephone: 304-847-5252
Fax: 304-847-7182
Email: webcosencitz@frontiernet.net
Phillip Cooper, Director

Wetzel County Committee on Aging (IIIB)
145 Paducah Drive
New Martinsville, WV 26155
Telephone: 304-455-3220
Fax: 304-455-0280
Email: wetzelccoa@suddenlinkmail.com
Mary Ash, Director

Wirt County Committee on Aging, Inc.
PO Box 370 (Washington St.)
Elizabeth, WV 26143
Telephone: 304-275-3158
Fax: 304-275-4631
Email: wccoa@suddenlinkmail.com
Lorraine Roberts, Director

Wood County Senior Citizens Association, Inc.
P. O. Box 1229 (914 Market Street)
Parkersburg, WV 26102
Telephone: 304-485-6748
Fax: 304-485-8755
Email: mdennis@suddenlinkmail.com
Michael Dennis, Director

Council on Aging (Wyoming County)
PO Box 130 (Old Itmann School Bldg., Rt. 10)
Itmann, WV 24847
Telephone: 304-294-8800; 800-499-4080
Fax: 304-294-8803
Email: gibsonj@wccoa.com

Website: www.wccoa.com
Jennifer Gibson, Director

Help at Home: http://www.wvseniorservices.gov/HelpatHome/tabid/56/Default.aspx

Help at Home

Helping people to remain in their homes and communities for as long as possible is the overarching goal of aging programs in our state. Services for those needing assistance in their homes vary from helping with housekeeping to more intensive personal care services such as help with bathing, dressing, and eating. Medical and financial eligibility for each program varies.

- Lighthouse
- FAIR (Family Alzheimer's In-Home Respite)
- Older Americans Act Programs/LIFE
- Medicaid Aged and Disabled Waiver
- Medicaid Personal Care
- West Virginia Transition Initiative

Family Alzheimer's In Home Respite (FAIR):
http://www.wvseniorservices.gov/HelpatHome/FAIRFamilyAlzheimersInHomeRespite/tabid/75/Default.aspx

FAIR (Family Alzheimer's In-Home Respite)

Caring for a loved one with Alzheimer's disease or a related dementia can be very stressful, and caregivers need a regular break from the demands of the job. The FAIR Program, available in every county of West Virginia, offers relief to family caregivers and, at the same time, provides one-on-one attention and individualized activities for persons with a written diagnosis of Alzheimer's disease or a related dementia.

FAIR gives caregivers the time to do things most of us take for granted—run errands, keep appointments, visit family and friends, shop for groceries, or even take a nap. FAIR clients (family caregivers) can receive up to sixteen hours of respite per week, based on need and availability of hours and trained staff. The fee for FAIR services depends on the income of the person with dementia. See FAIR Policies for more detailed information.

A FAIR brochure is available for printing, and a 30-second FAIR video can be viewed below.

For further information, please call your county aging provider or contact us at the Bureau of Senior Services.

Staying Healthy: http://www.wvseniorservices.gov/StayingHealthy/tabid/55/Default.aspx

Staying Healthy

Staying healthy is such an important focus of the Bureau of Senior Services that the words *Well and Vital* are part of our logo. Programs that help seniors get healthy and stay that way are very much a part of the array of services provided throughout the state.

- Disease Prevention and Management
- Food and Fitness
- Health Care Promotion
- Older Americans Act Programs/LIFE
- SHIP (Medicare)

SHIP (State Health Insurance Program*) Medicare*

Welcome to West Virginia SHIP: http://www.wvship.org/

Welcome To WV SHIP

Welcome to WV SHIP's website. SHIP stands for State Health Insurance Assistance Program and its goal is to provide reliable and up-to-date information to Medicare beneficiaries and their families. The purpose of this site is to offer information about Medicare to those individuals and families who are seeking answers. Additionally, it serves as an interactive resource for SHIP counselors from around the state to utilize for updates and training.

We are very proud of our nationally recognized SHIP services that are offered in West Virginia. Our site areas (About WV SHIP, SHIP Services, Find a SHIP Counselor, Publications, SHIP Partners, and Contact SHIP) are designed to help you find what you are looking for quickly and easily. We hope that you will find our website easy to navigate and full of useful information. If you have trouble finding what you are looking for, however, please give us a call or contact us via e-mail.

Nationwide, 77 million Baby Boomers will become eligible for Medicare starting in the year 2011. The number of West Virginians age 65 and older will increase by 27,000 each year. WV SHIP is positioned to continue to provide dependable services as the number of beneficiaries increases and as changes are introduced in Medicare to meet the demands of an aging population.

Lighthouse: http://www.wvseniorservices.gov/HelpatHome/Lighthouse/tabid/74/Default.aspx

Lighthouse

Lighthouse is designed to assist those seniors who have functional needs in their homes, but whose income or assets disqualify them for Medicaid services. The Lighthouse Program, available in each county, is funded entirely by state monies and provides support in four areas: personal care, mobility, nutrition, and housekeeping.

An individual may receive up to sixty hours of service per month, based on a client assessment and resources available. To participate in the program one must be at least sixty years of age and meet the functional eligibility need. Lighthouse has a sliding scale fee reimbursement in place. See <u>Lighthouse Policy and Procedures Manual</u> for more detailed information.

A <u>Lighthouse brochure</u> is available for printing, and a 30-second Lighthouse video can be viewed below.

For further information, please call your <u>county aging provider</u> or <u>contact us</u> at the Bureau of Senior Services.

Links to Helpful Sites:
http://www.wvseniorservices.gov/GettingAnswers/LinkstoHelpfulSites/tabid/64/Default.aspx

Links to Helpful Sites

There are many web sites of organizations throughout the country and the world that are related to the field of aging and the concerns of seniors. The following lists are divided into three categories—national and international private and public organizations, U.S. government and quasi-governmental organizations, and West Virginia government and private and public organizations.

The Bureau of Senior Services is not responsible for the contents of any of the sites referenced below; these links are provided only as an information service.

- National and International Private and Public Organizations
- U.S. Government and Quasi-Governmental Organizations
- West Virginia Government and Private and Public Organizations

West Virginia Government and Private and Public Organizations:
http://www.wvseniorservices.gov/GettingAnswers/LinkstoHelpfulSites/WVGovernmentandPrivateandPublicOrgs/tabid/104/Default.aspx

West Virginia Government and Private and Public Organizations

- Alzheimer's Association, WV Chapter
  As part of the national Alzheimer's Association, this chapter is a nonprofit group dedicated to improve the lives of families living with dementia.
- Americans with Disabilities Act Information Center
  Serving the Mid-Atlantic region which encompasses West Virginia, this information center provides both professionals and consumers with pertinent information regarding ADA.
- Appalachian Regional Commission
  Comprised of 13 states, the ARC was created to provide opportunities for self-sustaining economic development and improved quality of life in Appalachian communities.
- Appalachian Studies Association
  This organization's mission is to encourage study, disseminate information, and enhance communication between Appalachian peoples, their communities, governmental organizations, and educational institutions.

- Attorney General
  The WV Attorney General is responsible for protecting consumers from fraud and offering educational opportunities that increase awareness.
- Bureau of Business & Economic Research
  Working through West Virginia University, the BBER conducts business and economic research with a focus on West Virginia and the region. The Bureau disseminates research findings, data products and Census information.
- Healthcare at West Virginia University
  Operating under the authority of the WVU Robert C. Byrd Health Science Center, this site provides consumers with medical referrals and provides informational materials to consumers needing details on specific health care issues.
- Mission West Virginia
  Mission West Virginia is a non-profit organization that collaborates with public and private entities, particularly faith communities, equipping them to utilize existing resources to form new partnerships, encouraging innovative social change, and building stronger communities in West Virginia. Information on the Relatives as Parents Program (RAPP) is available.
- PayingForSeniorCare.com
  A free information website and comprehensive resource locator tool designed to help people find the financial resources required to pay for the long term care of their loved ones.
- Public Service Commission of WV
  The PSC supervises and regulates rates, services, operations and other activities of all public utilities including common and contract motor carriers of passengers. The PSC also receives consumer complaints.
- State Health Education Council of WV
  A nonprofit organization that works toward improving the health and wellness of West Virginians through networking, education and community involvement.
- WorkForce West Virginia
  In addition to the BEP's role concerning workers compensation, unemployment, and workforce enhancement initiatives, the agency maintains multiple data sets and resource information concerning employment trends.
- WV Alliance for Sustainable Families
  This organization was created to improve services receiving public assistance through research, education, advocacy and coalition building.
- WV Board of Examiners for Registered Professional Nurses
  This group is a legally constituted agency of state government that protects public health, safety and welfare through the regulation of the practice of registered professional nursing.
- WV Bureau for Behavioral Health and Health Facilities
  Part of DHHR and operating through the Bureau of Public Health, this office provides information on state-owned long-term care facilities and hospitals.
- WV Caregivers
  Sponsored by West Virginia University's Center on Aging, this site provides pertinent information to family caregivers needing additional support in caring for a loved one.
- WV Center for End-of-Life Care
  Operating through WVU's Center for Health Ethics and Law, this agency works towards helping families, individuals and health care organizations improve the quality of living during the final years of life.

- WV Commission for National and Community Service
  This organization coordinates the various national volunteer service programs such as Foster Grandparents, RSVP, and AmeriCorps through local and regional providers.
- WV Commission for the Deaf and Hard of Hearing
  Both an independent commission and part of DHHR, this Commission serves as a communication bridge between hearing persons and those who are deaf or hard of hearing.
- WV Department of Health and Human Resources
  DHHR is the lead agency for protecting the welfare, safety and health of West Virginians. Specific offices providing services to seniors are included separately within this section.
- WV Developmental Disabilities Council
  Both an independent council and part of DHHR, the Council serves as the lead advocate to represent the interests and needs of people with developmental disabilities.
- WV Directors of Senior and Community Services
  This site is the location of the association representing the county-based aging service programs.
- WV Division of Rehabilitation Services
  Working through the Department of Education and the Arts, Rehabilitation Services provides services, support, medical treatment and counseling for people with physical and/or mental limitations.
- WV Health Care Association
  This entity is a membership organization comprised of the various long-term care facilities across the state with a particular focus on the nursing home industry.
- WV Health Care Authority
  The HCA is responsible for constraining health care costs and access for West Virginians through hospital rate setting, certificates of need, financial disclosures, planning, and rural health system development.
- WV Hospital Association
  This organization represents the interests, needs and issues pertaining to the provision of medical care provided by West Virginia hospitals.
- WV Housing Development Fund
  This organization is the state's housing finance agency specializing in mortgages for homes for individuals and families of low and moderate incomes, including financing to rehabilitate and create affordable apartments.
- WV Legislature
  This site provides information concerning the State Legislature, including bill tracking information, legislative contacts, bills adopted into state law, WV Code, and interim committee information.
- WV Library Commission
  WV Bureau of Senior Services works in partnership with the Commission to maintain aging materials. Go to the online catalog and perform a search of "bureau of senior services collection" to access or borrow aging publications and films.
- WV Medical Institute
  WVMI is a nonprofit, physician-sponsored organization dedicated to improving health care. WVMI provides consumers with pertinent information concerning Medicare and serves as the entity for reviewing medical eligibility for Medicaid services.
- WV Nurses Association
  A membership organization that assists nurses in furthering their practice of nursing through professional and legislative endeavors and serves as an information resource center.

- WV Office of Community Health Systems and Health Promotions
  Part of DHHR and operating through the Bureau of Public Health, this office provides specific information regarding county health departments, health clinics, and hospitals.
- WV Office of Health Facility Licensure and Certification
  Part of DHHR and operating through the Bureau of Public Health, this office assures minimal standards in personal care, assisted living, and nursing homes including the investigation of care complaints.
- WV Poison Center

  The West Virginia Poison Center provides comprehensive emergency poison information, prevention, and educational resources to West Virginians 24 hours a day, 7 days a week, 365 days a year. Each call to the poison center is answered by a Specialist in Poison Information who is specially trained in the management of poisoning emergencies.

- WV Seniors
  This site is a free online community featuring news related to aging, senior events, question and answer column, chats, and an extensive database of WV senior service providers.
- WV State Bar
  The State Bar represents lawyers licensed to practice law in WV and exists to serve members, the legal profession and the public. Information regarding the law, legal referrals and access to pro bono services is provided.
- WV State Medical Association
  A physician-based organization that improves the quality of health care through education, physician communications and networking.
- WV Statewide Independent Living Council
  An independent organization funded by state government, the SILC works with disabled adults who are interested in programs, practices and help toward living independently.
- WVU Center for Excellence in Disabilities
  WVUCED was created to enhance the quality of life of individuals of all ages with disbilities in order that they can experience productive, independent, and totally integrated lives.
- WVU Center on Aging
  Under the Health Science Center, the Center on Aging seeks to initiate, facilitate, and disseminate programs committed to promoting quality of life in later years and provides education, consultations and services to communities.
- WVU Robert C. Byrd Health Sciences Center
  The HSC is comprised of the various medical schools operating through WVU, including the Schools of Dentistry, Medicine, Nursing, and Pharmacy along with a variety of specialty centers.

Medicaid Aged and Disabled Waiver:

http://www.wvseniorservices.gov/HelpatHome/MedicaidAgedandDisabledWaiver/tabid/77/Default.asp
x

Medicaid Aged and Disabled Waiver

The Medicaid Aged and Disabled Waiver (ADW) Program provides in-home and community services to individuals 18 years of age and older who are medically and financially eligible. Medical eligibility is based on a functional assessment by a medical professional. (A Medical Necessity Evaluation Request must be completed by applicant and the applicant's physician.) Financial eligibility is determined at the county Department of Health and Human Resources offices; assets cannot exceed $2,000 and income can be no more than $2,022 per month. Policies are described in the Bureau for Medical Services' Aged and Disabled Waiver Manual.

To apply to become a provider for the Medicaid Aged and Disabled Waiver program:

1. Review the Medicaid Program Manual chapters 100, 200, 300, 400, 501, 600, 700, and 800 located on the West Virginia Bureau for Medical Services website at www.wvdhhr.org.
2. Review the Site Monitoring Tool available on this website.
3. Complete the Certification Application and mail to:
   Julie McClanahan, Director
   Medicaid Aged & Disabled Waiver Program
   West Virginia Bureau of Senior Services
   1900 Kanawha Blvd., East
   Charleston, WV 25305-0160
4. Once the application is received by the Bureau of Senior Services, a representative will contact you to schedule an onsite review.
5. If you meet all certification requirements based on the onsite review, the Bureau of Senior Services will notify Molina Healthcare.
6. Molina Healthcare will send you a Medicaid Aged and Disabled Waiver Enrollment Application.
7. The Enrollment Application must be returned to Molina Healthcare.
8. Once Molina Healthcare determines the Enrollment Application is complete, they will notify you and provide you with a Medicaid provider number.

If you have any questions regarding this process, please contact the West Virginia Bureau of Senior Services at 304-558-3317.

Services provided in the ADW include:

- Case Management – development of a service and support plan by a case management agency that reflects the wishes and preferences of the ADW member. View Case Management agencies.
- Consumer-Directed Case Management – an ADW member may choose to direct his own case management
- Homemaker – long-term direct care and support services (assistance with personal hygiene, nutritional support, and environmental maintenance) that are necessary in order to enable an individual to remain at home rather than enter a long-term care facility. View Homemaker agencies and Homemaker Selection Forms.
- Transportation – an ADW member may be transported by the homemaker in order to gain access to services and activities in the community
- RN Assessment and Review – a registered nurse will complete assessments of the ADW member at regular intervals to ensure that the member's plan of care is meeting his/her needs

- Personal Options – ADW members have a monthly budget that they use to hire caregivers/employees and purchase needed ADW services to assist with activities of daily living. View Overview of Personal Options.

Quality Assurance and Improvement Advisory Council

The Aged and Disabled Quality Assurance and Improvement Advisory Council consists of fifteen members who are former or current Aged and Disabled Waiver members (or their legal representatives), providers, direct care workers, family members, advocates, or other individuals interested in quality home and community-based services.
The members meet quarterly from 10:00 a.m. to 3:00 p.m. An hour is reserved at each Council meeting from 2:00 p.m. to 3:00 p.m. for stakeholder input. Meetings are held at the Bureau of Senior Services Conference Room located at the Charleston Town Center Mall.

The Quality Assurance and Improvement Advisory Council meeting dates:
July 26, 2011; October 25, 2011; January 24, 2012; April 24, 2012
Please contact Cecilia Brown, Quality Assurance Program Manager at 304-558-3317 with any questions regarding the Council, Council membership or participating in any Council Work Groups.

Training Curriculum Materials
The Bureau has a collection of curriculum materials that would be beneficial to ADW providers for training their direct care workers. Although available as a resource, it is not mandatory that ADW providers use these materials. Here you will find a list of the materials and the request form used to check them out. Training materials can be checked out for a two-week period, and there is a limit of five items per checkout. If you have any questions, please contact Tammy Webb at 304-558-3317.

For more information about the ADW, please contact the Aging & Disability Resource Center in your area, call the Bureau of Senior Services' Medicaid helpline at 866-767-1575, view Waiver at a Glance and the ADW brochure, contact us online, or see contact information for Medicaid staff.

Older Americans Act Programs/Life:
http://www.wvseniorservices.gov/HelpatHome/OlderAmericansActProgramsLIFE/tabid/76/Default.aspx

-

Older Americans Act Programs/LIFE

Individuals age 60 and older may be eligible for a variety of in-home services through the Older Americans Act. These services are offered through county aging providers (senior centers). As they may vary by county, please contact the providers for further information. Examples of services include:

- Home-delivered meals – a healthful meal—usually lunch—is delivered to the home of an eligible homebound individual. See HDM Policy & Procedures. In August 2008, Governor Manchin presented 17 new hot/cold delivery trucks to county aging providers. (See additional photos.)

Then, in August 2009, the Governor presented 11 additional hot/cold trucks and announced that six combination passenger and hot/cold delivery system buses will be on the road in the next few weeks. (See photos from the Governor's Office and the Bureau of Senior Services.) Finally, in August 2010, the Governor presented 20 additional hot/cold trucks. With these additional trucks, seniors in all 55 counties who haven't been served before will now have access to meal delivery services. (See photos from the Governor's Office and the Bureau of Senior Services.)

- Assisted Transportation – assistance for those who have difficulties using regular vehicular transportation
- Chore – heavy cleaning and yard maintenance for seniors who are unable to handle such tasks on their own
- Homemaker – preparation of meals, shopping, managing medication, and laundry for seniors who are unable to handle such tasks on their own
- Caregiver Support – helping caregivers access information and assistance, formation of support groups, and respite services for caregivers

LIFE (Legislative Initiative for the Elderly) is a state-funded program and part of the senior center array of services. Services vary by county but are modeled after those provided by the Older Americans Act.

Wisconsin

Public Services: http://www.wisconsin.gov/state/core/public_services.html

- Elder Services
    - Aging
    - Community Options Program
    - Elderly Nutrition
    - Family Care Options for Long-Term Care
    - Health and Human Services (including elder services)
    - Nursing Homes
    - Reports on Nursing Homes and Facilities
    - SeniorCare
    - Wisconsin Affordable Assisted Living

- Disability Services
    - Assistive Technology
    - Career Resources
    - Disabilities and Health Conditions Links - **NEW!**
    - Services for People with Disabilities
    - Vocational Rehabilitation

Aging: http://www.dhs.wisconsin.gov/aging/

Services for the Elderly

From this page you can access a variety of information on programs and services in Wisconsin for older people and caregivers. A brief description of each service is available.

Aging and Disability Resource Centers (ADRCs) are the first place for help. If your county doesn't have an ADRC, go to your county or tribal aging agency.

- Abuse and Neglect Services
- Aging & Disability Resource Centers (ADRC)
- Alzheimer's Disease and Dementia Resources
- Area Agencies on Aging
- Bureau of Aging and Disability Resources Contact List
- Community Options Program
- Demographics of Aging in Wisconsin
- Elderly Benefits Specialist
- Elderly Nutrition
- Estate Recovery
- Falls Prevention

- Family Care, Partnership and PACE
- Family Caregiver Support
- Guardianship of Adults
- Healthy Aging (Evidence-Based Prevention Programs)
- IRIS (Include, Respect, I Self-Direct)
- Medigap Helpline
- Senior Employment Program (WISE)
- State Health Insurance Program (SHIP)
- Spousal Impoverishment
- Voting Rights and Resources

Forms

- Declaration to Physicians (Living Will) - F-00060
- Power of Attorney for Health Care - F-00085
- Power of Attorney for Finance and Property - F-00036
- Authorization for Final Disposition - F-00086

Volunteer Opportunities

- Foster Grandparents Program
- Retired Senior Volunteers Program
- Senior Companion Program
- SHIP Volunteers

Training Opportunities

- Aging, Disabilities and Long-Term Care Training Events (PDF, 75 KB)
- Webcasts

Family Care Options for Support: http://www.dhs.wisconsin.gov/LTCare/

Quick Links:
Family Care Partnership Program
Wisconsin Council on Long-Term Care
Other Links

General Information	Program Monitoring and Evaluatlon	Program Operations	State and Federal Requirements	History of Long-Term Care Redesign

Family Care is a comprehensive and flexible long-term care service system, which strives to foster people's independence and quality of life, while recognizing the need for interdependence and support.

Goals of the Family Care Initiative

:

CHOICE – Give people better choices about the services and supports available to meet their needs.

ACCESS – Improve people's access to services.

QUALITY – Improve the overall quality of the long-term care system by focusing on achieving people's health and social outcomes.

COST-EFFECTIVENESS – Create a cost-effective long-term care system for the future.

Where to find updated information:

We will continue to update and add to the information about Family Care on these web pages, so check back frequently. If you need information that is not published here, please contact:

Family Care Information
DHS-DLTC-OFCE
1 West Wilson Street, Room 518
P.O. Box 7851
Madison WI 53707-7851
hollister.chase@wisconsin.gov

General Information

Quick Links:
Family Care Partnership Program
Wisconsin Council on Long-Term Care
Other Links

Because of frailties of aging or a developmental or physical disability, many people need help accomplishing activities of daily living and caring for their health. This help, referred to as long-term care, includes many different services, such as personal care, housekeeping or nursing. Long-term care is provided in people's homes, in small and large residential care facilities or group homes, in nursing facilities and in the workplace.

Most long-term care is actually provided by family members, and people pay directly for a lot of the care they receive. Yet the government in Wisconsin still spends more than a billion dollars a year paying for care that Wisconsin residents themselves cannot afford.

To help determine how to improve long-term care, the Wisconsin Department of Health Services spent more than two years during the mid-1990s gathering information not only from people who need long-term care, but also their relatives and service providers, as well as experts and taxpayers.

A new plan called **Family Care** was proposed in 1998 for consideration by citizens and their elected representatives. In his February 2006 State of the State speech, Governor Doyle announced plans to expand Family Care statewide and eliminate waiting lists for community-based long-term care programs during the next five years.

Select a link to the right for more general information about Family Care.

What is Family Care?
Who does Family Care serve?
Aging and Disability Resource Centers
Managed Care Organizations
Where in Wisconsin can you find Family Care?
How do you apply?
Consumer resources for questions
Real life stories
Why Family Care?
Being a Full Partner in Family Care

Aging and Disabled Resource Centers:
http://www.dhs.wisconsin.gov/ltcare/adrc/

Aging and Disability Resource Centers Customer Page

WHAT IS AN ADRC?

The place for information and assistance!

Aging and Disability Resource Centers (ADRCs) are the first place to go to get accurate, unbiased information on all aspects of life related to aging or living with a disability. ADRCs are friendly, welcoming places where anyone -- individuals, concerned families or friends, or professionals working with issues related to aging or disabilities -- can go for information specifically tailored to their situation. The ADRC provides information on broad range of programs and services, helps people understand the various long term care options available to them, helps people apply for programs and benefits, and serves as the access point for publicly-funded long term care. These services can be provided at the

ADRC, via telephone, or through a home visit, whichever is more convenient to the individual seeking help.

For additional information, see:

- ADRC Brochure(English, PDF 98 KB)
- ADRC Brochure (Spanish, PDF 104 KB)
- Video: Introduction to Aging and Disability Resource Centers 9 minute video (Webcast help)

HOW TO FIND AN ADRC

ADRCs are available in most, but not all, Wisconsin counties. Check the following links to find an ADRC in your area:

- **Finding an ADRC:** A directory or ADRCs, by county (PDF 51 KB) Updated August 2011
- **ADRC Map:** Map indicating which counties are served by an ADRC. (PDF, 304 KB) Updated March 2011

Note: If your county is not yet served by an ADRC, information about local Long Term Care Resources may be available through other sources.

SERVICES PROVIDED BY THE ADRC

An Aging and Disability Resource Center provides the following services and more:

Information and Assistance:

- Information about local services and resource
- Assistance in finding services to match your needs
  - In-home care
  - Housekeeping and chore services
  - Home modifications, safety and maintenance
  - Health (healthy lifestyles, management of chronic conditions, dementia, etc)
  - Respite
  - Transportation
  - Nutrition, home delivered meals
  - Housing, including senior and low income housing
  - Assisted Living, nursing homes and other long term care facilities
  - Financial assistance (e.g., Social Security, SSI, Disability, Medicare, Medicaid and other benefit programs)
  - Legal issues (guardianship, power of attorney, client rights advocacy)

- o   Abuse, neglect and financial exploitation
- o   Mental health, alcohol and drug abuse, crisis intervention
- o   Employment, vocational services, volunteer work
- o   Adaptive equipment
- o   Other

Long Term Care Options Counseling:

- Information about the choices you have when making decisions about where to live, what kind of help you need, where to receive that care and help, and how to pay for it.
- One-on-one consultation to help you think through the pros and cons of the various options in light of your situation, values, resources and preferences.

Benefit Counseling:

- Benefit specialists provide information about government and other benefits that you may be entitled to receive, such as Medicare, Medicaid, Social Security, Disability, low income housing, etc.
- Benefit specialists advocate for you when you have problems with Medicare, Social Security, and other benefits.
- Elderly Benefit Specialists serve people age 60 years of age and older.
- Disability Benefit Specialists serve adult with a disability under age 60. This includes people with a physical disability, people with a developmental disability, people with mental illness or substance use issues.

Access to Funding for Long Term Care:

- The ADRC can determine if you will be eligible for public funding for your long term care.
- The ADRC can help you prepare your Medicaid application, if eligible.
- The ADRC can explain the program choices you have that will provide your long term care. These programs include Family Care, IRIS and in some areas Partnership and PACE.

Health and Wellness:

- ADRC can connect you to wellness programs to help keep you healthy and independent.

Please don't hesitate to contact your local ADRC if you have questions or need help with any issue relating to aging or disability. Contact

information for the ADRCs can be found at **Finding an ADRC.** :
http://www.dhs.wisconsin.gov/ltcare/adrc/customer/adrccontactlist.pdf

Elderly Benefit Specialists:
http://www.dhs.wisconsin.gov/aging/EBS/benspecs.htm

Elderly Benefit Specialists

Locate your County and Tribal Benefit Specialists

Elderly Benefit Specialist Program Services Summary Report (PDF 111 KB)

State Health Insurance Assistance Program (SHIP)

Trainings for Elderly Benefit Specialists

Technical Assistance (PDF 655 KB)

Policies(see Chapter 9 for EBS policies starting on page 211)

What is an Elderly Benefit Specialist?

- Who Should Seek Help From An Elderly Benefit Specialist?
- What Elderly Benefit Specialists Can Do?
- Who is Eligible for Elderly Benefit Specialist Services?
- What does the Elderly Benefit Specialist Services cost?
- Who provides Elderly Benefit Specialist Services?

An elderly benefit specialist is a person trained to help older persons who are having a problem with their private or government benefits. They receive ongoing training and are monitored by attorneys knowledgeable in elder law. The attorneys are also available to assist older persons in need of legal representation on benefit matters.

Who Should Seek Help From An Elderly Benefit Specialist?

- Older persons who just want to know more about any private or public benefit.
- Older persons who need help in organizing the paperwork to apply for benefits.
- Older persons who have been denied a benefit that they think they are entitled to receive.

Return to top of page.

What can an Elderly Benefit Specialists Do?

- Provide accurate and current information on your benefits.
- Suggest alternative actions that you can take to secure benefits or appeal denials of benefits.
- Advocate on your behalf with other parties.
- Explain what legal action or other possible solution is required.
- Refer you to an appropriate attorney when necessary.

Benefit specialists can help you with a variety of programs and issues, including:

- Medicare; Medicare Part D
  - Medicare Health plan decisions need to be made between **October 15th - December 7th**. Contact an Elderly Benefit Specialist for more information. Also visit: www.medicare.gov (exit DHS)
- Medicare Supplemental Insurance;
- Supplemental Security Income (SSI);
- Social Security;
- Medical Assistance;
- Consumer problems;
- Age discrimination in employment;
- Homestead Tax Credit;
- Housing problems;
- Supportive Home Services;
- Food Stamps;
- Other legal and benefit problems.

Return to top of page.

Who Is Eligible For Elderly Benefit Specialist Services?

Anyone 60 years of age or older who is having a problem in securing a public or private benefit is eligible for the Elderly Benefit Specialist Program.

Return to top of page.

What Does the Elderly Benefit Specialist Service Cost?

The program is supported with funds from the State of Wisconsin and the federal Older Americans Act. Most Elderly Benefit Specialist programs also receive federal funds through the State Health Insurance Assistance Program. There is no charge for the service, but persons assisted by the program are encouraged to make a donation towards the cost. All donated funds will be used to expand the program. Services will not be refused or limited in any way if a contribution is not made.

Return to top of page.

Who Provides Elderly Benefit Specialist Services?

Services are either provided directly by county or tribal aging units or they are contracted by these entities to another agency. The area agencies on aging contract for training and support of the benefit specialists by attorneys. The State Bureau on Aging and Disability Resources in the Wisconsin Department of Health Services coordinates the program statewide.

For more information, contact the county or tribal benefit specialist nearest you. Ask specifically for the benefit specialist when calling. To receive the best service, it is advisable to schedule an appointment in advance.

Disability Benefit Specialist Program:
http://www.dhs.wisconsin.gov/disabilities/benspecs/program.htm

Disability Benefit Specialist Program

What is a disability benefit specialist?

Disability benefit specialists (DBS) help answer questions and solve problems related to Social Security, Medicare, health insurance and other public and private benefits for people with disabilities.

They serve people **ages 18-59** witha physical or a developmental disability, a mental illness or a substance abuse disorder. Services are free and confidential. Similar services are available to people age 60 or older through the Elderly Benefit Specialist program.

View a webcast in American Sign Language about disability benefit specialist services. (*Duration: 5 min.*)

Program brochures are available in English (PDF, 96 KB), Hmong(PDF, 159 KB) and Spanish(PDF, 110 KB).

Program statistics are available for 2003 through 2010.

Where can I find a disability benefit specialist?

Aging and Disability Resource Centers offer DBS services in 59 of Wisconsin's 72 counties. Find a benefit specialist in your county of residence. : http://www.dhs.wisconsin.gov/aging/EBS/counties.htm

Deaf or hard of hearingpersons may opt to seek DBS services for people who use sign language through the Office for the Deaf and Hard of Hearing.

Enrolled tribal members who live on or near a reservation in Wisconsin may opt to work with a tribal benefit specialist.

Questions about how working might affect your disability benefits? Contact a work incentives benefit specialist (exit DHS).

Wyoming

Department of Health: http://www.health.wyo.gov/

Aging Division: http://www.health.wyo.gov/aging/index.html

Aging Division Mission

The Wyoming Department of Health's Aging Division exists to provide a flexible and responsive continuum of services that enables Wyoming's older adults to age-in-place with maximum dignity and independence.

The Aging Division has the challenge to meet this mission in a state that is sparsely populated, and geographically diverse. Human services are thinly spread and often not available in individual communities. The division gladly rises to meet that challenge with an ever growing list of providers of Older American Act, Medicaid, and grant-funded services.

To the left are links to various areas within the division. Click on those links that are of interest to you.

Aging Division Programmatic Goals and Priorities

1. Empower Wyoming's older adults, their families, and other consumers to make informed personal decisions about, and to be able to identify and easily access existing social, legal, health and long-term care options and services.

2. Enable Wyoming's older adults to remain in their own homes and communities with high quality of life for as long as possible through the provision of home and community-based services, including support for family caregivers.

3. Empower Wyoming's older adults to stay active and healthy through programs and services administered by and funded through the Aging Division, including evidence-based health promotion and disease prevention programs.

4. Ensure the rights of Wyoming's older adults and prevent their abuse, neglect, and exploitation.

5. Commit to a culture of staff and provider excellence, clearly demonstrating impact and program effectiveness, and a strong sense of contribution in the provision of services to Wyoming's older adults.

6. Continually expand our knowledge of new and changing issues facing Wyoming's older adults, and properly respond to those issues.

7. Maintain consistent, effective, accountable and responsive management and stewardship of the public's resources.

About Aging

We continually work to provide a flexible and responsive continuum of services to Wyoming's older adults who wish to be independent and self-reliant. The Aging Division does this through a diverse and full spectrum of services. These services are funded through:

- The Older Americans Act (Administration on Aging)
- Medicaid
- State General Funds
- Private Grant Funding

Services we provide can be viewed by clicking on the "Services" link to the left. Providers of these varied services can be located by clicking on the "Service Providers and Provider Information" link, also to the left.

Many of our staff travel often visiting and assessing the providers, making sure seniors in Wyoming have quality services. If you want to speak with one of our staff members, The "Contact Us" link takes you to our index of staff members.

Aging Division
Wyoming Department of Health
6101 Yellowstone Road, Suite 259B
Cheyenne, WY 82002
(307) 777-7986
Toll Free 1-800-442-2766
Fax (307) 777-5340
E-mail: wyaging@wyo.gov
http://www.wyomingaging.org

Aging Division Services: http://www.health.wyo.gov/aging/services/index.html

Aging Division Services

The Aging Division provides many services for older adults. Some are funded through Medicaid, and the Older Americans Act, while others are funded through grants the Division pursues. Below are the services the Division administers. For more information on each service, including who and where the service is being provided, click on the name of the service.

Supportive Services

Nutrition Services

Community Based In Home Services

Mental Wellness Coordination Services

Disease Prevention & Health Promotion Service

Community Service Employment For Older Americans

Allotments For Vulnerable Elder Rights Protection Activities

Long Term Care Home and Community Based Waiver Services

Assisted Living Facility Waiver Services

National Family Caregiver Support Program

Home Health Services

Nursing Home Services

Hospice Services

State-Licensed Shelter Care

Centenarian Program

Information and Referral Service

FIND SERVICES AND SERVICE PROVIDERS BY CALLING 800-442-2766

Supportive Services: http://www.health.wyo.gov/aging/services/supportive.html

Supportive Services

Supportive services are provided to assist older adults to remain independent and enjoy a healthier lifestyle and social interaction. If you would like to see what supportive services are in which county, please view the OAA services provider index.

Transportation - Provision of a means of going from one location to another. Does not include any other activity.

Outreach

- Intervention initiated by an agency or organization for the purpose of identifying potential clients and encouraging their use of existing services and benefits.

Counseling -

professional counseling provided through the OAA provider by a contract or volunteer professional counselor, either individual or group.

Shopping assistance

- Providing assistance in the purchase of food, clothing, medical supplies, household items, and/or recreational materials for a client.

Nutrition education

- A program to promote better health by providing accurate and culturally sensitive nutrition, physical fitness, or health information and instruction to participants (and their care-givers, if applicable) in a group or individual setting overseen by a dietitian or individual of comparable expertise.

Chore services -

Providing assistance to persons having difficulty with one or more of the following instrumental activities of daily living; heavy housework, yard work or sidewalk maintenance.

Eligibility for these services

: A client must be over 60 years of age.

Community Based In-Home Services Page: http://www.health.wyo.gov/aging/services/cbihs.html

Community-Based In-Home Services Page

The Community Based In Home Services program (CBIHS) is used to provide services to those qualified individuals who are at risk of premature institutionalization. These services are designed to keep people in the least restrictive environment for as long as possible. If you would like to see what CBIHS services are in which county, please view the OAA services provider index.

Case management - Assistance either in the form of access or care coordination in circumstances where the person and/or their care-givers are experiencing diminished functioning capacities, personal conditions or other characteristics which require the provision of services by formal service providers. Activities of case management include assessing needs, developing care plans, authorizing services, arranging services, coordinating the provision of services among providers, follow-up and reassessment as required.

Personal care - Providing personal assistance, stand-by assistance, supervision or cues for persons with the inability to perform with one or more of the following activities of daily living; eating, dressing, bathing, toileting, transferring in and out of bed/chair, or walking.

Chore services - Providing assistance to persons with the inability to perform one or more of the following instrumental activities of daily living; heavy housework, yard work, or sidewalk maintenance.

Homemaker services - Providing assistance to persons with an inability to perform one or more of the following instrumental activities of daily living; preparing meals, shopping for personal items, managing money, using the telephone, or doing light housework.

Respite care - Respite care services offer temporary, substitute supports, or living arrangements for older persons in order to provide a brief period of relief or rest for family members or other caregivers.

Personal Emergency Response Systems - Electronic warning devise informing emergency personnel of an accident or safety hazard to a client in their home.

Adult day care - Provision of personal care for dependent adults in a supervised, protective, congregate setting during some portion of a twenty-four-hour day.

Hospice - Services provided to the terminally ill, allowing him/her to remain at home with their family.

Eligibility for these services: A client must be 18 years of age or older, and, through an ongoing evaluation, to be at risk of premature institutionalization.

Senior Employment, Ombudsmen, Centenarian & Information and Referral Services Page:
http://www.health.wyo.gov/aging/services/other.html

Senior Employment, Ombudsmen, Centenarian & Information and Referral Services Page

Community Service Employment for Older Americans is also known as senior employment. This program reintroduces older workers to the labor market. *This program is now administered by Wyoming Department of Workforce services.* The new link to information on these services is http://dwsweb.state.wy.us/community/scsep.asp

Allotments for vulnerable elder rights protection activities has several components: the Long-Term Care Ombudsman program, the Legal Assistance Developer program, and the Legal Services program.

The Long Term Care Ombudsman advocates on behalf of older persons in institutions or receiving long term care in -home services and their families.

The Legal Assistant Developer program provides, on a statewide basis, the protection of rights of vulnerable older persons.

The Legal Services program provides legal assistance services to older Americans.

Eligibility for these services: A client must be over 60 years of age, a spouse of an individual over 60 years of age, or a disabled person living in senior housing attached to a congregate meals site.

Centenarian program recognizes those individuals who have reached the age of 100.

Information and Referral services - Information and referral provides current information on opportunities and services available to individuals in their community. Information and Referral questions may be answered by calling either: toll free (800) 442-2766, or (307) 777-7986

FIND SERVICES AND SERVICE PROVIDERS THROUGH CONNECT WYOMING

http://windweb.uwyo.edu/wind/pathways/seniors/

National Family Caregiver Support Program Services Page:
http://www.health.wyo.gov/aging/services/nfcp.html

National Family Caregiver Support Program Services Page

The National Family Caregiver Support program (NFCSP) is available to those qualified individuals who provide care for the elderly at home, and grandparents raising grandchildren the age of eighteen and under. If you would like to see what NFCSP services are in which county, please view the OAA services provider index.

Assistance - Assistance, for this program, is help with accessing services for the caregiver, either in a group setting or one to one contact.

Case management - Over-site either in the form of access or care coordination in circumstances where the person and/or their care-givers are experiencing diminished functioning capacities, personal conditions or other characteristics which require the provision of services by formal service providers. Activities of case management include assessing needs, developing care plans, authorizing services, arranging services, coordinating the provision of services among providers, follow-up and reassessment as required.

Counseling/Education - Counseling/education is organized activities related to the support, training and counseling for caregivers to help deal with the stress of caring for a elderly adult or child.

Information - Information includes outreach, group education and health fairs to relay information to those caregivers not aware of services out there for them.

Respite care - Respite care services offer temporary, substitute supports, or living arrangements for older persons in order to provide a brief period of relief or rest for family members or other caregivers.

Supplemental Services - Durable services to aid the caregiver in keeping their care receiver in the home.

Eligibility for these services: A client must be over 60 years of age if caring for a child 19 and younger or a person of any age caring for a qualified care receiver who is 60 years or older.

FIND SERVICES AND SERVICE PROVIDERS THROUGH CONNECT WYOMING

http://windweb.uwyo.edu/wind/pathways/seniors/

Home Health, Hospice, Nursing Home, & State Licensed Shelter Care Services Page:
http://www.health.wyo.gov/aging/services/Medicaid.html

Nutrition Services: **http://www.health.wyo.gov/aging/services/nutrition.html**

Nutrition Services

The Nutrition Program provides hot nutritious meals meeting the one-third Recommended Dietary Allowance. These meals are available at community focal points or they are delivered to an individual's home if they are unable to attend a congregate meal site. If you would like to see what Nutrition services are in which county, please view the OAA services provider index.

Congregate Nutrition Services - Meals available at a community focal point.

Home Delivered Services - Meals delivered to an individual's home.

Eligibility for these services: A client must be over 60 years of age, a spouse of an individual over 60 years of age, or a disabled person living in senior housing attached to a congregate meals site.

FIND SERVICES AND SERVICE PROVIDERS THROUGH CONNECT WYOMING

http://windweb.uwyo.edu/wind/pathways/seniors/

For Seniors Main Page: http://www.health.wyo.gov/aging/seniors.html

Links to Sites of Interest to Seniors

While searching for things to put on the Division's Web page, we came across several links to sites that may be of interest to seniors. Some are fun, some serious, and some contained a wealth of knowledge we could not even begin to delve into on these web pages. Below is just a beginning. Dive in and click on a site, watch where it takes you! Don't worry about getting lost - you can always click on the "HOME" button at the top and it will take you back to your home page and you can start all over again! (Don't think of it as getting lost, but as taking a Sunday drive through the internet!)

Since starting this page, the Division has been given so many sites, that it was decided to split sites up into sections. Below are the sections decided upon.

Please note: The authorized use of these links is limited to informational and educational purposes only. To review the State's full disclaimer, go to the State of Wyoming's Copyright and Disclaimer page.

Adult/Child Abuse Mandatory Reporting -
Department of Family Services home page where you can access information about the Mandatory Reporting laws for Adult and Child Abuse. Includes information on how and where to report.

Aging Associations & Organizations -
Sites for organizations and associations dedicated to the Older Adult.

Disease-Related Organizations & Associations -
Sites for organizations and associations dedicated to promoting awareness for diseases.

Health-Related Sites -
Websites dedicated to the health and well being of Older Americans.

Home Care/Cargiving and Association Sites -
Websites dedicated to those entities that provide care in the home and for caregivers.

Multi-Layered Sites-
Websites geared for Older Americans, with several layers of information.

Miscellaneous Sites -
Sites that don't really fit into any of the above categories.

Ombudsman Map -
Wyoming Long-Term Care Ombudsman map

Wyoming Services -
Different sites that provide the ability to search for services across the State of Wyoming.

Senior Articles

Evalyn Hoover Award

The Evalyn Hoover Lifetime Achievement Award is presented every other year at the Wyoming
Governor's Conference on Aging to honor a Wyoming.

New Internet Search for Older Adult Services

Tired of running around looking for long-term care information in your community? Well, now senior
services in the state can be accessed from just one Internet address. This free service was created by the
University of Wyoming's INstitute for Disabilities (WiND), the Department of Health's Division on Aging,
and AARP Wyoming. Log on to get information sorted by city or county, or by type of service. The
internet address is: http://windweb.uwyo.edu/wind/connect/

Note: If you have any problems with site including data content (or lack of data content) , or
accessibility, please contact this web designer or the senior pathways web designer. This search engine
can only be as good as the data in it.

Calling All Seniors!

The Senior Companion Program is looking for caring individuals who are low income, over 60 and willing
to visit the frail elderly and homebound. The Program will pay a non-taxable hourly stipend, as well as

mileage and meal reimbursements. The Senior Companion Program serves all counties in Wyoming. Please call 307-634-1010 for more information.

Advanced Directives

Per a mandate from the Wyoming Legislature, the Aging Division is to make available the most current approved version of the State's Advanced Directives.

Advances Directives describe two kinds of legal documents, an individual's instruction and a power of attorney for health care. These documents allow a person to give instructions about future medical care inc ase they are unable to participate in medical decisions due to serious illness or incapacity.

Advanced Directives form - The form to be completed by a person to out line their wishes.

WyAHCD form guide & glossary - This document provides guidance and deifinitions of terms in the Advance Directives form.

www.ingramcontent.com/pod-product-compliance
Lightning Source LLC
Chambersburg PA
CBHW080406290526
45791CB00008BA/2169